Yasushi Naito

Pediatric Ear Diseases

Diagnostic Imaging Atlas and Case Reports

242 figures, 7 in color and 5 tables, 2013

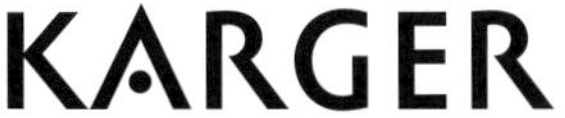

Basel · Freiburg · Paris · London · New York · New Delhi · Bangkok ·
Beijing · Tokyo · Kuala Lumpur · Singapore · Sydney

Dr. Yasushi Naito
Kobe City Medical Center General Hospital
Kobe City Hospital Organization
Kobe, Japan

Library of Congress Cataloging-in-Publication Data
Naito, Yasushi.
  Pediatric ear diseases : diagnostic imaging atlas and case reports /
Yasushi Naito.
       p. ; cm.
  Includes bibliographical references and index.
  ISBN 978-3-318-02232-2 (hardcover : alk. paper) -- ISBN 978-3-318-02233-9
(e-ISBN)
  I. Title.
  [DNLM: 1. Ear Diseases--diagnosis--Atlases. 2. Ear
Diseases--diagnosis--Case Reports. 3. Adolescent. 4. Child. 5. Ear,
Inner--abnormalities--Atlases. 6. Ear, Inner--abnormalities--Case Reports.
WV 17]
  RF291.5.C45
  618.92'0978--dc23
                          2013002892

Bibliographic Indices. This publication is listed in bibliographic services, including Current Contents® and PubMed/MEDLINE.

© Copyright 2013 by S. Karger AG, P.O. Box, CH–4009 Basel (Switzerland)
www.karger.com
Printed in Germany on acid-free and non-aging paper (ISO 97069) by Kraft Druck, Ettlingen
ISBN 978–3–318–02232–2
eISBN 978–3–318–02233–9

Contents

Preface

This book consists of two sections: a pediatric temporal bone imaging atlas, followed by case reports on a variety of typical pediatric ear diseases. As an atlas, this book shows complete contiguous temporal bone CT sections of an infant and of an older child, listing detailed anatomic names of the structures, including very fine ones, that appear in each image. In addition, developmental changes in the size, shape, location and orientation of the primary components of the temporal bone are also shown to demonstrate how the temporal bone grows with age. This book will be of great help to those who are interested in pediatric ear diseases, since accurate assessment of the disorders is very difficult without this sort of atlas, which has not been published so far.

The section following the atlas contains a collection of case reports. In this section, case images are shown alongside normal reference images of a child in the same age range as the patient, allowing readers to identify the key findings for diagnosing the disorder without needing to refer to an atlas of normal images. Images taken before and after treatment are also displayed side by side, to clearly illustrate the point of the post-treatment follow-up. Such layout is unique to this book, and is very effective for learning image diagnosis. To obtain a complete perspective of a disease, it is necessary to know not only the steps leading up to its diagnosis but also the treatment and the results following it. This is why I made the latter half of this book a collection of case reports, not simply a display of the diseases' key images.

I hope that this book will be of use to those who are involved in the medical care of children suffering from ear diseases.

Yasushi Naito
Kobe, Japan, 2013

Most of the images shown in this book are temporal bone CTs, but in some cases MRIs are also employed to observe structures such as the inner ear, internal auditory canal, and posterior cranial fossa. The temporal bone imaging parameters described below pertain to the majority of the images contained herein. Although different parameters are employed in a portion of the CT and MR images, a detailed explanation of each would be of little clinical significance. As most readers who are not radiologists are likely unfamiliar with the values described below, we recommend that, when asked for direction regarding temporal bone CT or MRI examination procedures by radiologists either at your own facility or at an outsourced imaging lab, you photocopy this page and present it as an example. However, regarding the voxel size values shown below, please be aware that these are the sizes of the minimum units comprising the image and structures smaller than this cannot be isolated and depicted, so represent the maximum resolution of the images shown herein.

As a general rule, the images shown are rectangular with an aspect ratio of 3:4. The axial cross-sections display the area indicated inside the box in figures 1 (CT) and 2 (MRI) below, centered on the inner ear and tympanic cavity. The coronal cross-sections generally display the area from the inferior margin of the mastoid process to the superior margin of the anterior semicircular canal.

A number of problems arise when attempting to display in print form clinical images normally viewed either as backlit transparencies or on a computer display. It is difficult in actual printed images to fully satisfy the conflicting objectives of losing as little information included in the image as possible while preventing the display of data that should not have been shown in the original image. We have made an effort to fulfill both objectives as much as possible but, in some images, areas that were originally air are sometimes depicted as slightly shaded, or structures such as tympanic membranes or tendons that should be delicately expressed with intermediate gradations become difficult to distinguish. We hope that you will take the above difficulties into consideration when viewing the images presented in this book.

Temporal Bone Target CT Imaging Parameters

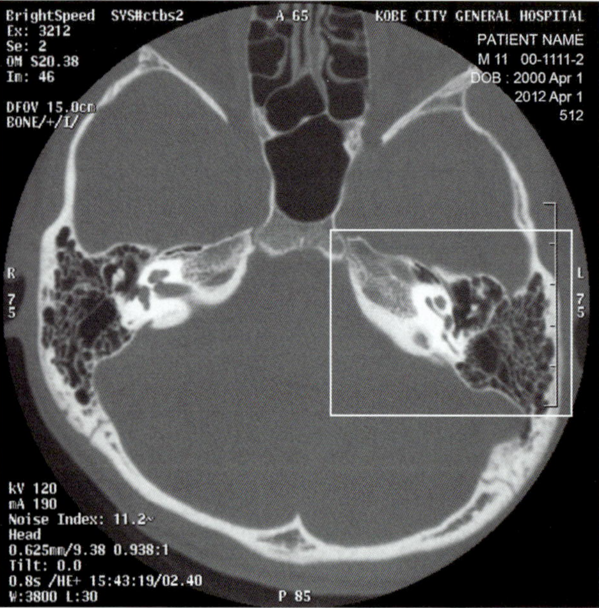

Fig. 1. Temporal bone CT image

Principal equipment used: GE BrightSpeed (16 MD CT), 120 kV, helical pitch of 0.562, "Bone" reconstruction algorithm. Axial cross-sections: bilateral simultaneous imaging, FOV: 150 mm, matrix size: 512 × 512, slice thickness: 0.625 mm, no gap (voxel size: 0.29 × 0.29 × 0.63 mm). Coronal cross-sections: unilateral imaging, FOV: 96 mm, matrix size: 512 × 512, slice thickness: 0.625 mm, no gap. Display window width is 3800, window level is 30.

Temporal Bone MR Imaging Parameters

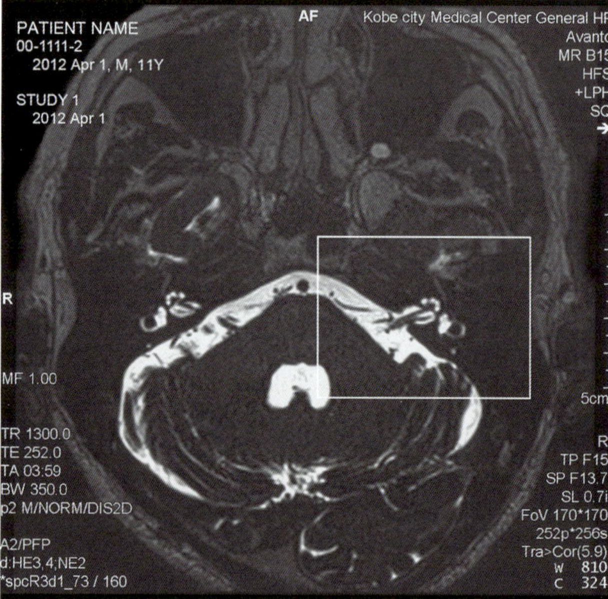

Fig. 2. Temporal bone MRI

Equipment used: Siemens Avanto 1.5T MRI system, SPACE (Sampling Perfection with Application optimized Contrasts using different flip angle Evolution) pulse sequence, Turbo Spin Echo, 3D T2-weighted images. Imaging parameters: FOV: 170 mm, slice thickness: 0.7 mm, matrix size: 256 × 256 (voxel size: 0.66 × 0.66 × 0.7 mm), TR: 1300 ms, TE: 253 ms, flip angle: 160 deg (variable), number of excitations: 2. GRAPPA used for parallel imaging.

Pediatric Ear Diseases
Diagnostic Imaging Atlas and Case Reports

Normal CT Images of the Temporal Bone

The foundation for temporal bone imaging diagnosis lies in obtaining a thorough understanding of the ear's normal anatomical structures and their three-dimensional relationship. Through repeated comparison and identification of the details of normal structures and the anatomical terms that describe them, one gradually forms a mental image of the temporal bone's overall three-dimensional orientation. When one concurrently views clinical case images, one's eyes are drawn naturally to those forms that differ from the norm, which can then be compared to various known disease findings to arrive at an accurate diagnosis. This process also applies to pediatric cases but, with the exception of minor ailments such as otitis media, encounters with infant diseases in everyday clinical practice are infrequent, and examples of imaging diagnosis even rarer. Consequently, pediatric images are usually Interpreted with normal adult anatomy in mind. However, the temporal bone of infants in particular differs from that of an adult's with respect to the sizes and relative ratios of each component, so caution is required in reading and interpreting findings.

This chapter displays a complete series of serial cross-section and descriptive images, without omission, of temporal bone CT axial sections and coronal sections from both infants and older children. By examining the images from infants and older children, first separately and then in comparison, we will be able to develop a mental image of the anatomy of the temporal bone and its postnatal development.

Chapter 1

❶ Infant
❷ Older Child

❶ Infant

Figure 1 shows the basic anatomy of the ear. All the anatomical components shown in this figure exist from birth; however their sizes and locations change with age. The inner ear and ossicles in an infant's temporal bone are the same size as an adult, but the external auditory canal, internal auditory canal, and mastoid air cells are still small and grow with age. Roughly speaking, the cochlea, vestibule, semicircular canals, and tympanic cavity are at the center and change little, while the periphery expands anteroposteriorly, laterally, and vertically. Horizontal expansion, both laterally and front to back, can be observed through axial sections and vertical expansion through coronal sections. Of the various structures of the temporal bone, normal development of the mastoid air cells is suppressed by otitis media. Consequently when viewing pediatric temporal bone images, along with age, one must also take previous middle ear diseases into consideration.

In order to avoid surgical complications during ear surgery, it is necessary to have an accurate grasp of the positions of major anatomical structures within the temporal bone. However, an infant's temporal bone is smaller and more delicate than an adult's and its anatomical orientation during surgery is different. When performing temporal bone surgery under a microscope, even an error of 1 mm may result in injury to the facial nerve, the semicircular canals, or the stapes. Common preoperative checkpoints for most otological surgical procedures include: 1) degree of mastoid air cell development and the height of the base of the middle cranial fossa lateral to the epitympanum (attic); 2) lateromedial width and air cell development of the facial recess region; 3) distance between the sigmoid sinus and the posterior wall of the external auditory canal; 4) pneumatization (=air cell development) in the direction of the mastoid process; and 5) thickness of the cranial wall in the temporoparietal region. If any of these are narrower or smaller than normal, one must plan ahead to determine how to overcome the difficulties presented to secure sufficient surgical field visibility and achieve one's objective.

The images shown are of a 4-month-old female infant who underwent CT examination for bilateral hearing loss. They are presented here as normal temporal bone CT images as no clear abnormal findings were discovered in them. The coronal section images were reconstructed from data taken in the axial section images, with no direct images taken from a supine hanging-head position. For display purposes, coronal section images have been magnified to approx. 1.7 times the axial section images. Also, the images are arranged from bottom to top (inferior to superior) for the axial sections and from front to back (anterior to posterior) for the coronal sections. Images of the same cross sections are arranged side by side, with the right image annotated to indicate each anatomical structure. (Scale shown in images indicates 1 cm)

The base line for the CT images was set based on the plane that includes bilateral OM lines, the line that passes through the outer canthus of the eye and the center of the external auditory canal.

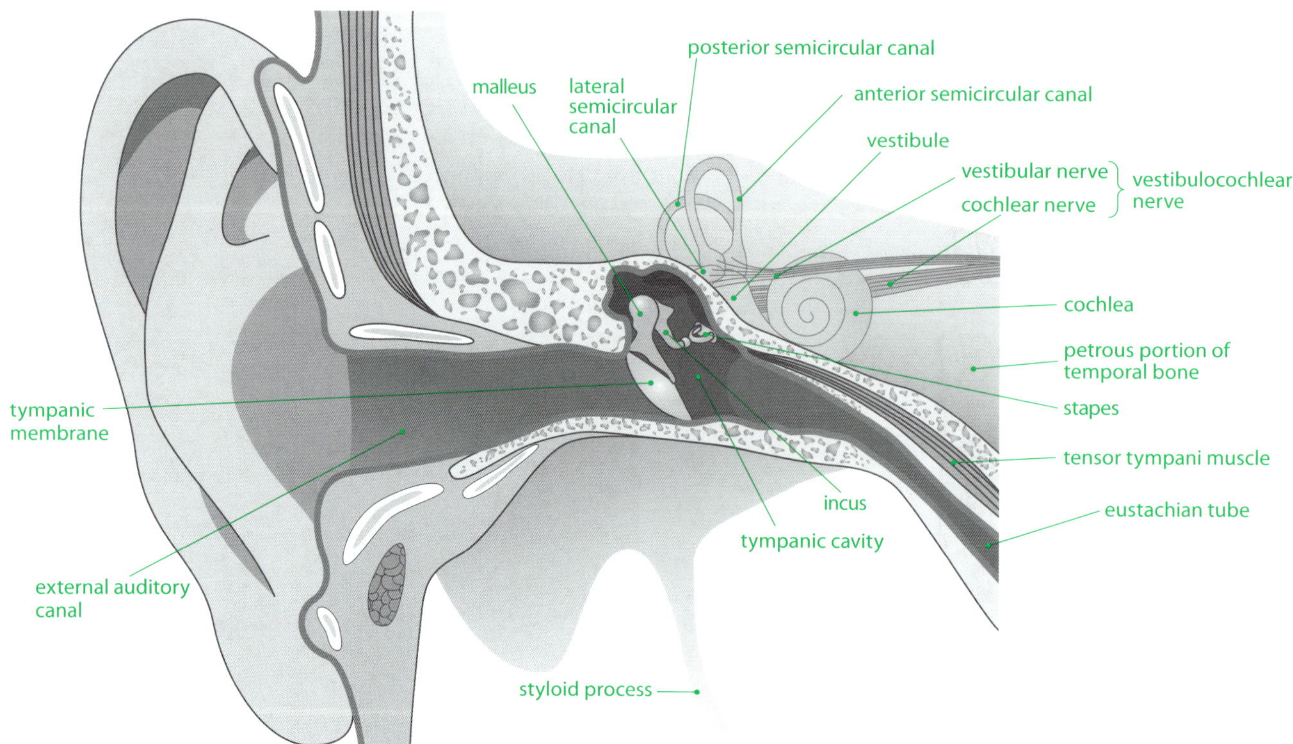

Fig. 1. The anatomy of the ear.

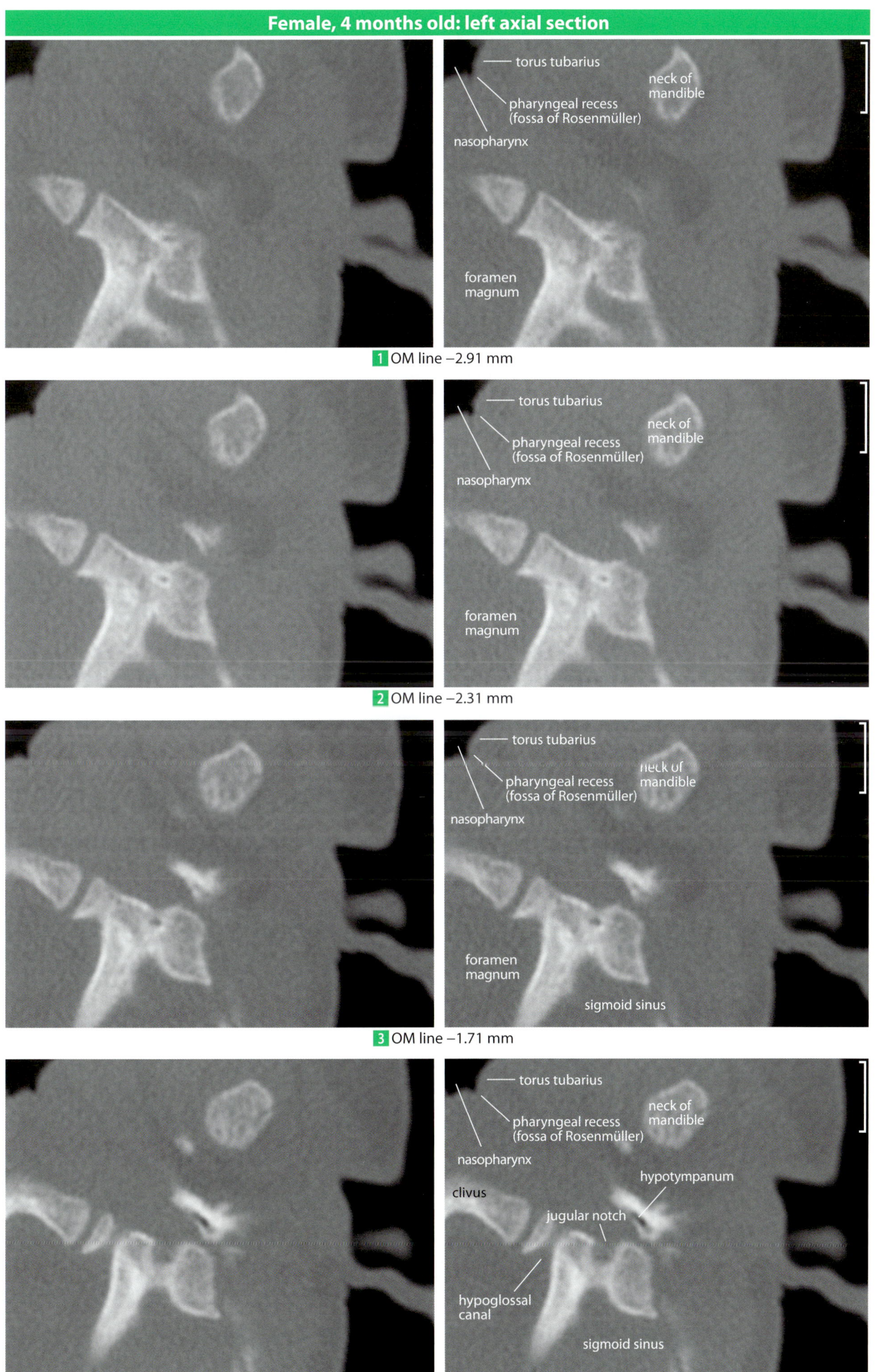

1 OM line −2.91 mm

2 OM line −2.31 mm

3 OM line −1.71 mm

4 OM line −1.12 mm

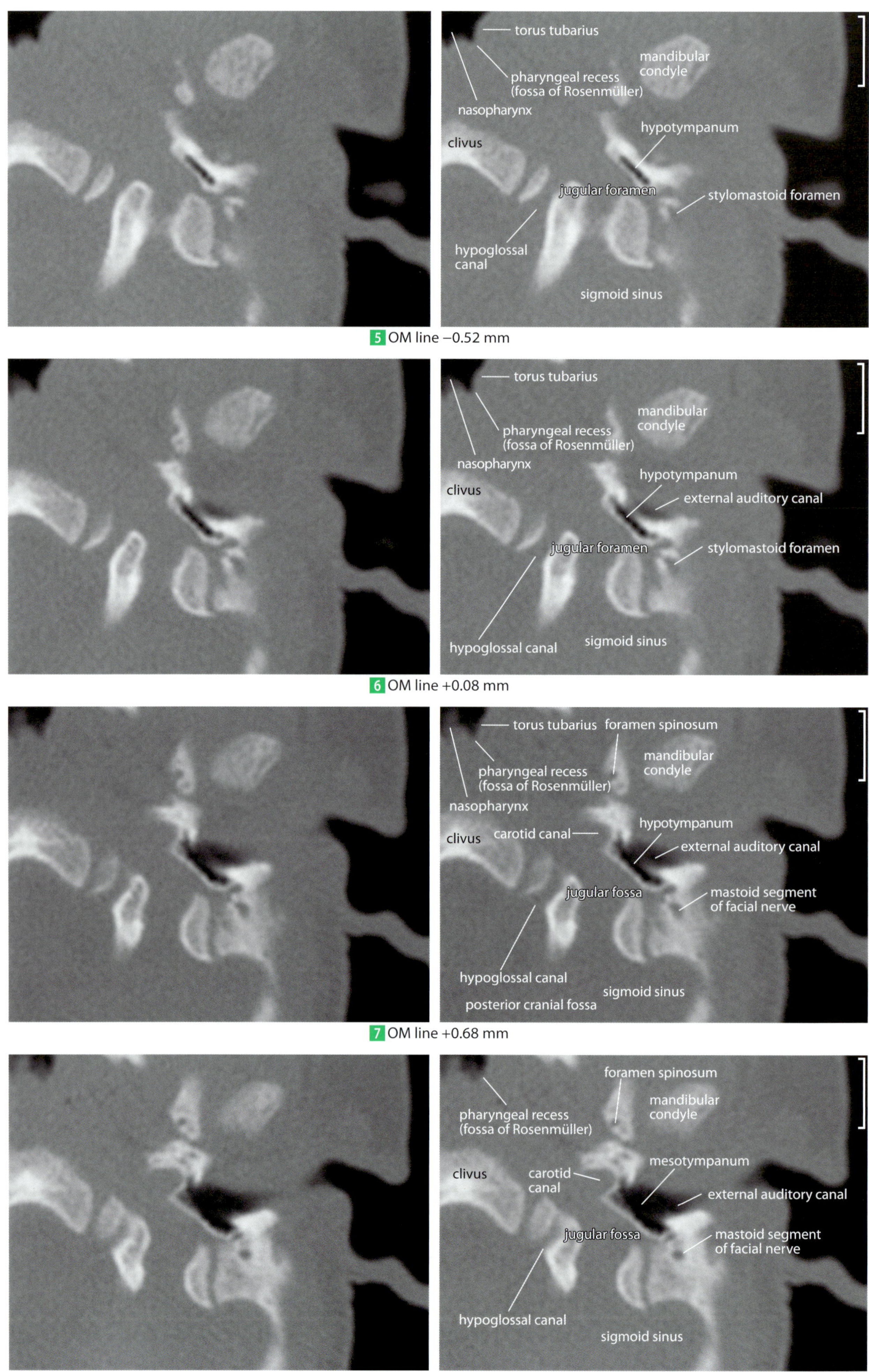

5 OM line −0.52 mm

6 OM line +0.08 mm

7 OM line +0.68 mm

8 OM line +1.28 mm

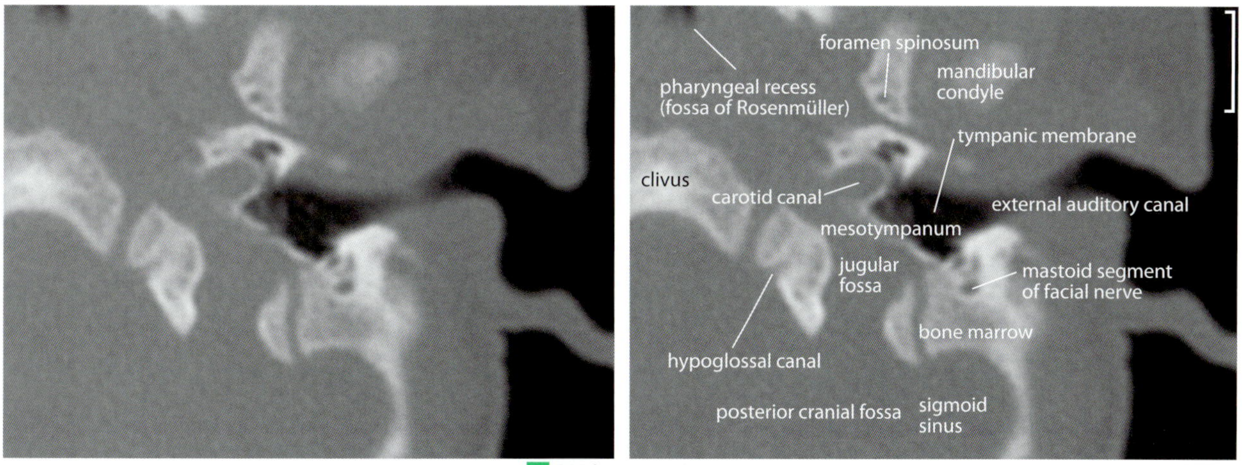

9 OM line +1.88 mm

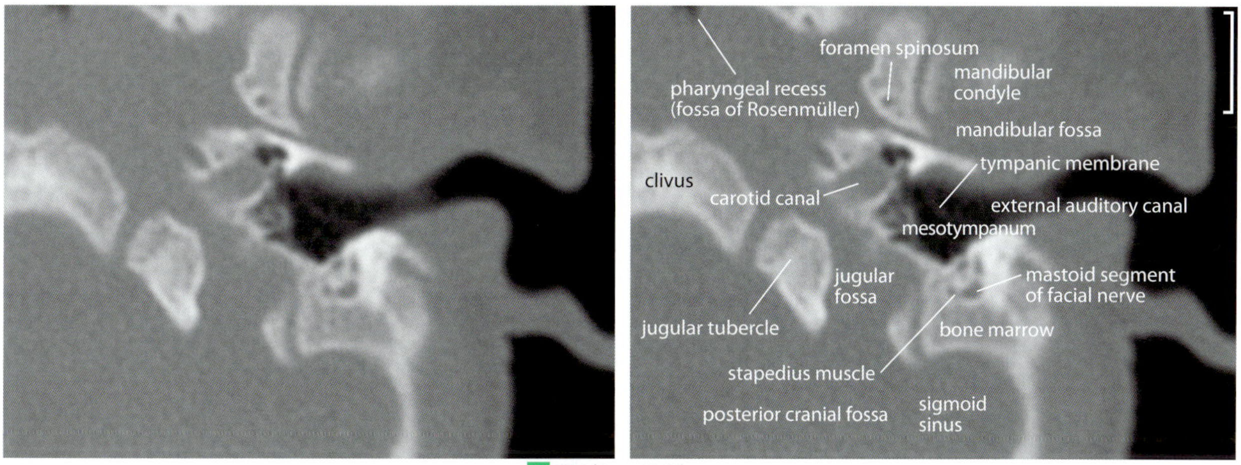

10 OM line +2.48 mm

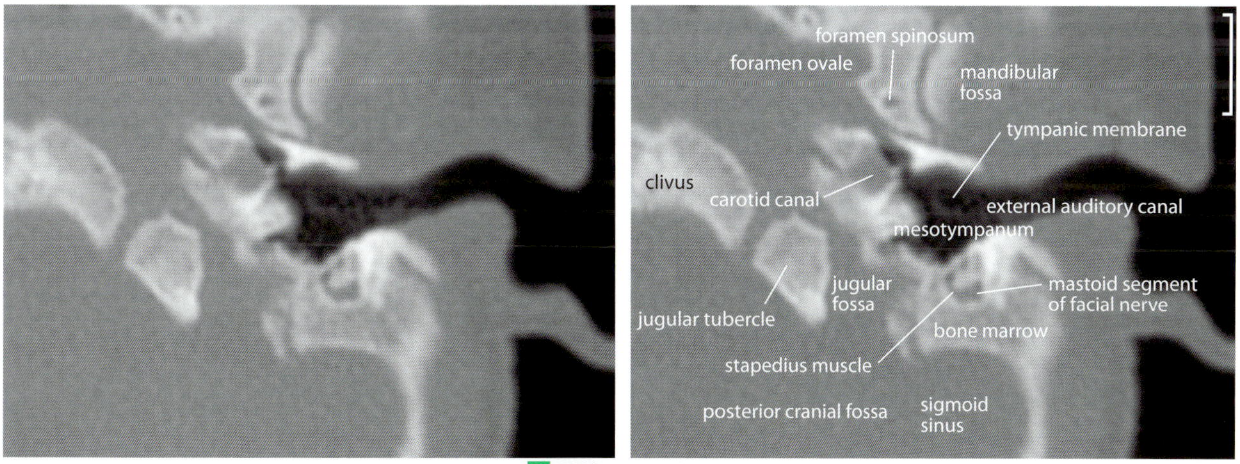

11 OM line +3.08 mm

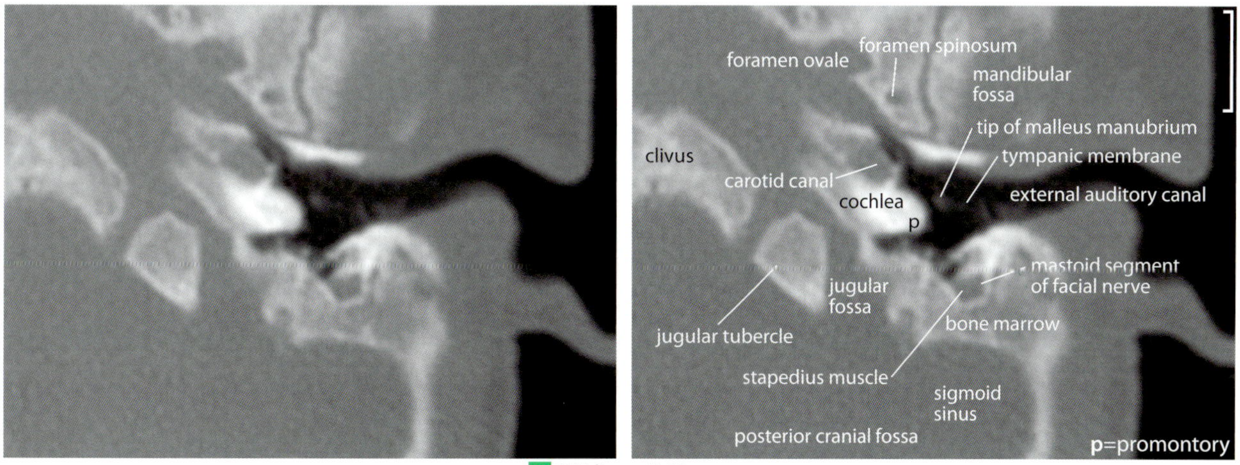

12 OM line +3.68 mm

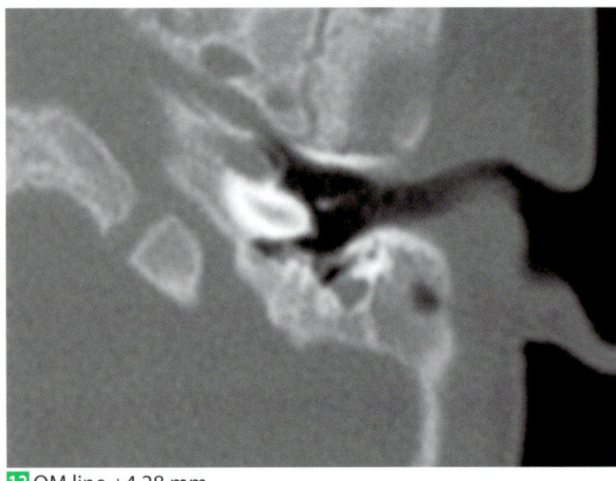

13 OM line +4.28 mm

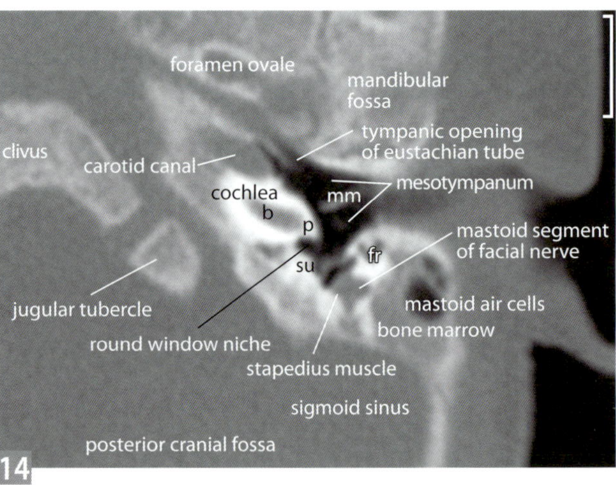

b=basal turn of cochlea; **p**=promontory;
mm=manubrium of malleus;
su=subiculum of promontory; **fr**=facial recess

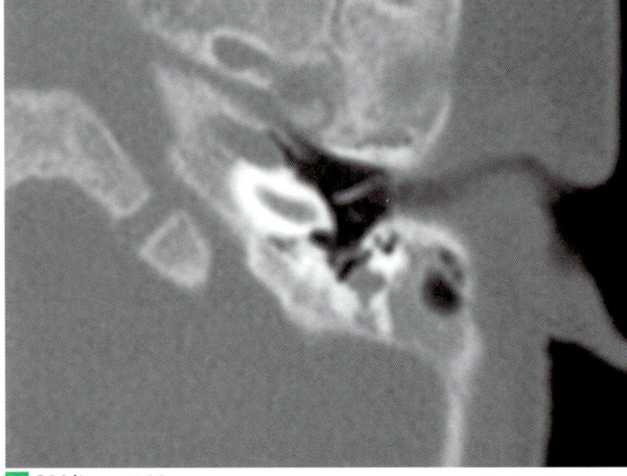

14 OM line +4.88 mm

b=basal turn of cochlea; **p**=promontory;
mm=manubrium of malleus; **le**=lenticular process of incus;
h=head of stapes; **su**=subiculum of promontory;
ts=tympanic sinus; **fr**=facial recess

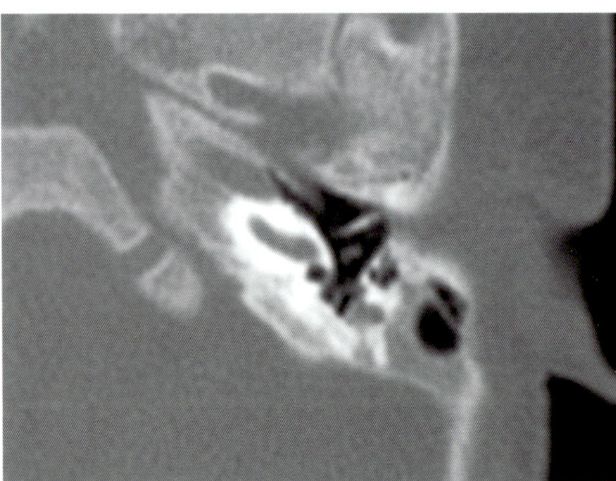

16 OM line +6.08 mm

b=basal turn of cochlea; **o**=osseous spiral lamina; **p**=promontory;
n=neck of malleus; **le**=lenticular process of incus;
=incudostapedial joint; **h**=head of stapes; **ts**=tympanic sinus;
fr=facial recess

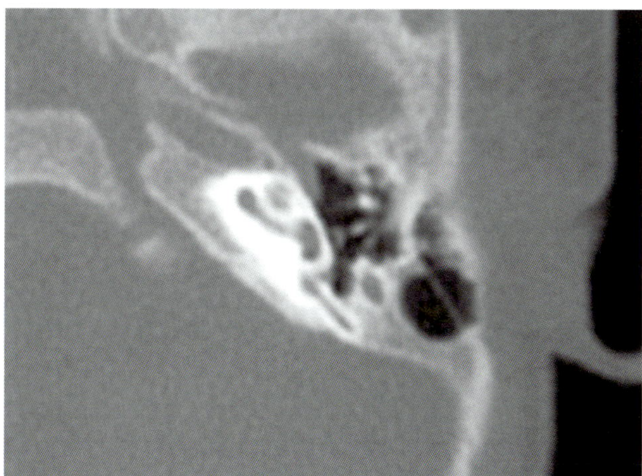

17 OM line +6.68 mm

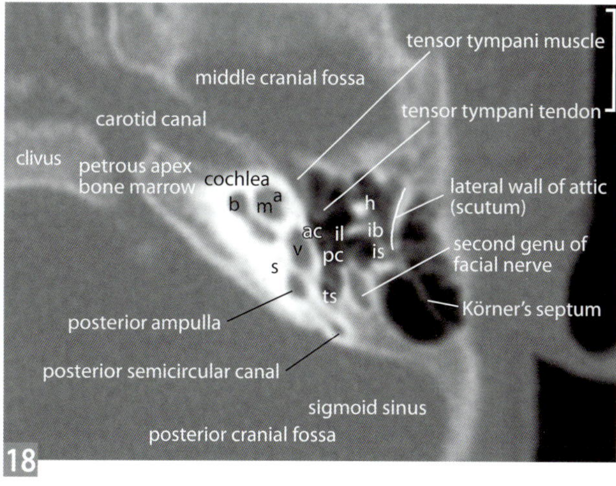

18

a=apical turn of cochlea; **m**=middle turn of cochlea;
b=basal turn of cochlea; **v**=vestibule; **s**=singlar canal;
h=head of malleus; **ib**=body of incus; **il**=long process of incus;
is=short process of incus; **ac**=anterior crus of stapes;
pc=posterior crus of stapes; **ts**=tympanic sinus

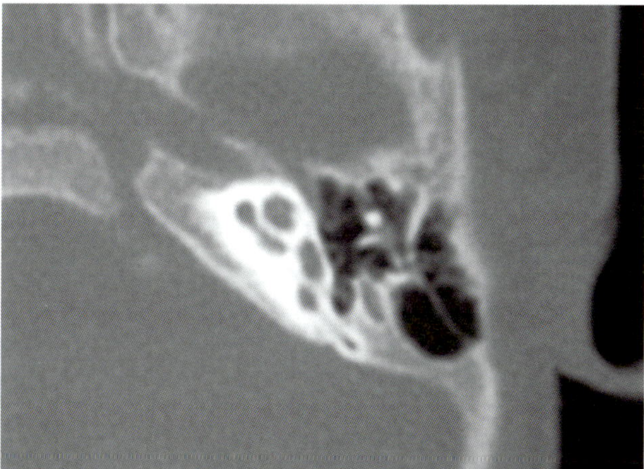

18 OM line +7.28 mm

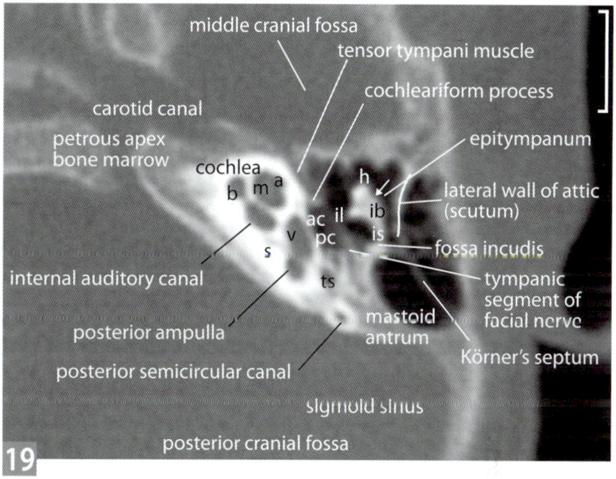

19

a=apical turn of cochlea; **m**=middle turn of cochlea;
b=basal turn of cochlea; **v**=vestibule; **s**=singlar canal;
h=head of malleus; ✐=malleoincudal joint; **ib**=body of incus;
il=long process of incus; **is**=short process of incus;
ac=anterior crus of stapes; **pc**=posterior crus of stapes;
ts=tympanic sinus

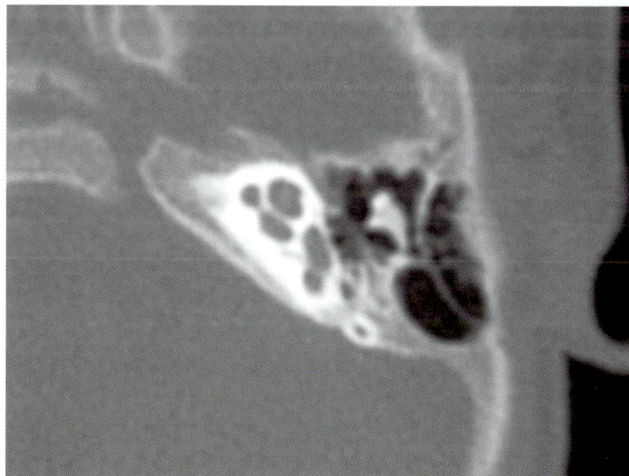

19 OM line +7.88 mm

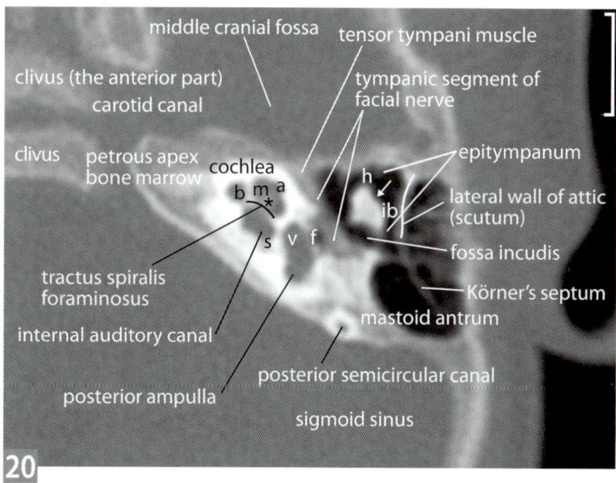

20

a=apical turn of cochlea; **m**=middle turn of cochlea;
b=basal turn of cochlea; ✶=modiolus; **f**=footplate of stapes;
v=vestibule; **s**=singlar canal; **h**=head of malleus;
✐=malleoincudal joint; **ib**=body of incus

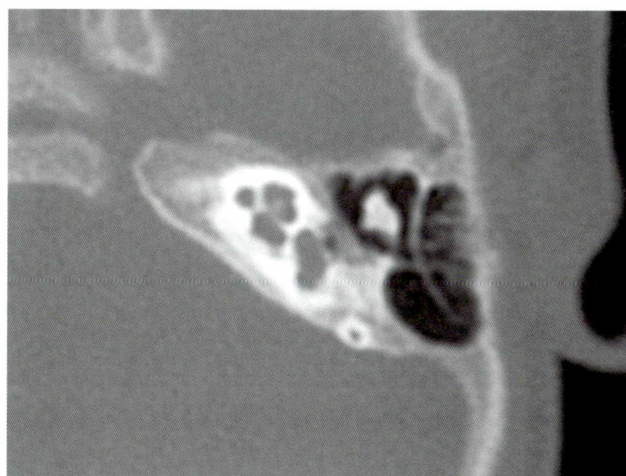

20 OM line +8.48 mm

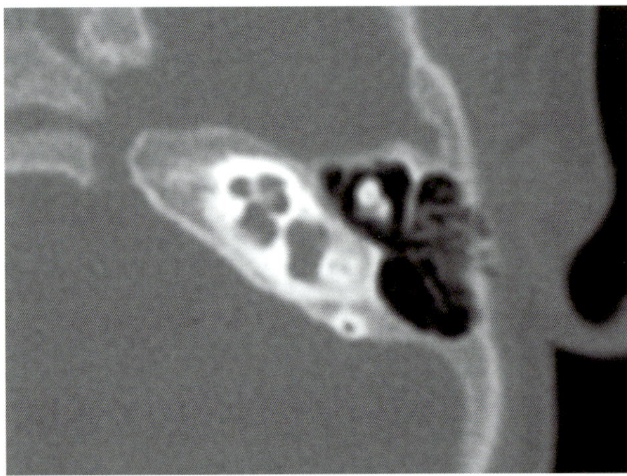

21 OM line +9.08 mm

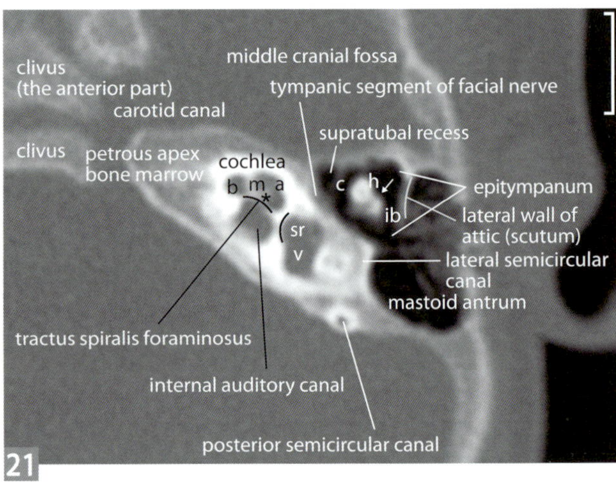

a=apical turn of cochlea; **m**=middle turn of cochlea;
b=basal turn of cochlea; *=modiolus; **v**=vestibule;
sr=spherical recess; **c**=anterior attic bony plate (cog);
h=head of malleus; =malleoincudal joint; **ib**=body of incus

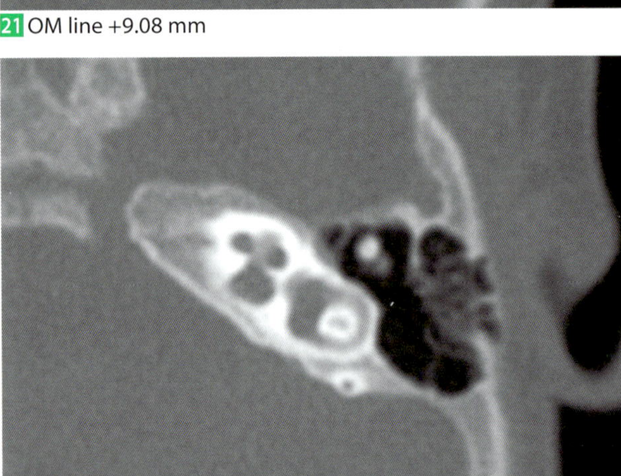

22 OM line +9.68 mm

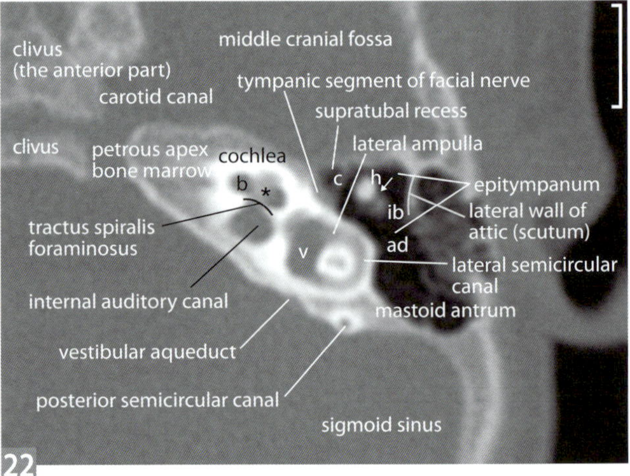

b=basal turn of cochlea; *=modiolus; **v**=vestibule;
c=anterior attic bony plate (cog); **h**=head of malleus;
=malleoincudal joint; **ib**=body of incus; **ad**=aditus ad antrum

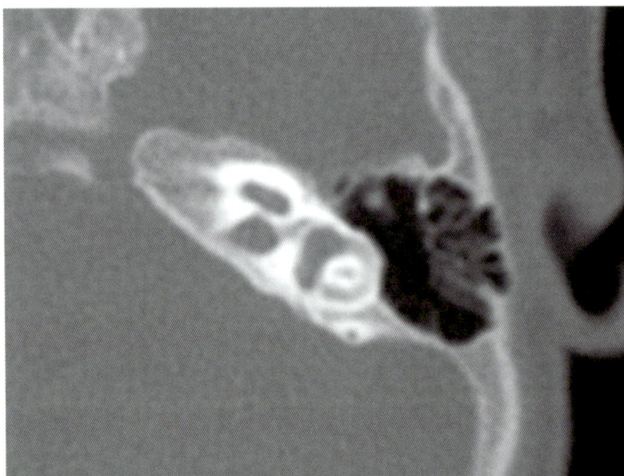

23 OM line +10.28 mm

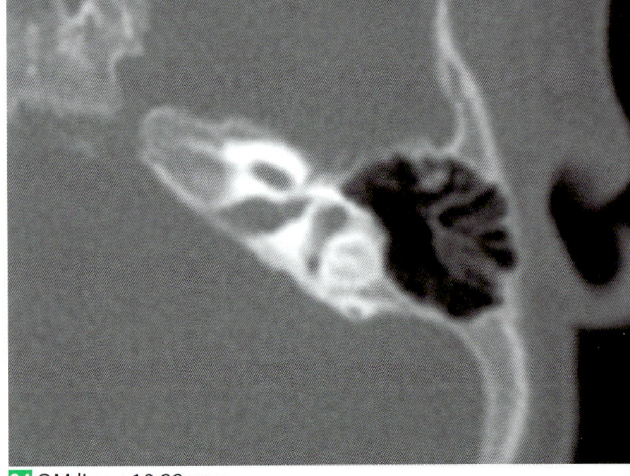

24 OM line +10.88 mm

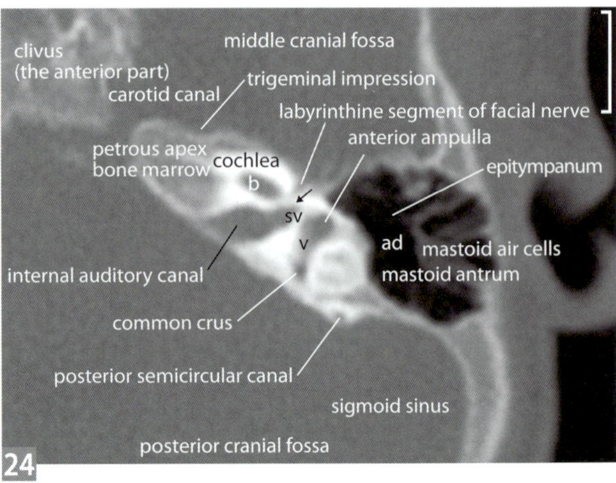

b=basal turn of cochlea; =Bill's bar;
sv=superior vestibular nerve; **v**=vestibule; **ad**=aditus ad antrum

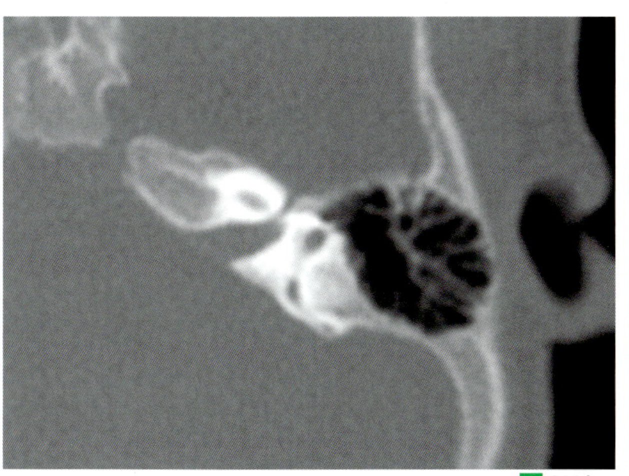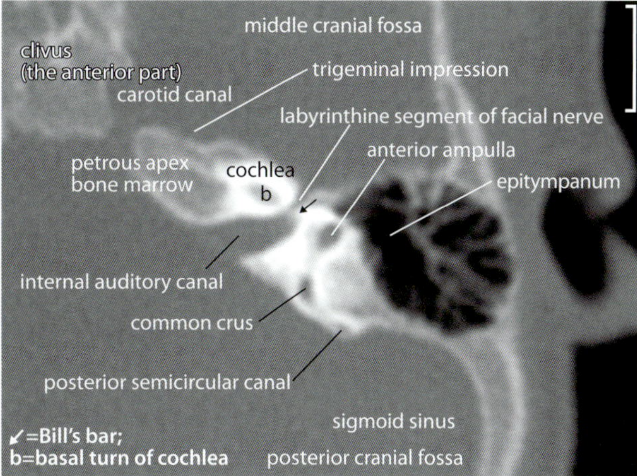

25 OM line +11.48 mm

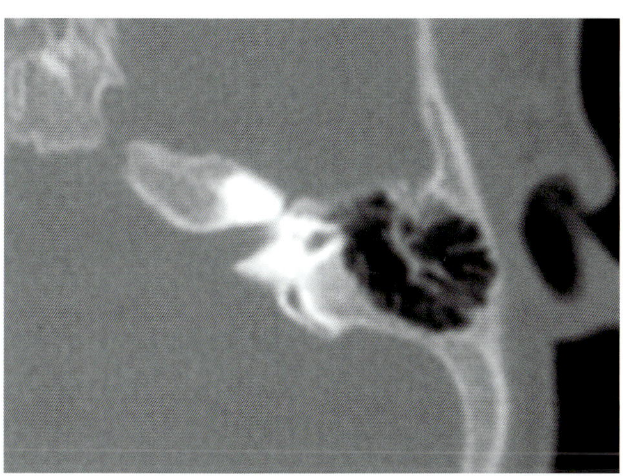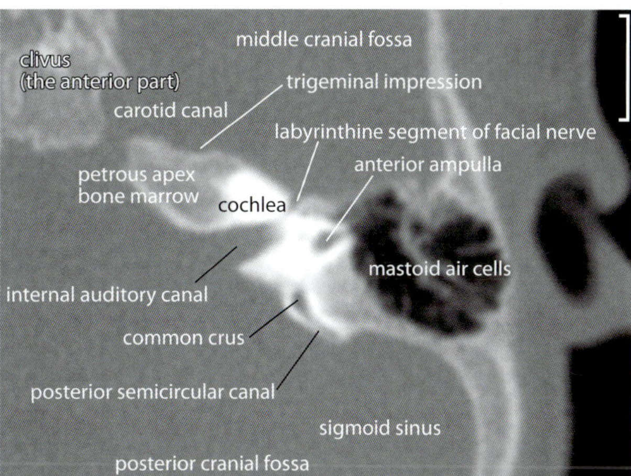

26 OM line +12.08 mm

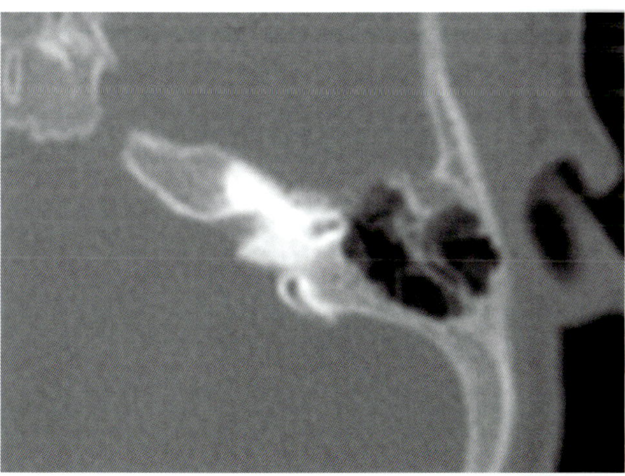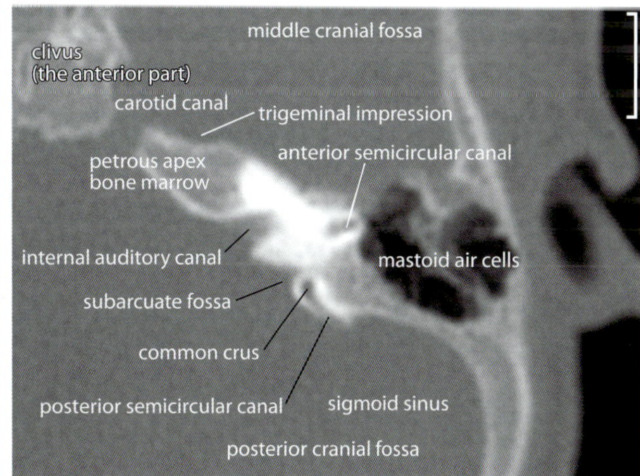

27 OM line +12.68 mm

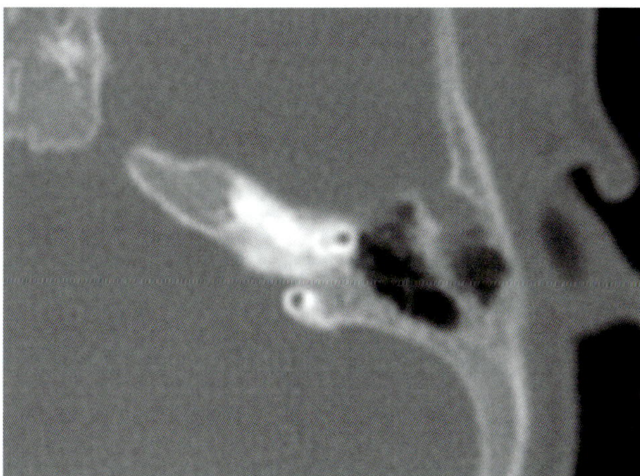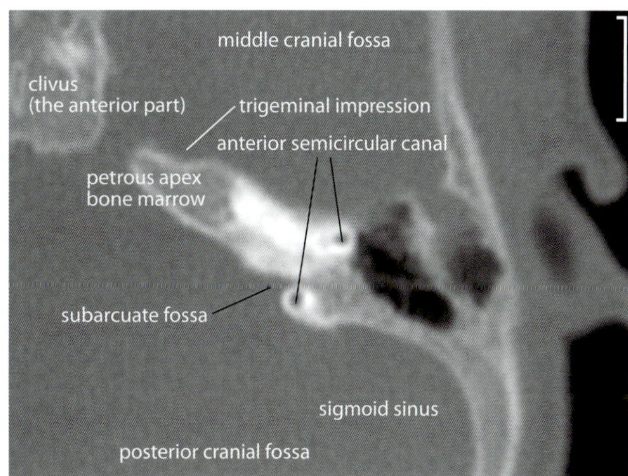

28 OM line +13.28 mm

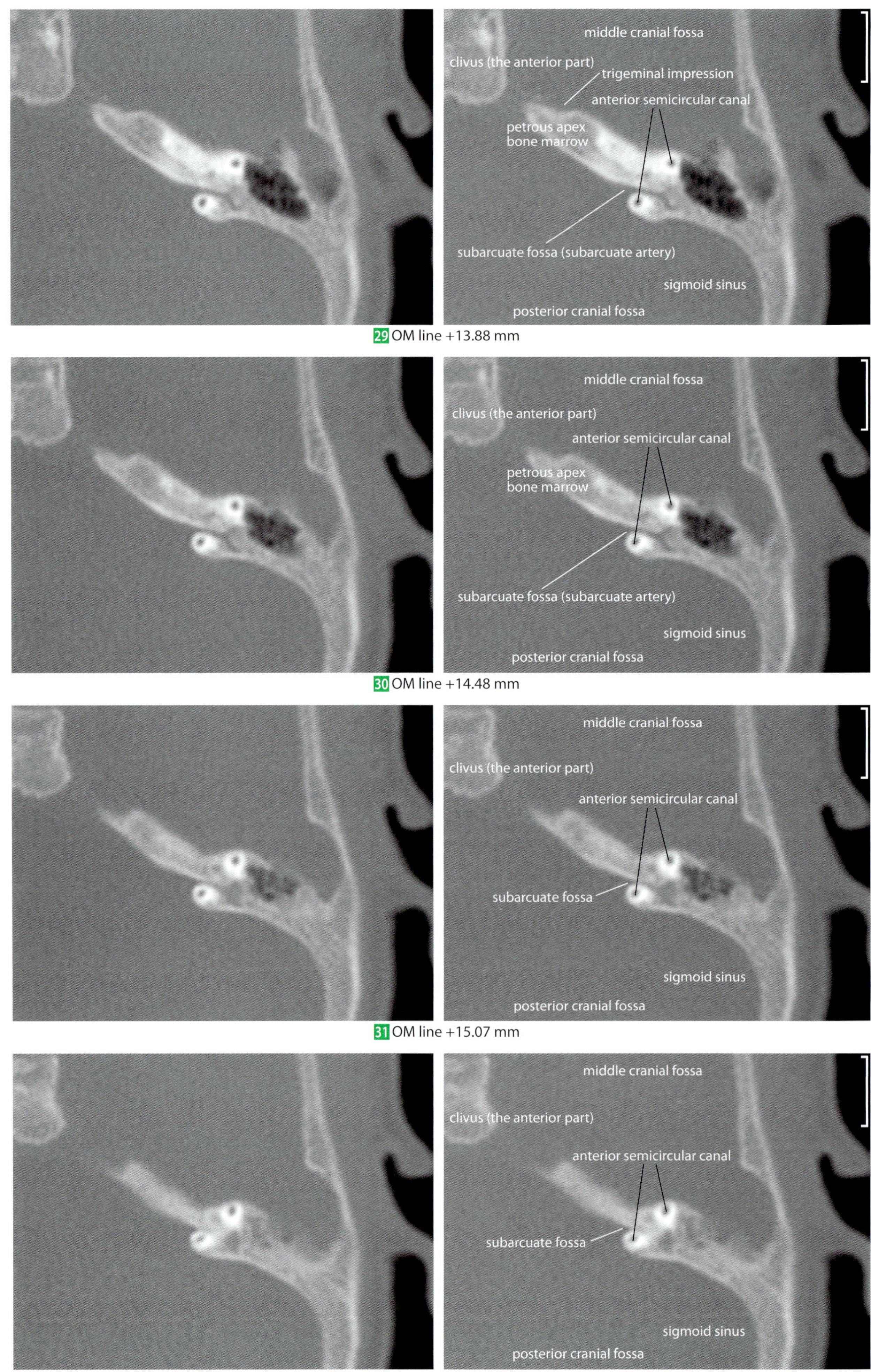

middle cranial fossa
clivus (the anterior part)
trigeminal impression
anterior semicircular canal
petrous apex
bone marrow
subarcuate fossa (subarcuate artery)
sigmoid sinus
posterior cranial fossa
29 OM line +13.88 mm
middle cranial fossa
clivus (the anterior part)
anterior semicircular canal
petrous apex
bone marrow
subarcuate fossa (subarcuate artery)
sigmoid sinus
posterior cranial fossa
30 OM line +14.48 mm
middle cranial fossa
clivus (the anterior part)
anterior semicircular canal
subarcuate fossa
sigmoid sinus
posterior cranial fossa
31 OM line +15.07 mm
middle cranial fossa
clivus (the anterior part)
anterior semicircular canal
subarcuate fossa
sigmoid sinus
posterior cranial fossa
32 OM line +15.67 mm

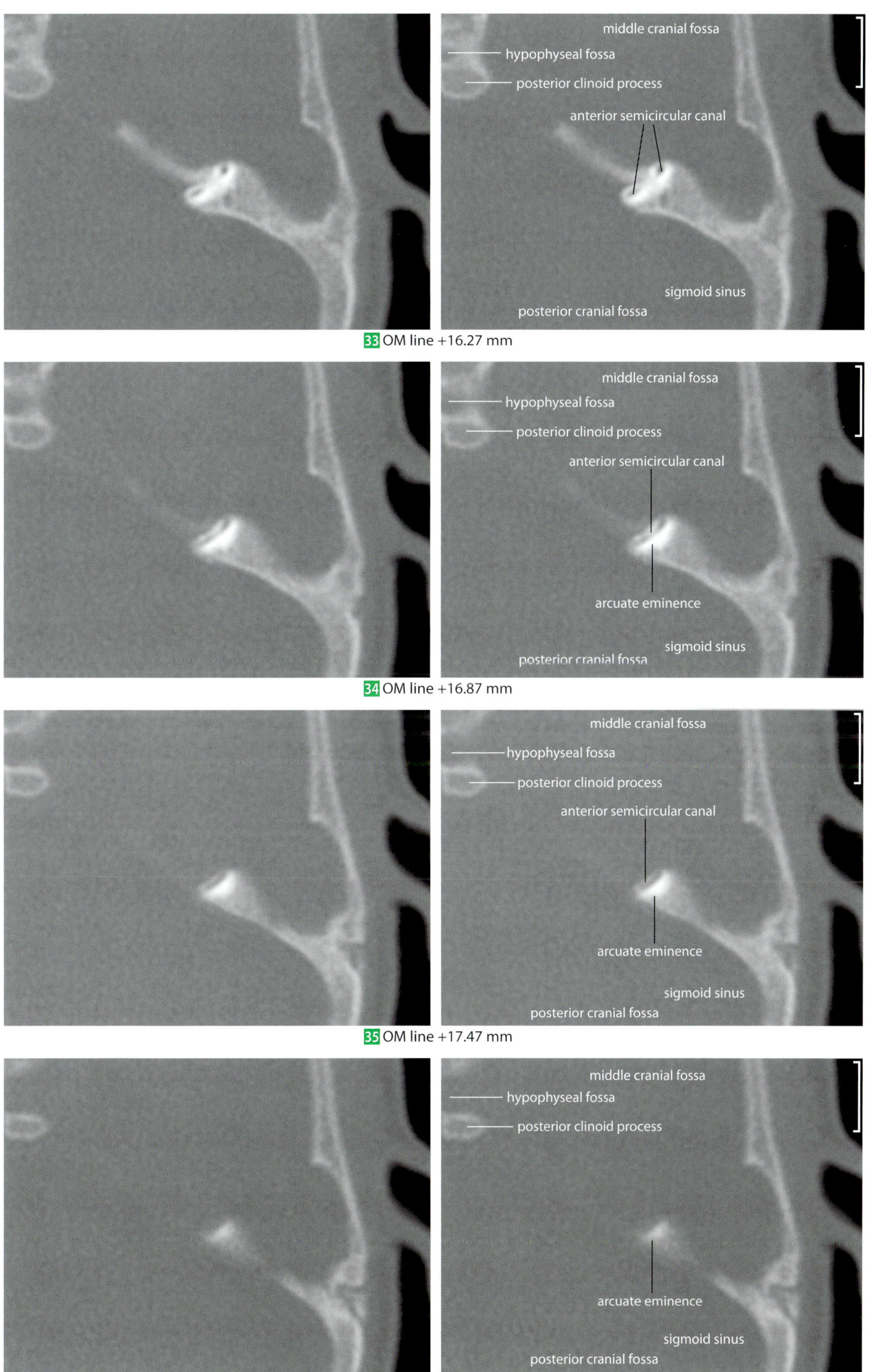

33 OM line +16.27 mm

34 OM line +16.87 mm

35 OM line +17.47 mm

36 OM line +18.07 mm

Female, 4 months old: left coronal section

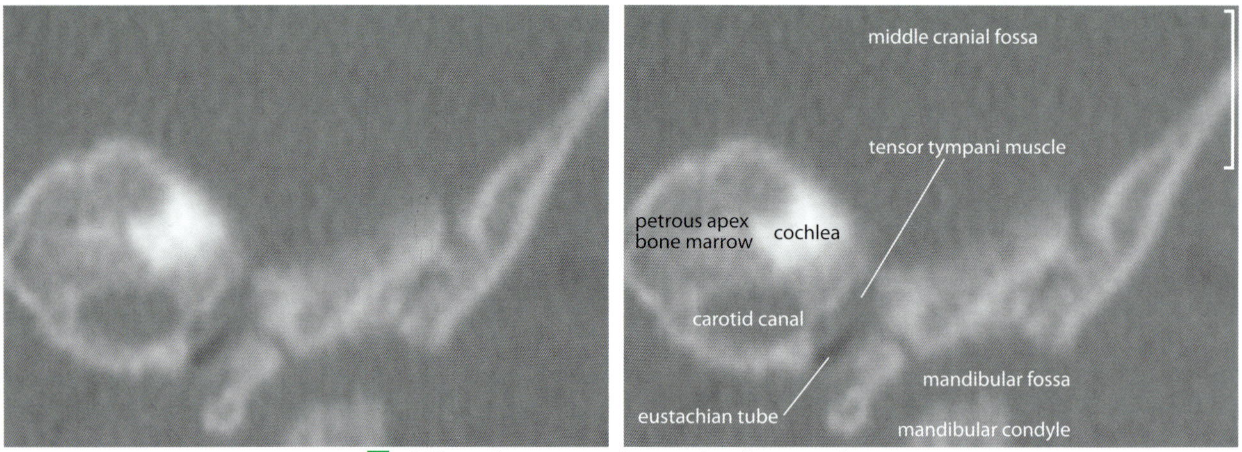

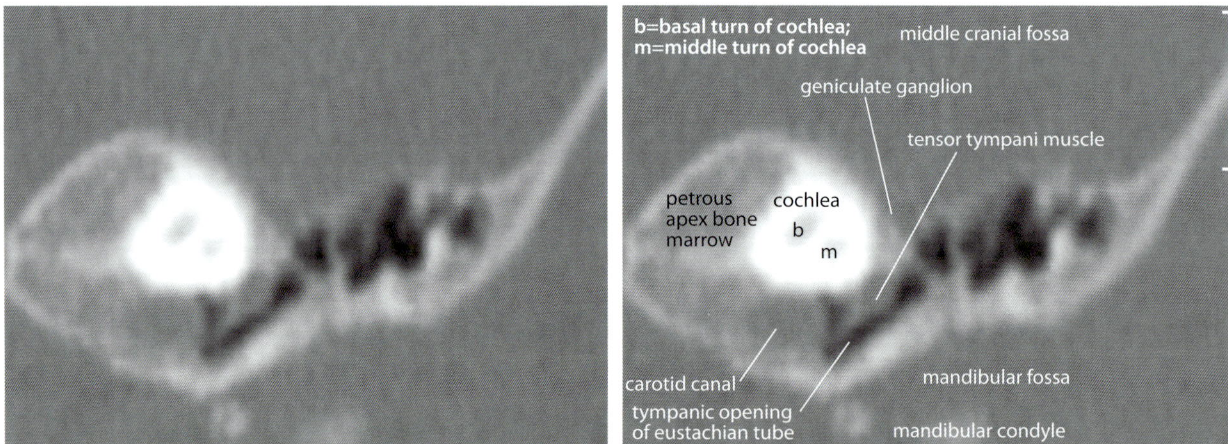

1 +4.00 mm from center of external auditory canal

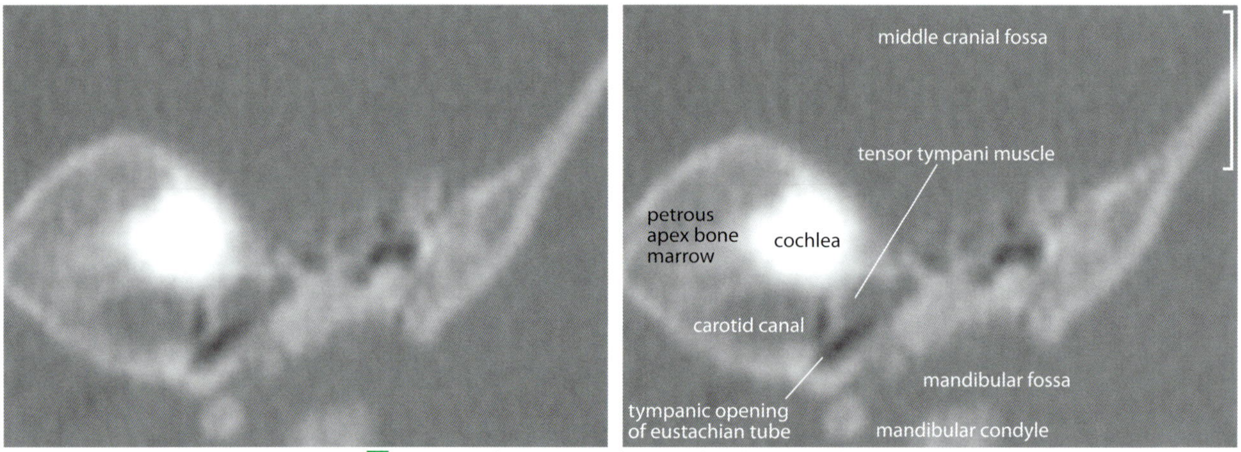

2 +3.35 mm from center of external auditory canal

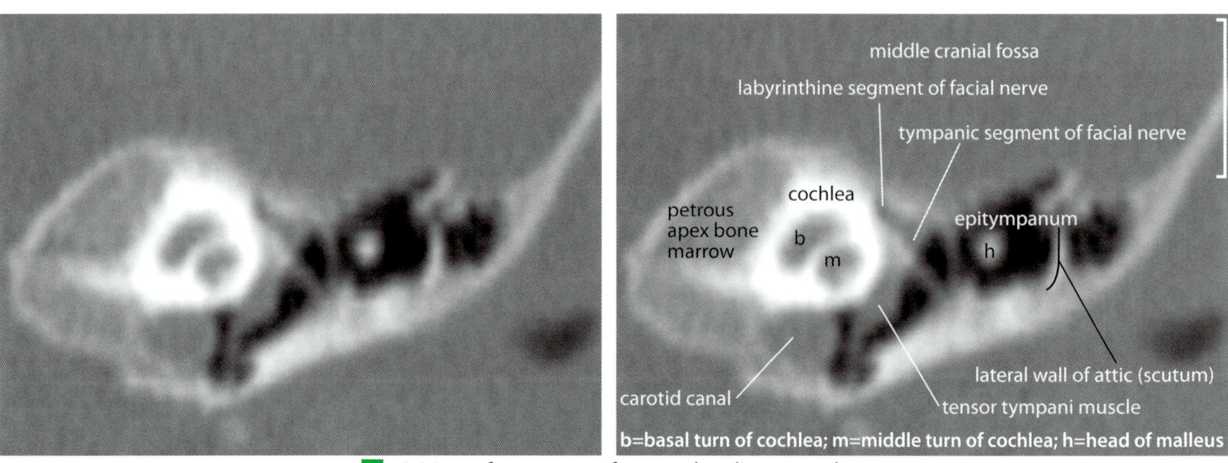

3 +2.70 mm from center of external auditory canal

4 +2.04 mm from center of external auditory canal

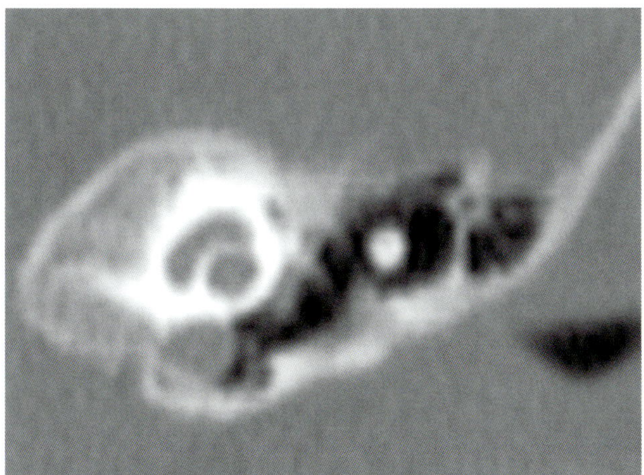

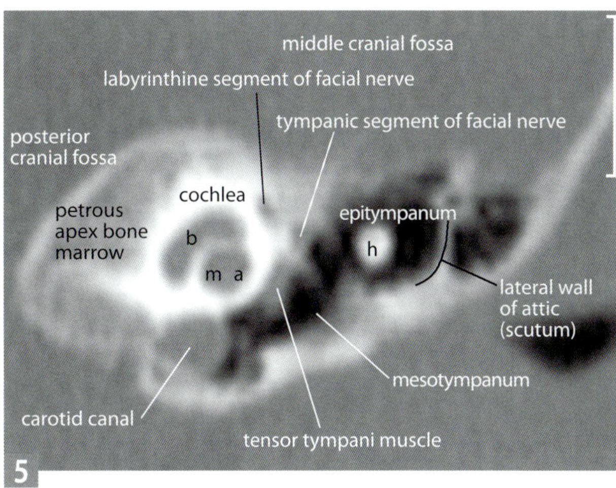

b=basal turn of cochlea; **m**=middle turn of cochlea; **a**=apical turn of cochlea; **h**=head of malleus

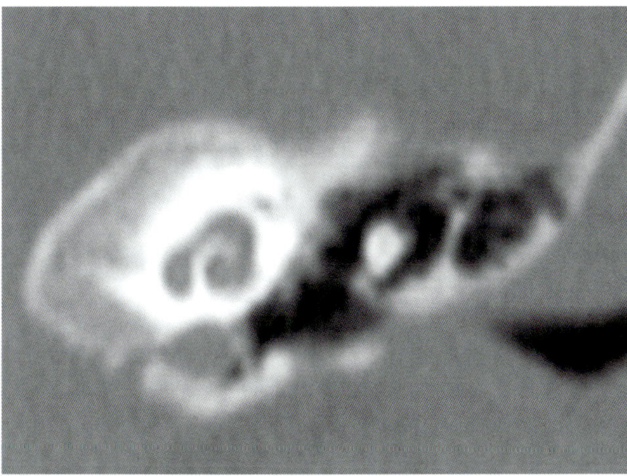

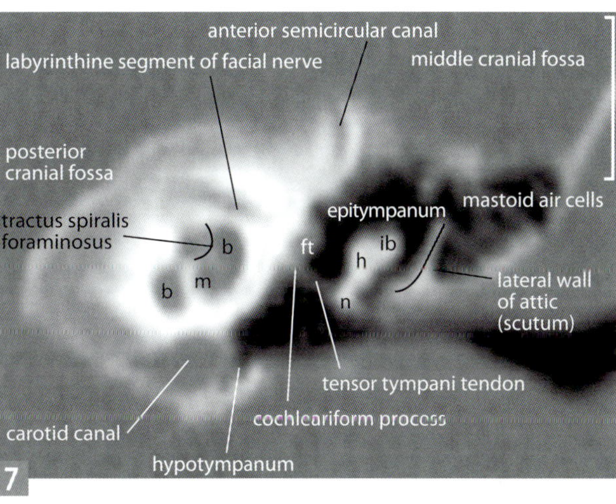

ft=tympanic segment of facial nerve; **b**=basal turn of cochlea; **m**=middle turn of cochlea; **ib**=body of incus; **h**=head of malleus; **n**=neck of malleus

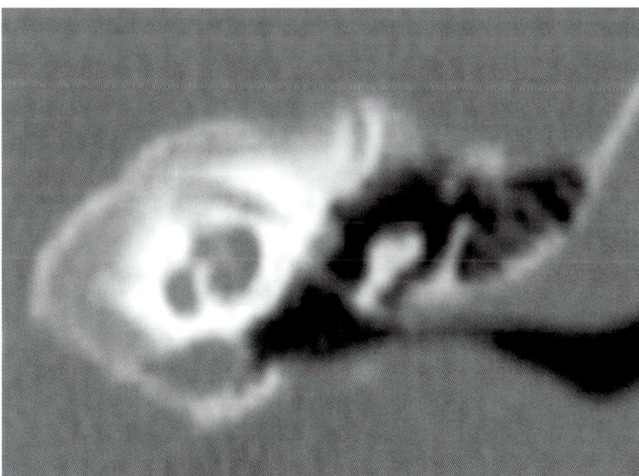

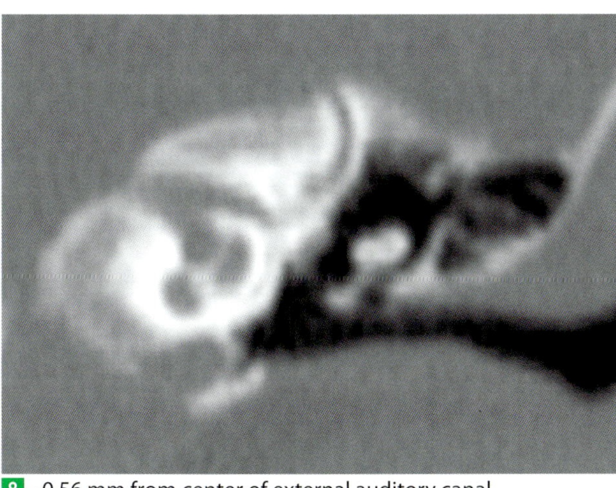

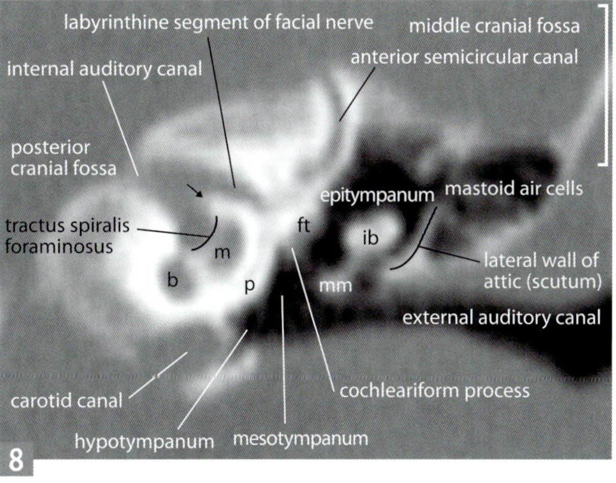

ft=tympanic segment of facial nerve; **b**=basal turn of cochlea; **m**=middle turn of cochlea; **p**=promontory; ↘=transverse crest; **ib**=body of incus; **mm**=manubrium of malleus

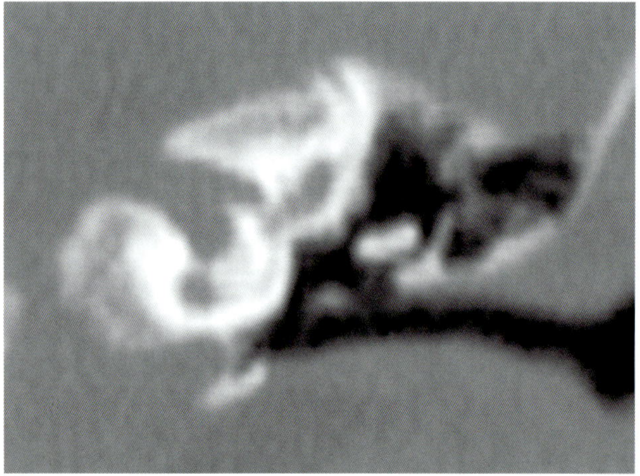

9 −1.22 mm from center of external auditory canal

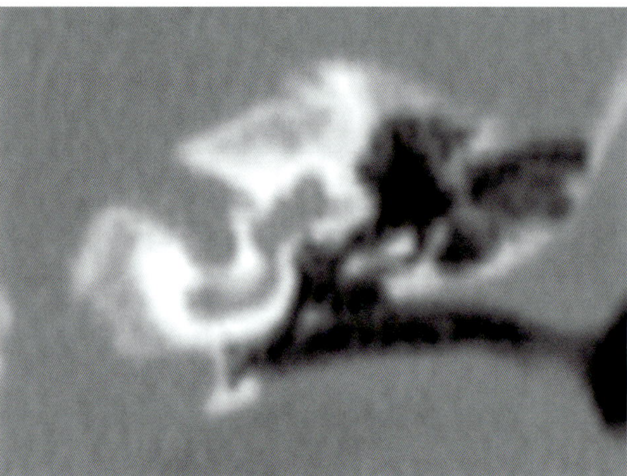

10 −1.87 mm from center of external auditory canal

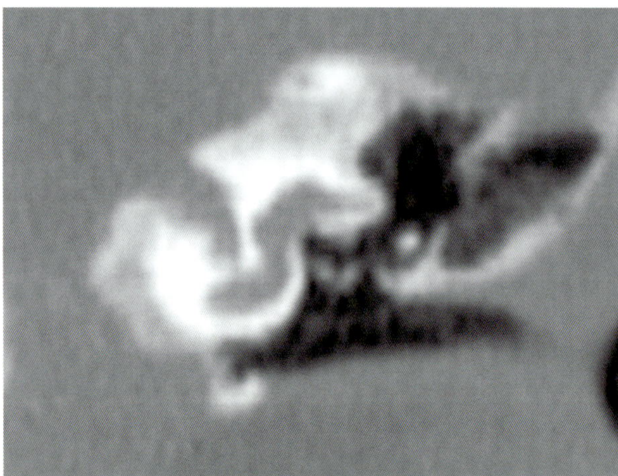

11 −2.52 mm from center of external auditory canal

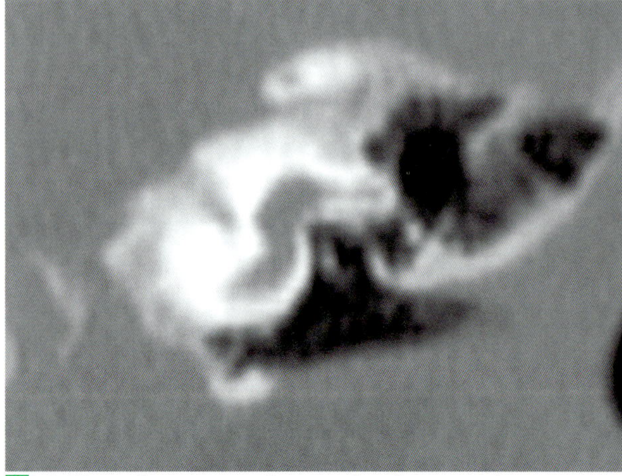

12 −3.17 mm from center of external auditory canal

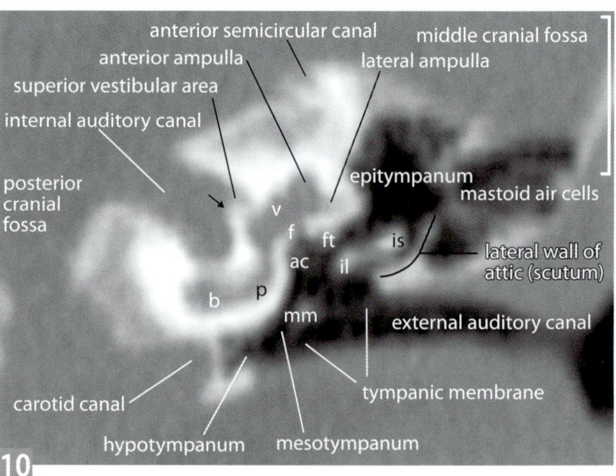

ft=tympanic segment of facial nerve; **v**=vestibule; **b**=basal turn of cochlea; **p**=promontory; ↘=transverse crest; **is**=short process of incus; **il**=long process of incus; **mm**=manubrium of malleus; **ac**=anterior crus of stapes; **f**=footplate of stapes

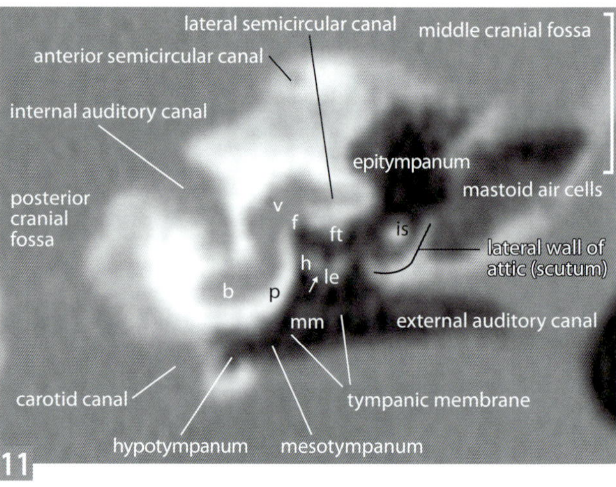

ft=tympanic segment of facial nerve; **v**=vestibule; **b**=basal turn of cochlea; **p**=promontory; **is**=short process of incus; **le**=lenticular process of incus; ↗=incudostapedial joint; **h**=head of stapes; **f**=footplate of stapes; **mm**=manubrium of malleus

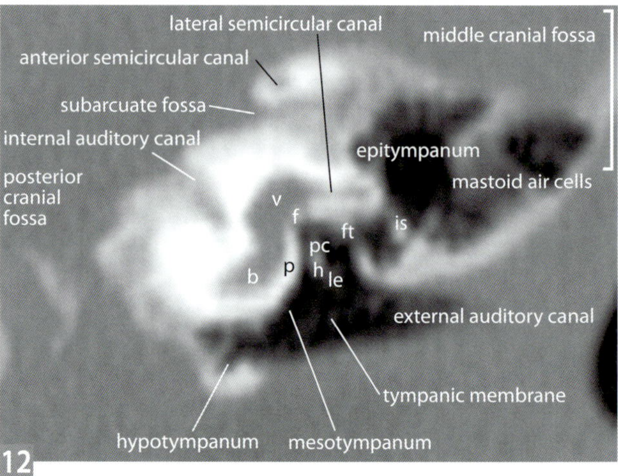

ft=tympanic segment of facial nerve; **v**=vestibule; **b**=basal turn of cochlea; **p**=promontory; **is**=short process of incus; **le**=lenticular process of incus; **h**=head of stapes; **pc**=posterior crus of stapes; **f**=footplate of stapes

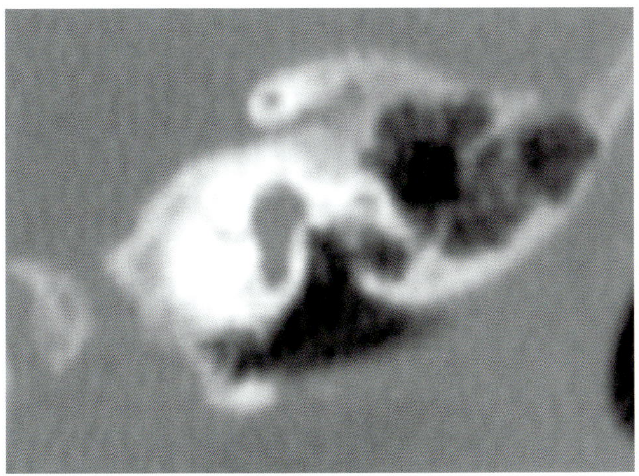

13 −3.82 mm from center of external auditory canal

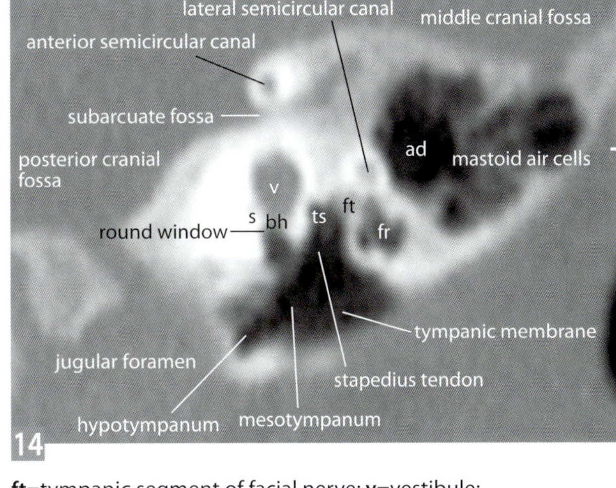

ft=tympanic segment of facial nerve; **v**=vestibule;
bh=basal turn of cochlea (hook portion); **s**=singlar canal;
ad=aditus ad antrum; **fr**=facial recess; **ts**=tympanic sinus

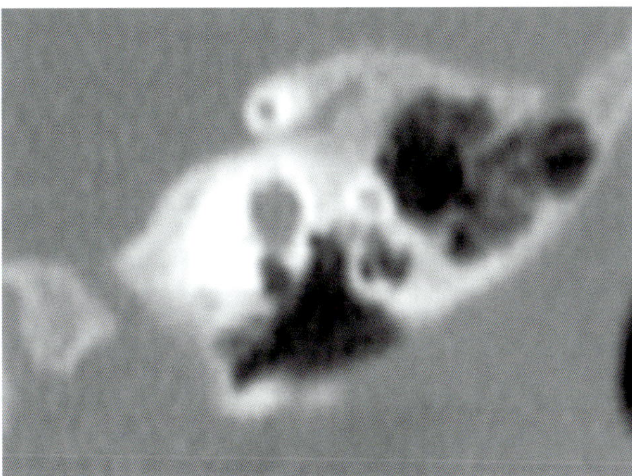

14 −4.47 mm from center of external auditory canal

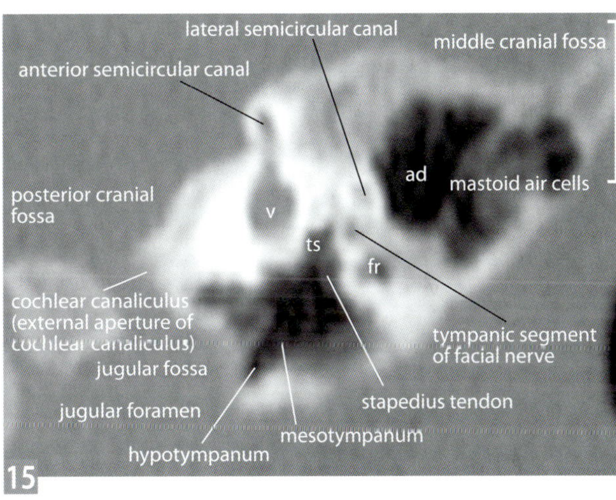

v=vestibule; **ad**=aditus ad antrum; **fr**=facial recess

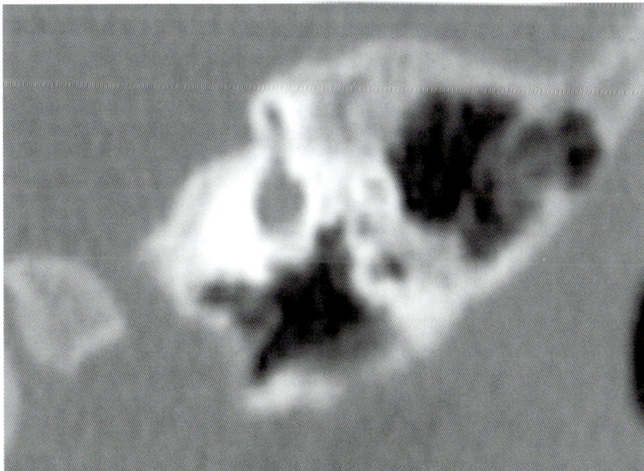

15 −5.13 mm from center of external auditory canal

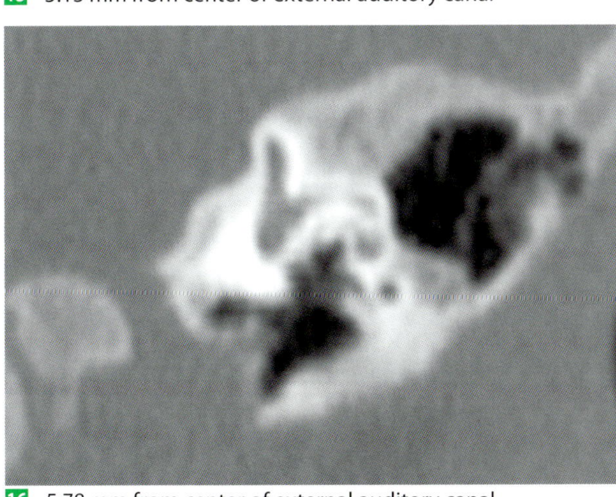

16 −5.78 mm from center of external auditory canal

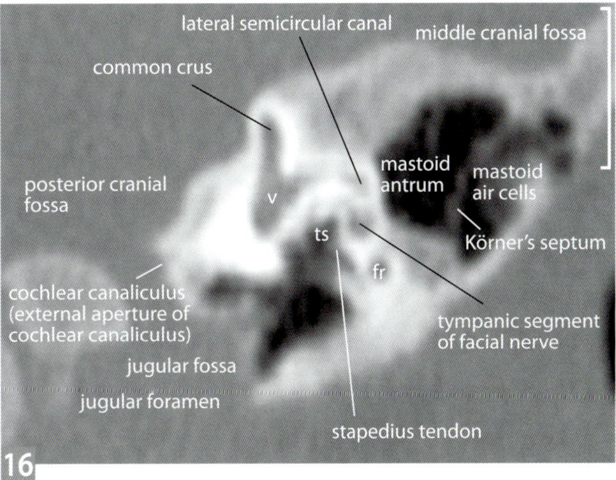

v=vestibule; **ts**=tympanic sinus; **fr**=facial recess

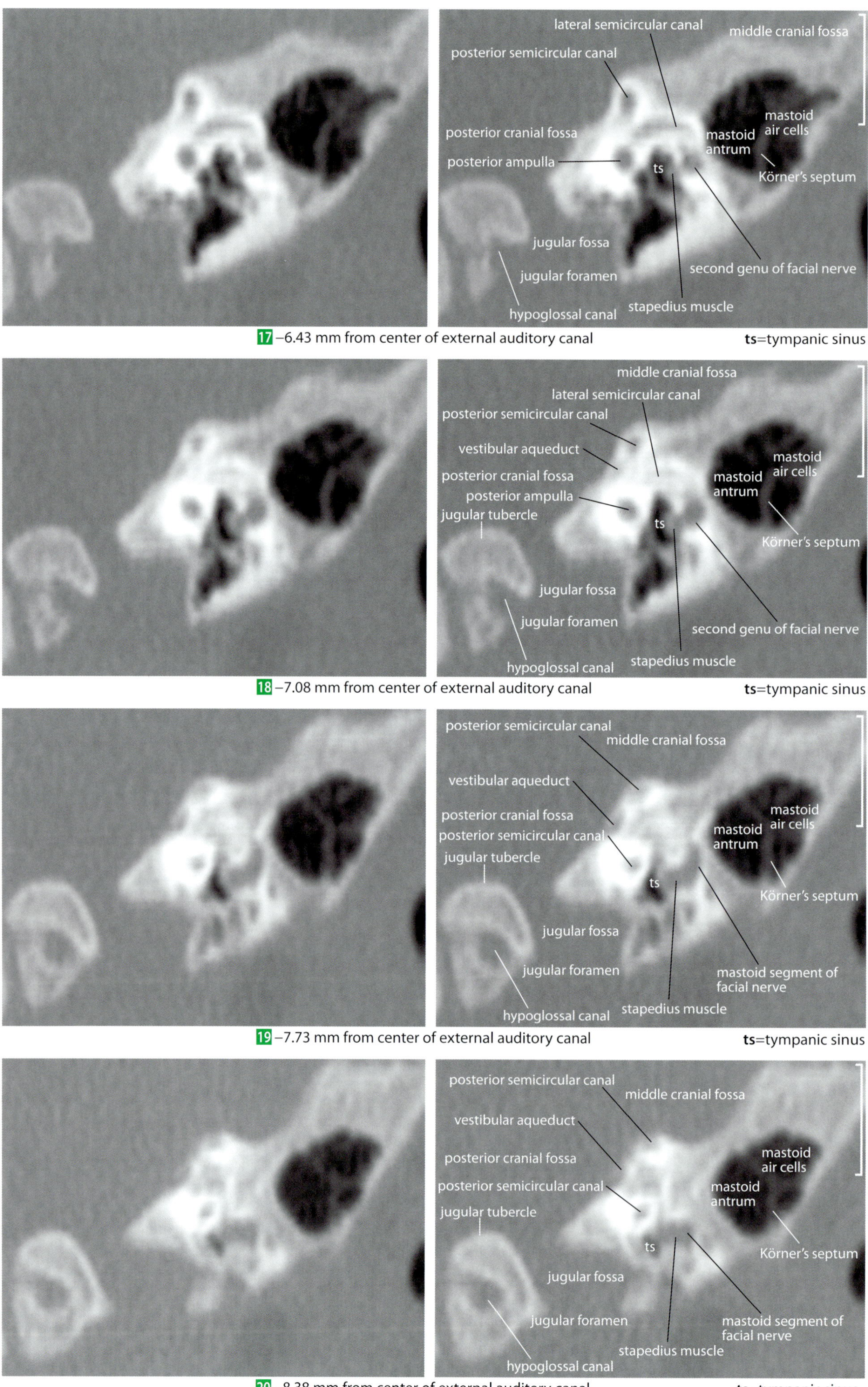

17 −6.43 mm from center of external auditory canal — **ts**=tympanic sinus

18 −7.08 mm from center of external auditory canal — **ts**=tympanic sinus

19 −7.73 mm from center of external auditory canal — **ts**=tympanic sinus

20 −8.38 mm from center of external auditory canal — **ts**=tympanic sinus

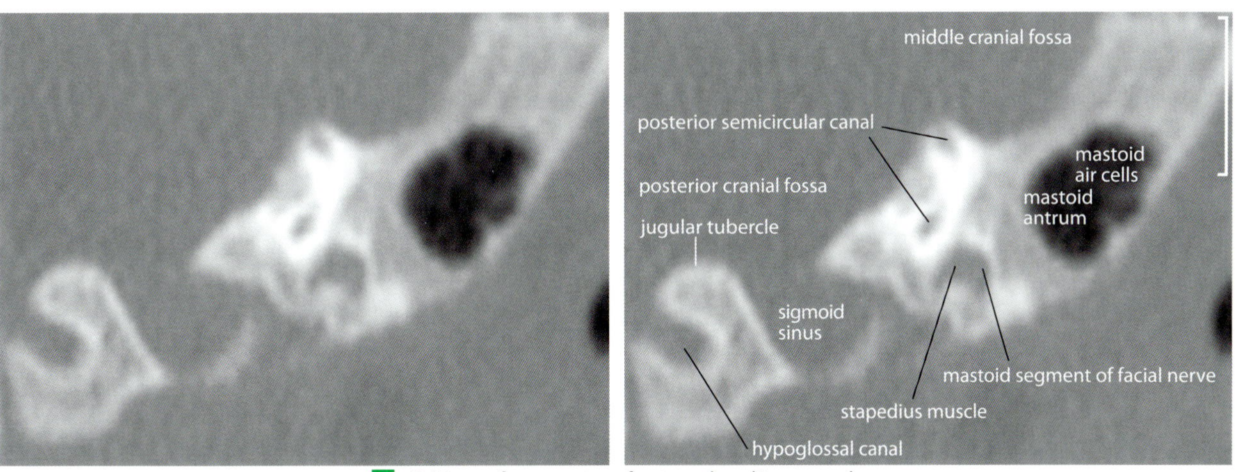

21 −9.04 mm from center of external auditory canal

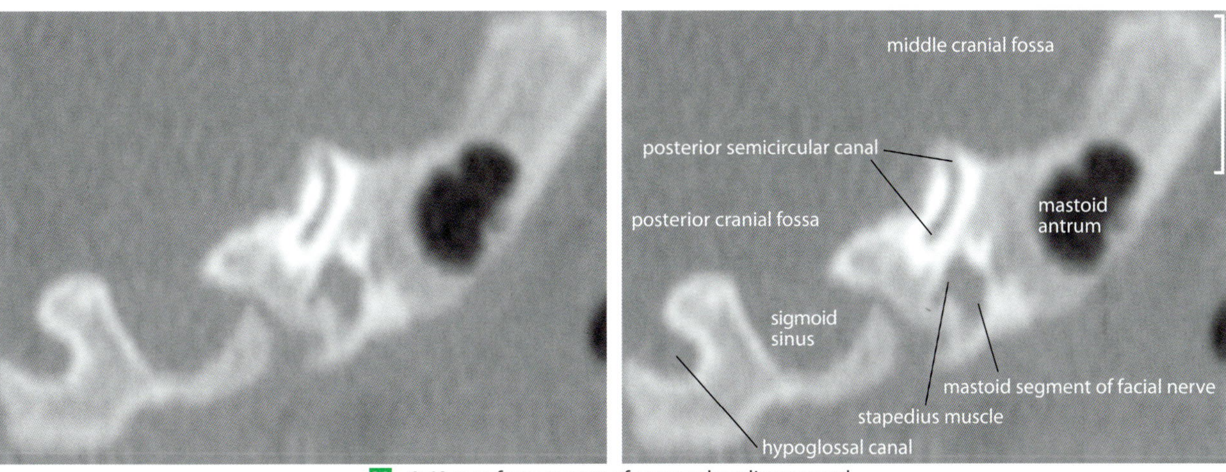

22 −9.69 mm from center of external auditory canal

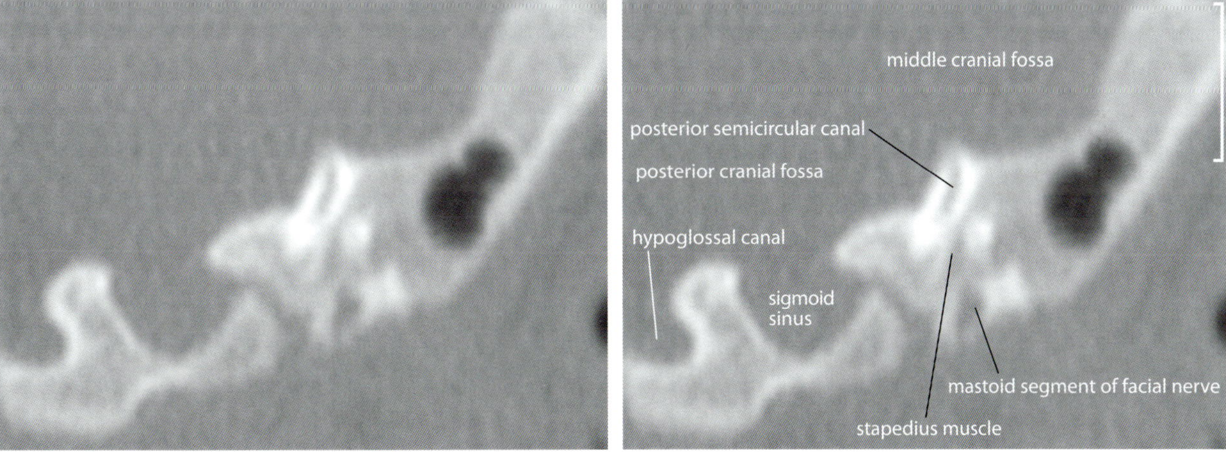

23 −10.34 mm from center of external auditory canal

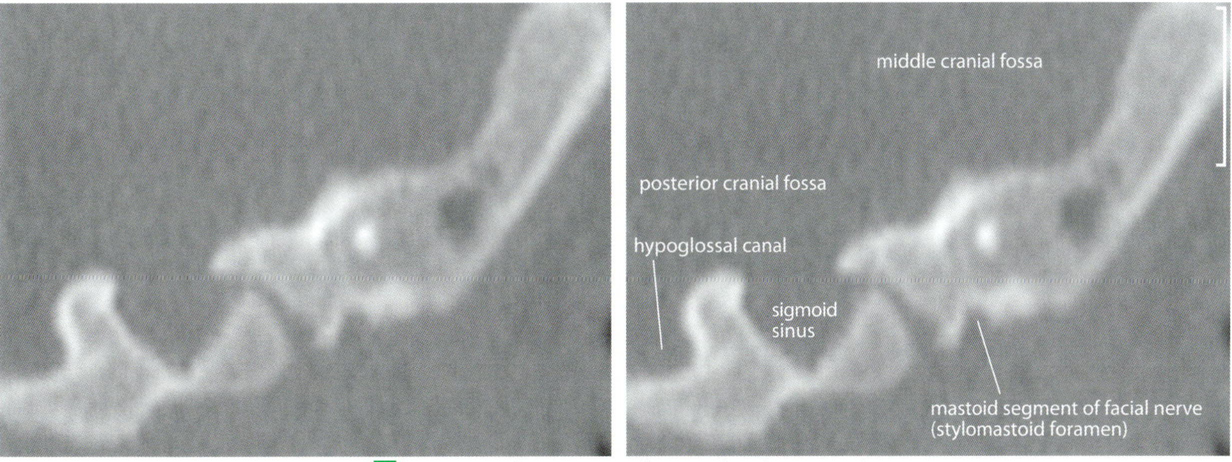

24 −10.99 mm from center of external auditory canal

❷ Older Child

Postnatal growth of the temporal bone is extremely rapid in the first three years, then continues at a gradually decreasing rate until at puberty it has just about reached adult size. The temporal bone of a child at puberty has almost completed growing and is basically no different from that of an adult.

Compared to the infant images, the temporal bone of the older child is larger overall and displays dramatic development and expansion of the air cells. The bone forming the external auditory canal has also developed and elongated. The internal auditory canal is also longer, but its internal diameter does not appear to have changed significantly. There is almost no change to the inner ear or tympanic cavity. The mastoid segment of the facial nerve is longer due to the growth of the mastoid process.

While infant temporal bone imaging is often conducted to scrutinize congenital abnormalities, in older children as a rule the diagnosis of congenital disease has already been established and imaging is used to test for acquired disease. In this volume as well, the majority of cases concerning congenital disease were diagnosed before five years old, whereas over half the cases of inflammatory disease are of children ten years or older.

In other words, in pediatric ear imaging diagnosis, inflammatory and infectious diseases or injuries become more common the older the child, and insufficient development of mastoid air cells, granulation and fluid retention due to inflammation, osteolytic lesions, and so on are subject to observation. By comparing the normal images shown here with the various cases cited later on in the chapter on inflammatory diseases in children, one may attain an understanding of how these diseases influence temporal bone development and which areas are vulnerable to harm.

The images shown are of a male, sixteen years, ten months old, who underwent CT examination for functional hearing loss. They are presented here as normal temporal bone CT images as no clear abnormal findings were discovered in them. The coronal section images were reconstructed from data taken in the axial section images. For display purposes, coronal section images have been magnified to approx. 1.7 times the axial section images. Also, the images are arranged from bottom to top (inferior to superior) for the axial sections and from front to back (anterior to posterior) for the coronal sections. Images of the same cross sections are arranged side by side, with the right image annotated to indicate each anatomical structure. (Scale shown in images indicates 1 cm)

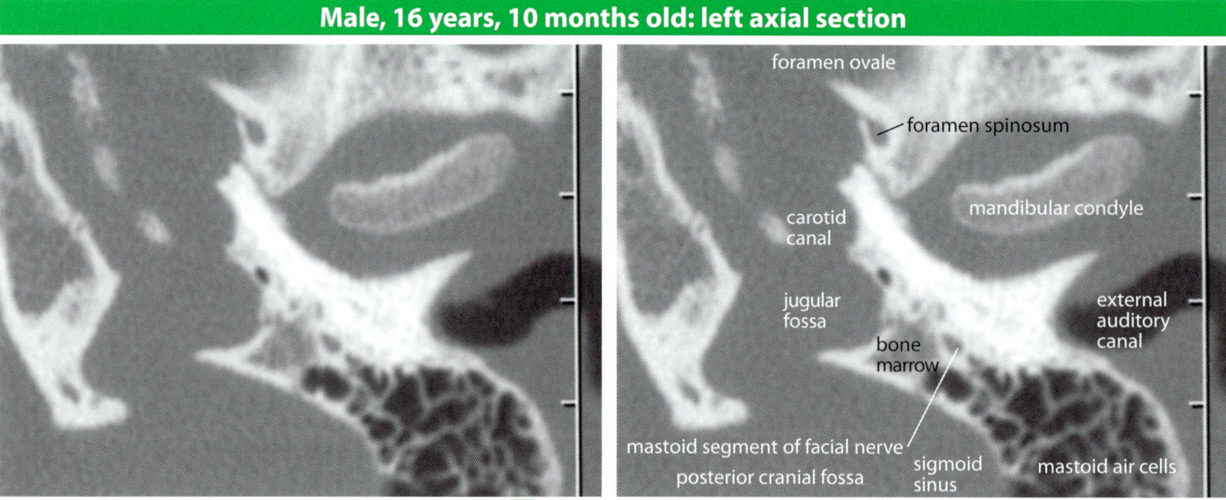

1 OM line +8.49 mm

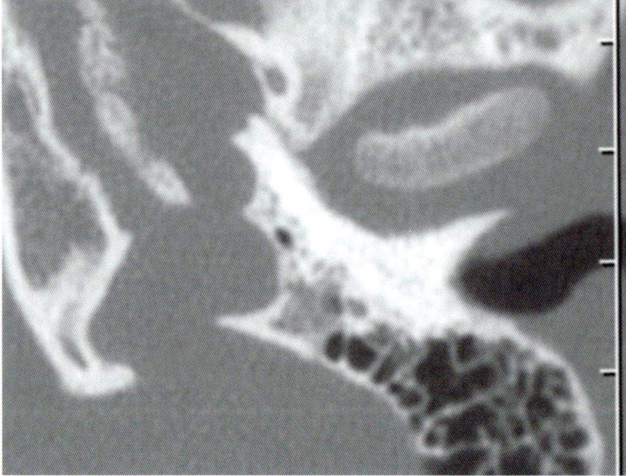

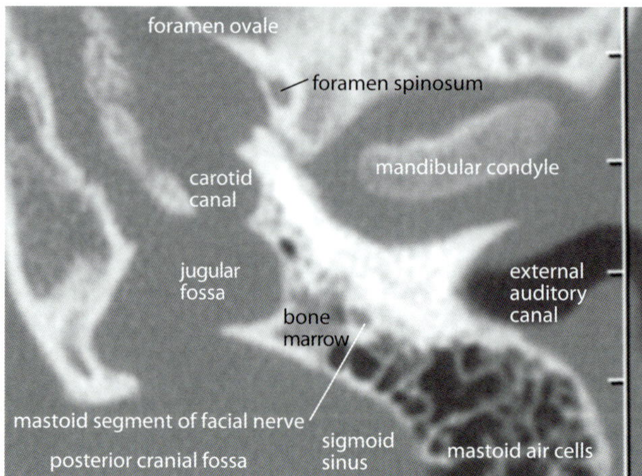

2 OM line +9.12 mm

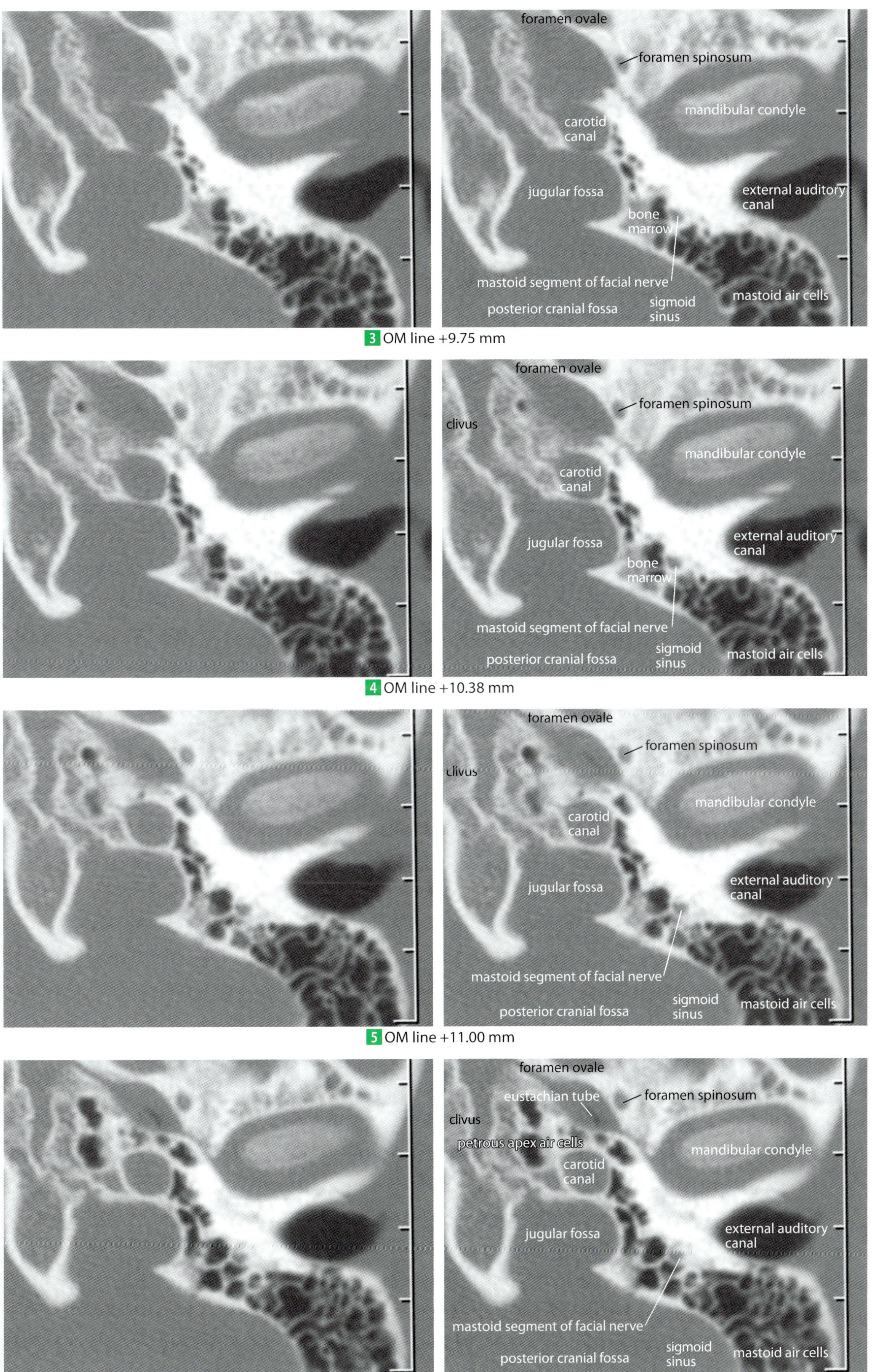

3 OM line +9.75 mm

4 OM line +10.38 mm

5 OM line +11.00 mm

6 OM line +11.62 mm

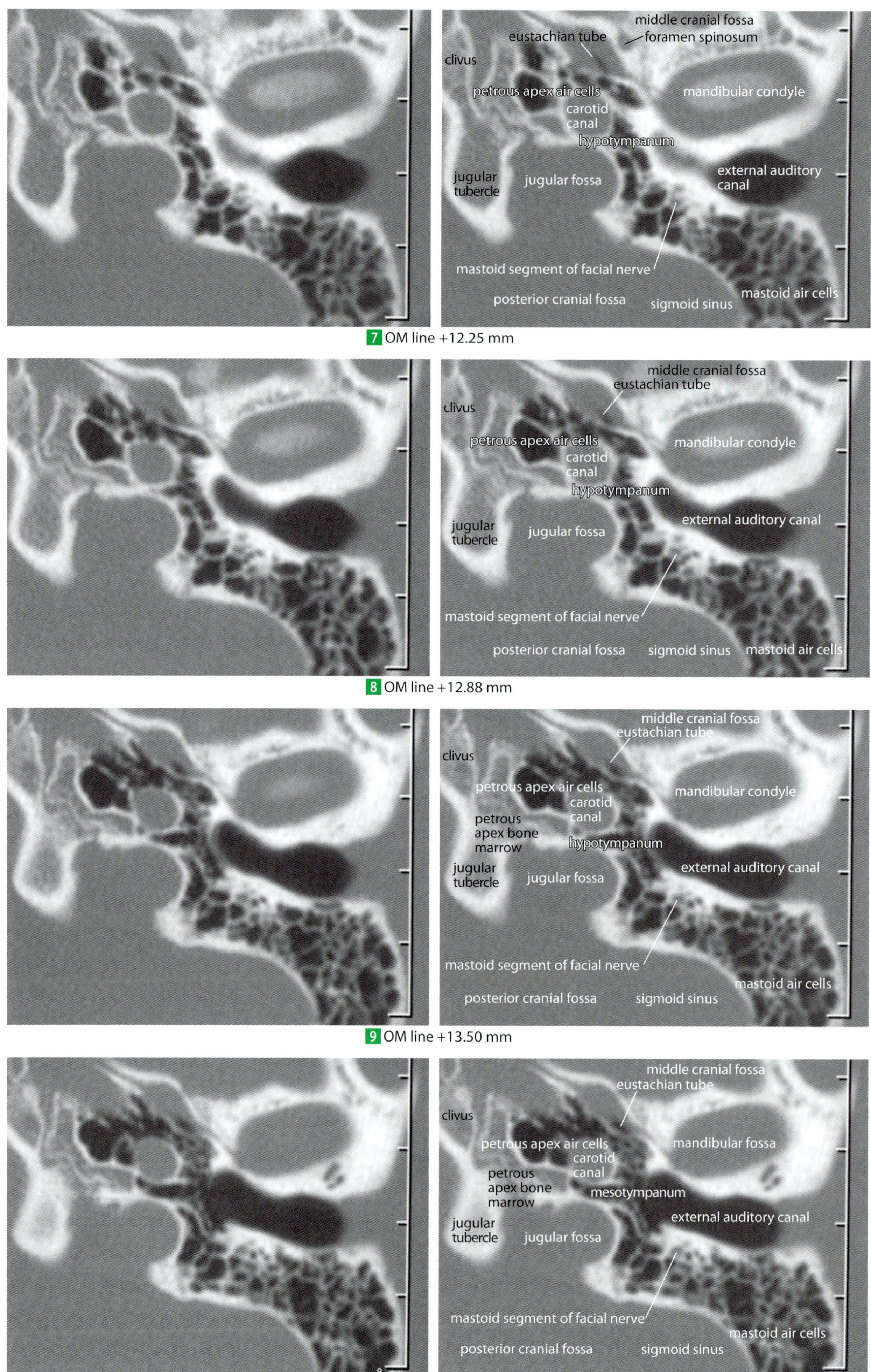

7 OM line +12.25 mm

8 OM line +12.88 mm

9 OM line +13.50 mm

10 OM line +14.13 mm

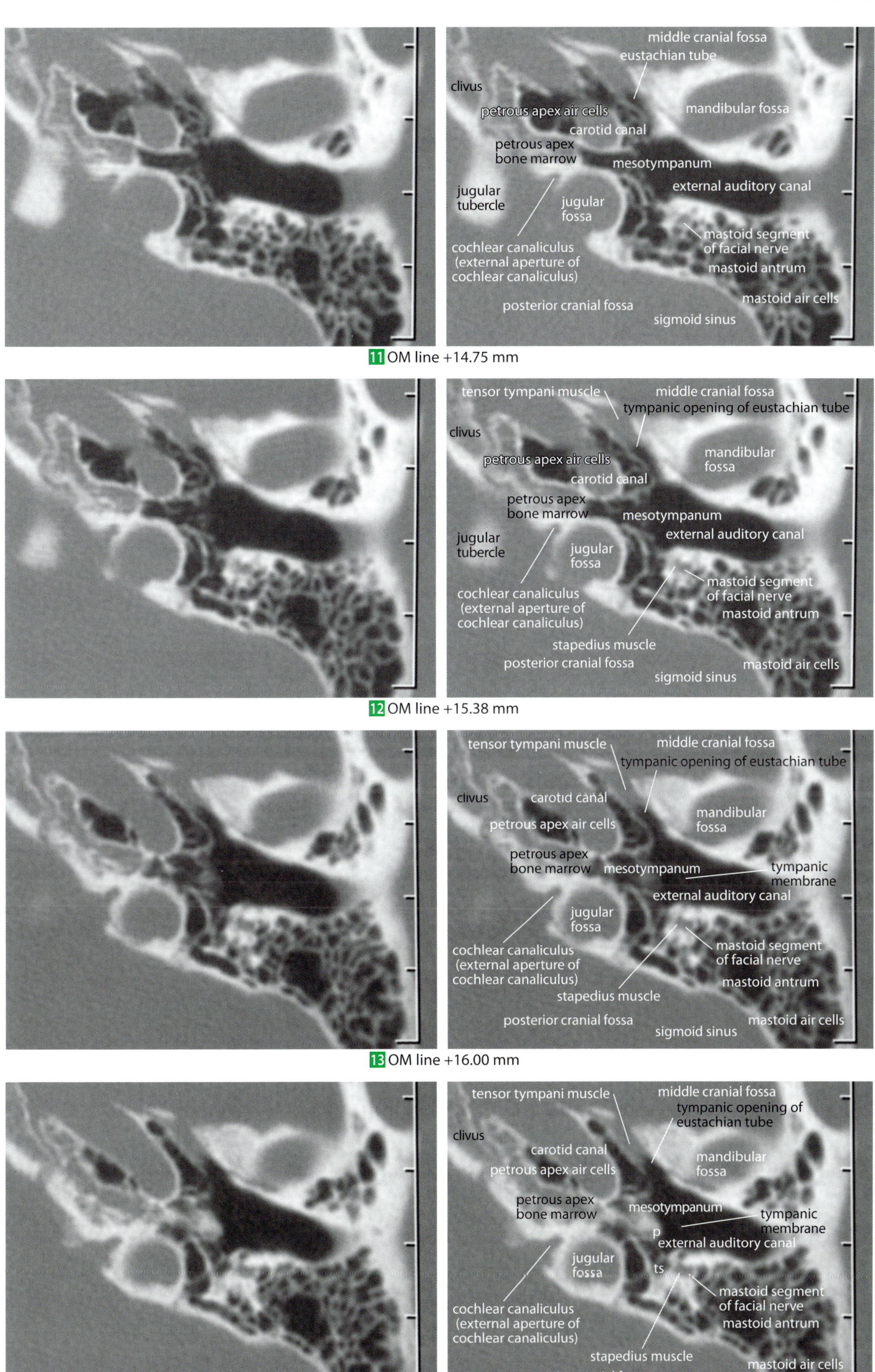

11 OM line +14.75 mm

12 OM line +15.38 mm

13 OM line +16.00 mm

14 OM line +16.62 mm

p=promontory; **ts**=tympanic sinus

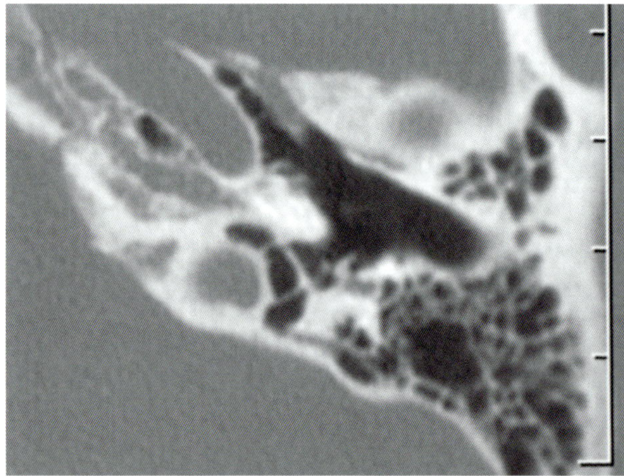

15 OM line +17.25 mm

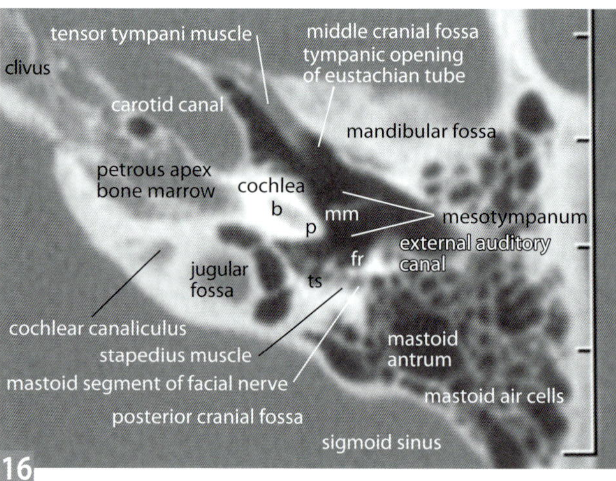

b=basal turn of cochlea; **p**=promontory;
mm=manubrium of malleus; **ts**=tympanic sinus; **fr**=facial recess

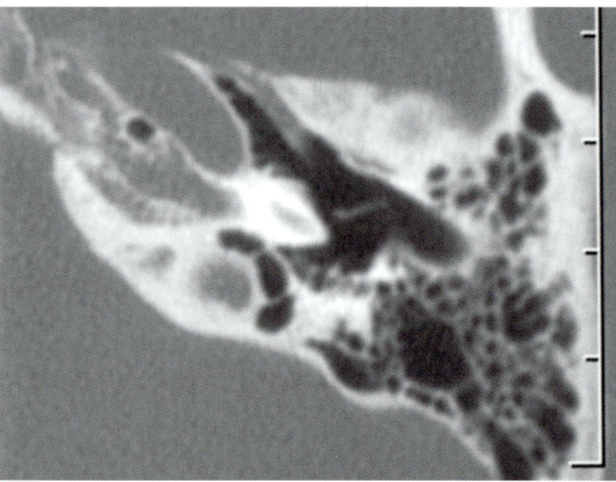

16 OM line +17.88 mm

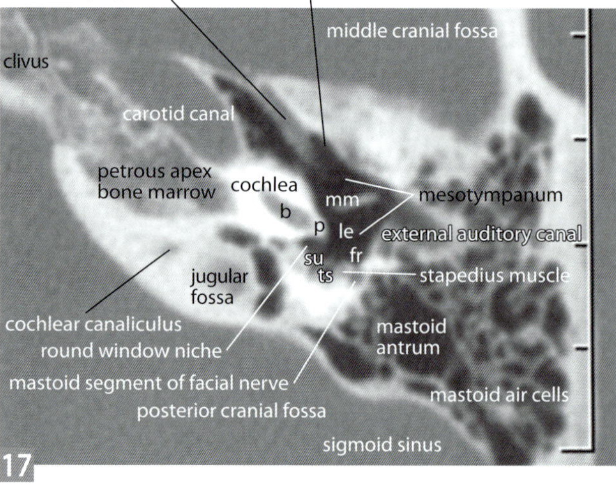

b=basal turn of cochlea ; **p**=promontory;
mm=manubrium of malleus; **le**=lenticular process of incus;
su=subiculum of promontory; **ts**=tympanic sinus; **fr**=facial recess

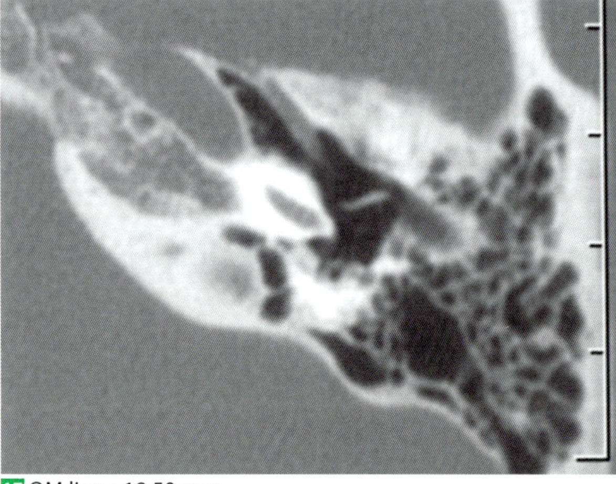

17 OM line +18.50 mm

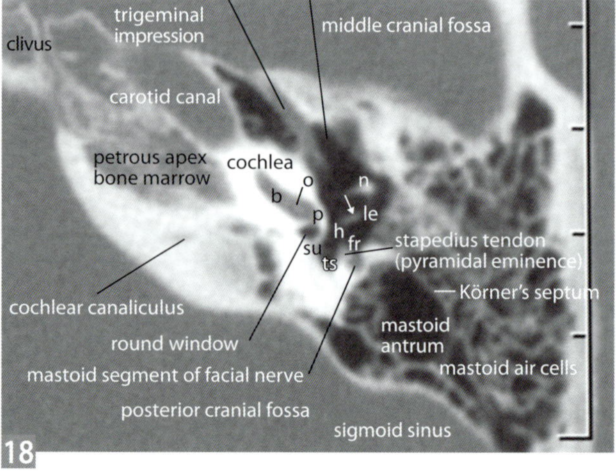

b=basal turn of cochlea; **o**=osseous spiral lamina; **p**=promontory;
n=neck of malleus; **le**=lenticular process of incus;
↘=incudostapedial joint; **h**=head of stapes;
su=subiculum of promontory; **ts**=tympanic sinus; **fr**=facial recess

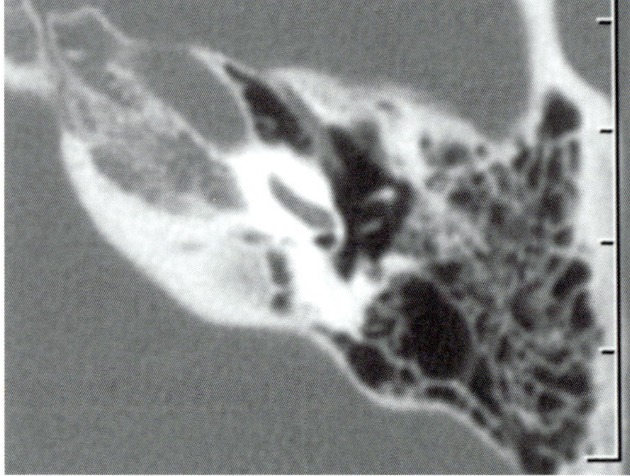

18 OM line +19.12 mm

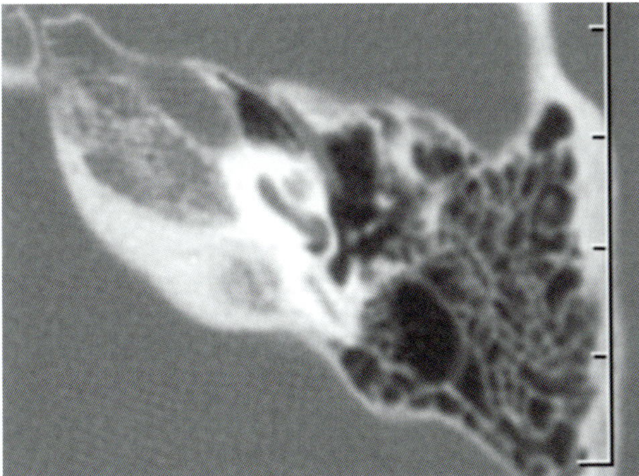

19 OM line +19.75 mm

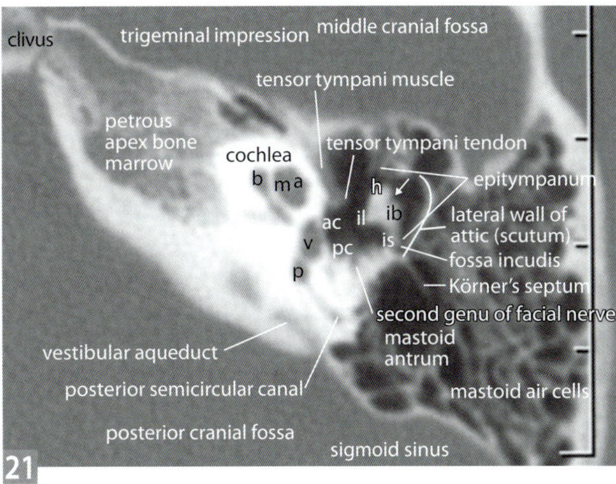

21

a=apical turn of cochlea; **m**=middle turn of cochlea;
b=basal turn of cochlea; **v**=vestibule; **h**=head of malleus;
⟋=malleoincudal joint; **ib**=body of incus; **il**=long process of incus;
is=short process of incus; **ac**=anterior crus of stapes;
pc=posterior crus of stapes; **p**=posterior ampulla

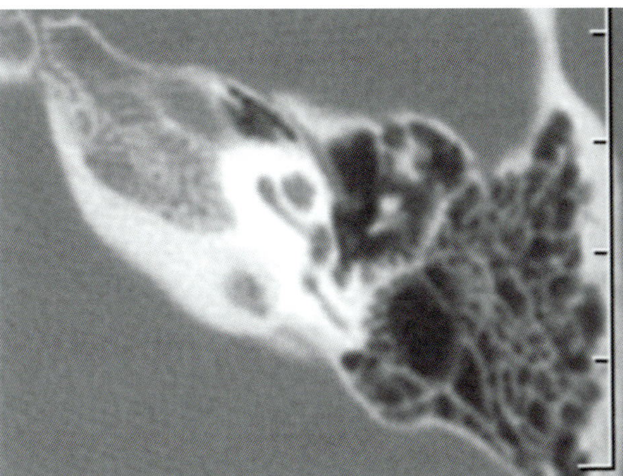

20 OM line +20.38 mm

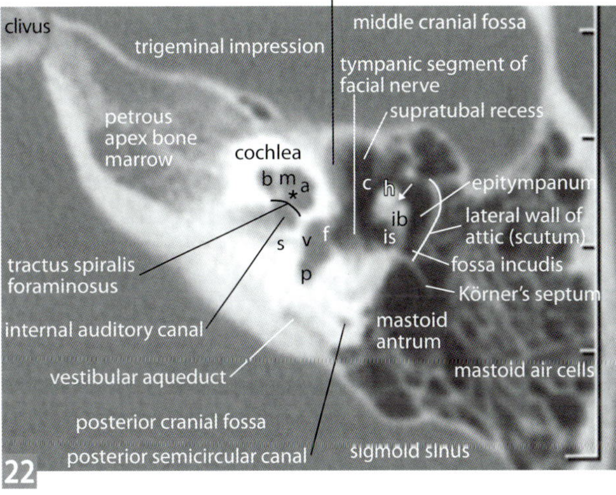

22

a=apical turn of cochlea; **m**=middle turn of cochlea;
b=basal turn of cochlea; ∗=modiolus; **v**=vestibule;
f=footplate of stapes; **c**=anterior attic bony plate (cog);
h=head of malleus; ⟋=malleoincudal joint; **ib**=body of incus;
is=short process of incus; **s**=singlar canal; **p**=posterior ampulla

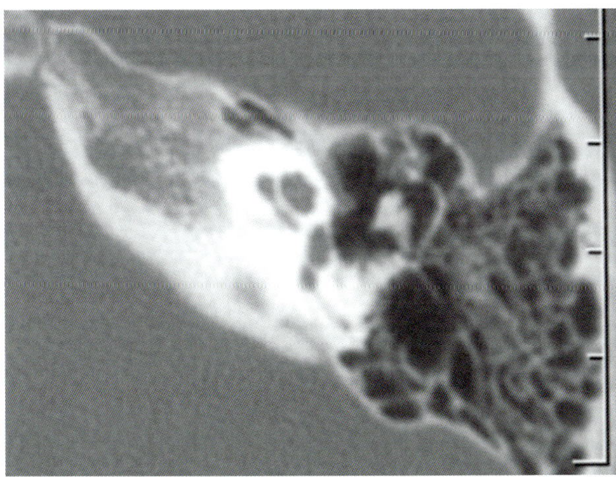

21 OM line +21.00 mm

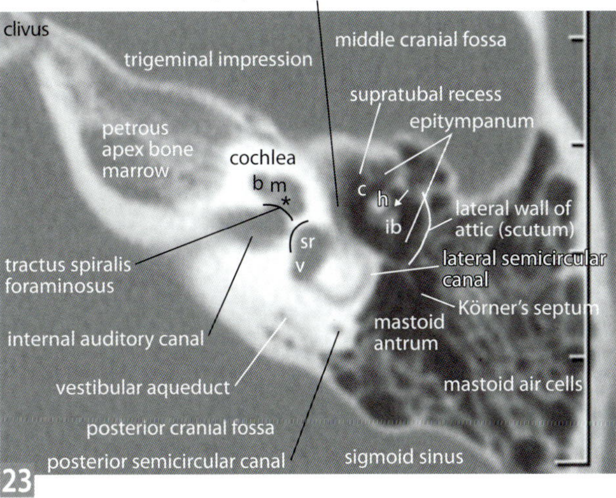

23

m=middle turn of cochlea; **b**=basal turn of cochlea; ∗=modiolus;
v=vestibule; **sr**=spherical recess; **c**=anterior attic bony plate (cog);
h=head of malleus; ⟋=malleoincudal joint; **ib**=body of incus

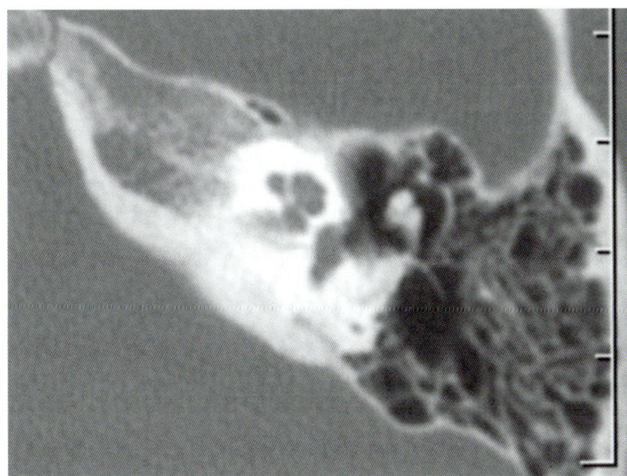

22 OM line +21.63 mm

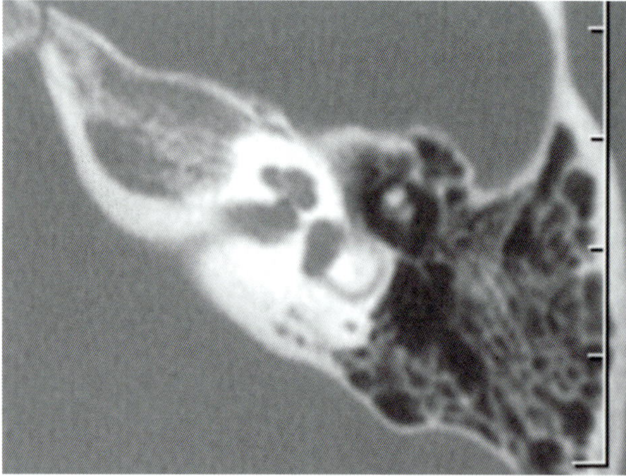

23 OM line +22.25 mm

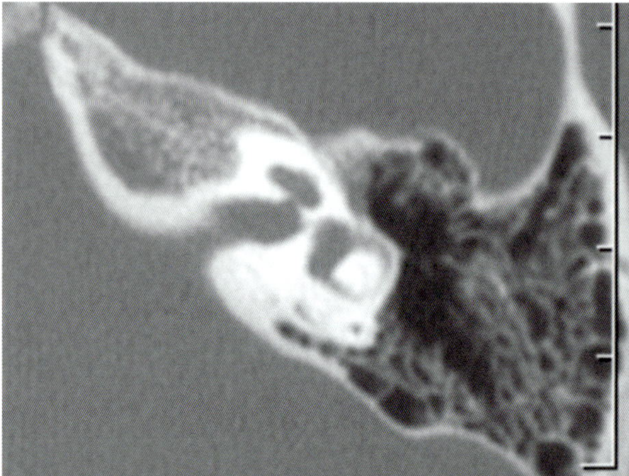

24 OM line +22.88 mm

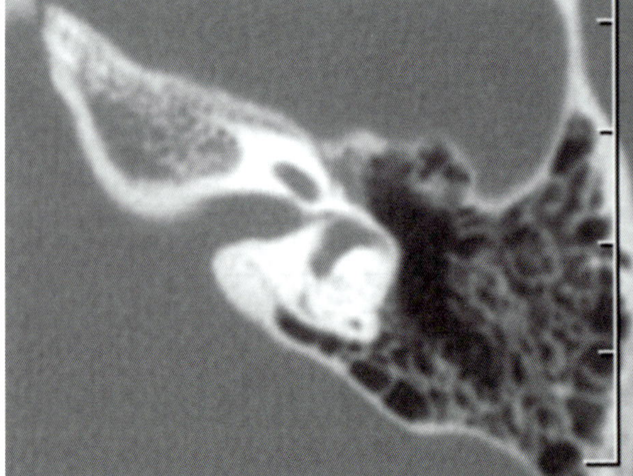

25 OM line +23.50 mm

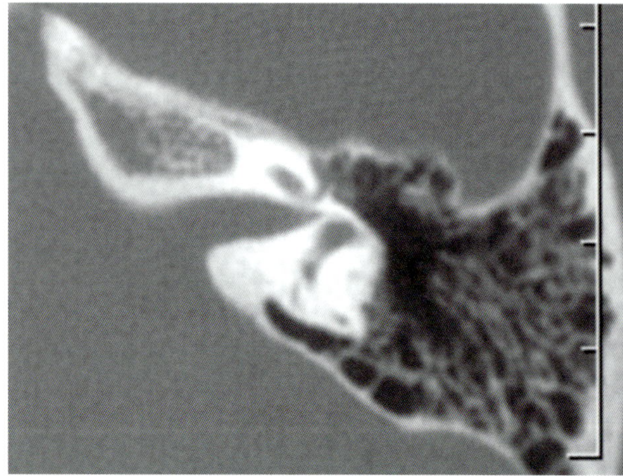

26 OM line +24.12 mm

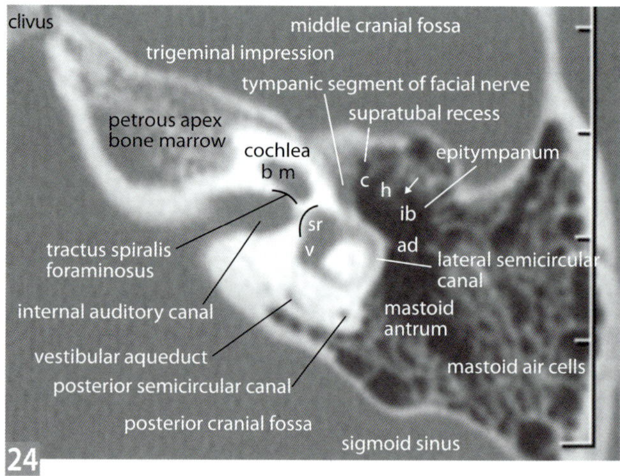

m=middle turn of cochlea; **b**=basal turn of cochlea ; **v**=vestibule; **sr**=spherical recess; **c**=anterior attic bony plate (cog); **h**=head of malleus; =malleoincudal joint; **ib**=body of incus; **ad**=aditus ad antrum

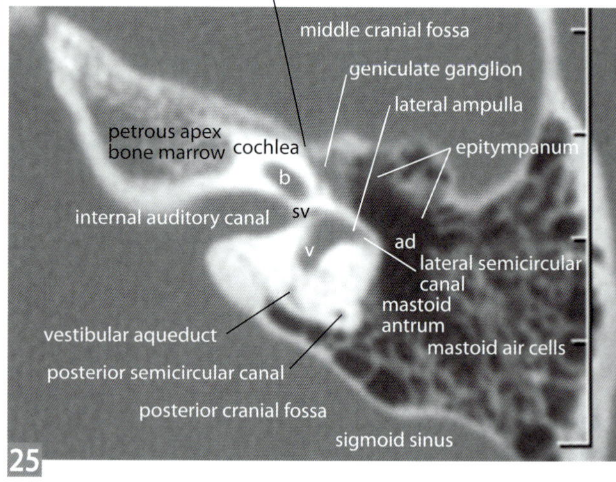

b=basal turn of cochlea; **sv**=superior vestibular nerve; **v**=vestibule; **ad**=aditus ad antrum

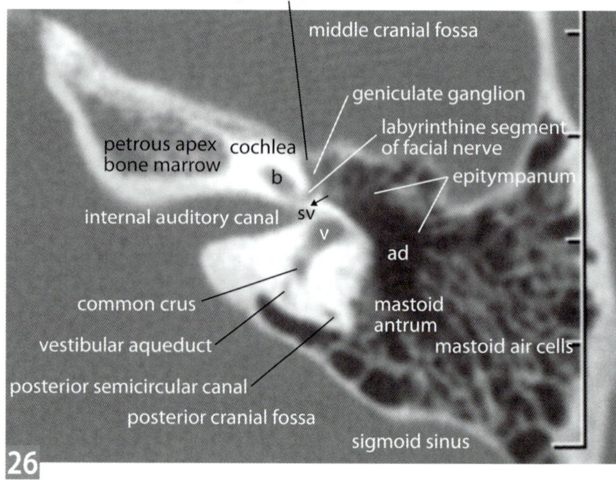

b=basal turn of cochlea; =Bill's bar; **sv**=superior vestibular nerve; **v**=vestibule; **ad**=aditus ad antrum

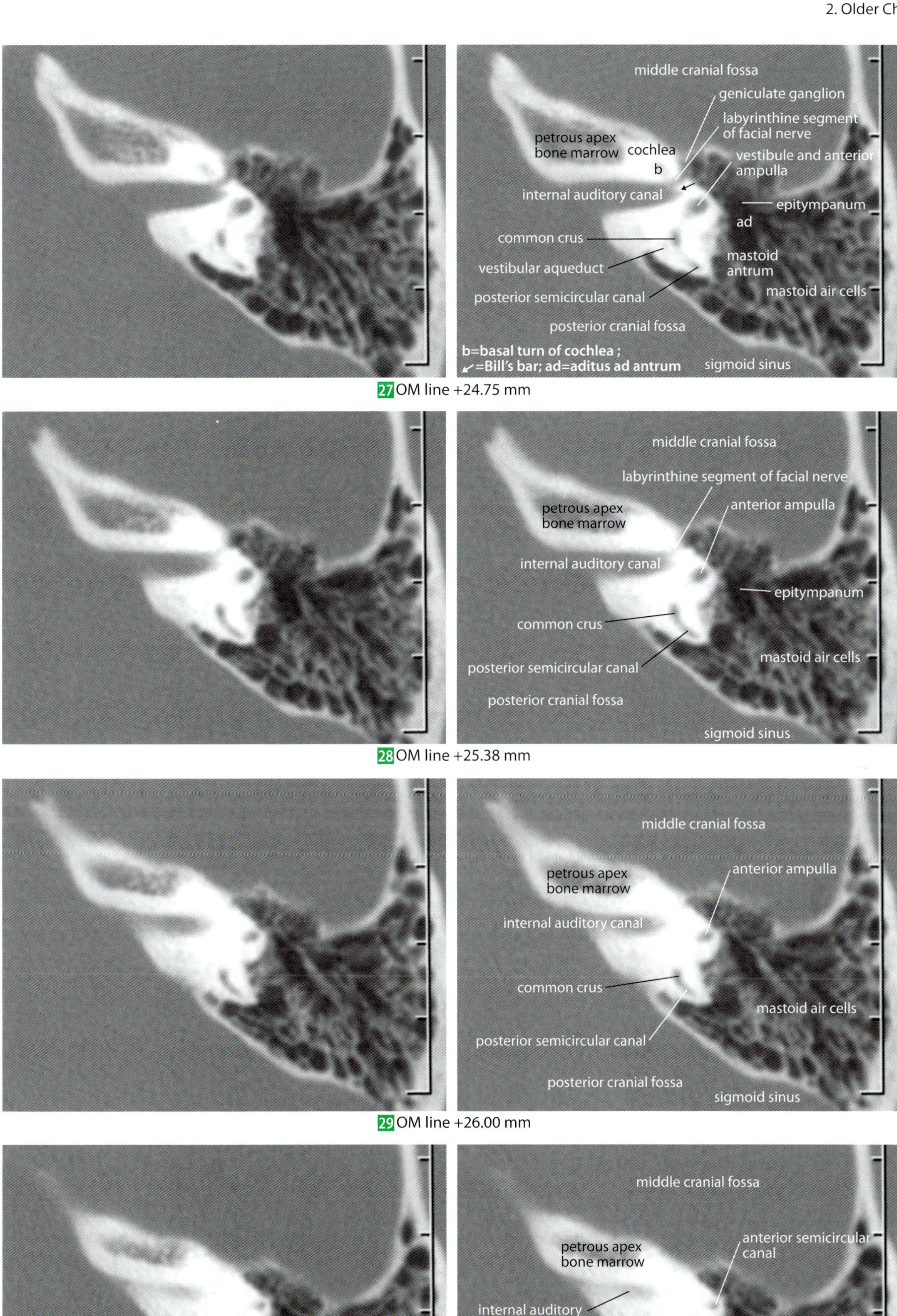

27 OM line +24.75 mm

28 OM line +25.38 mm

29 OM line +26.00 mm

30 OM line +26.62 mm

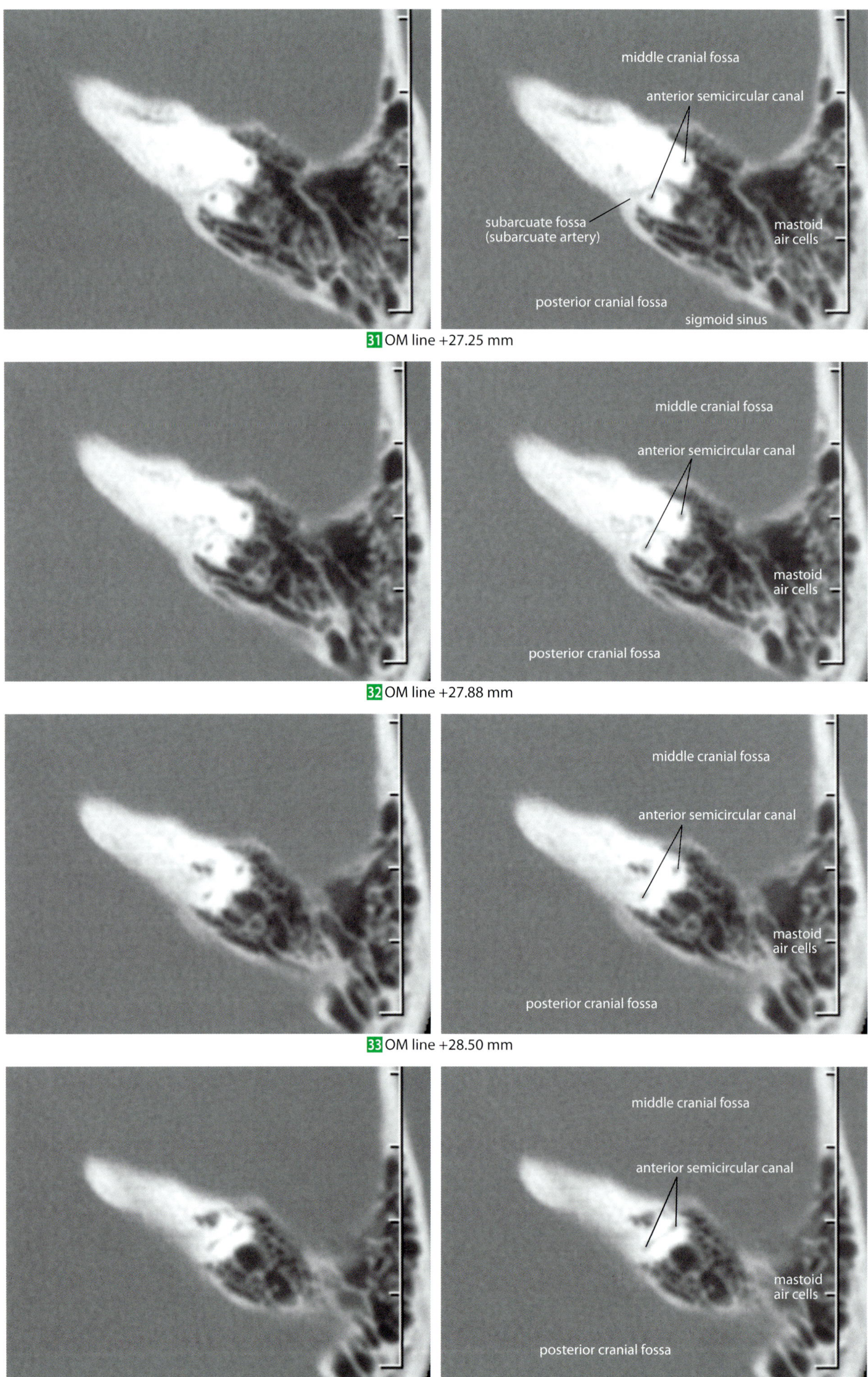

31 OM line +27.25 mm

32 OM line +27.88 mm

33 OM line +28.50 mm

34 OM line +29.13 mm

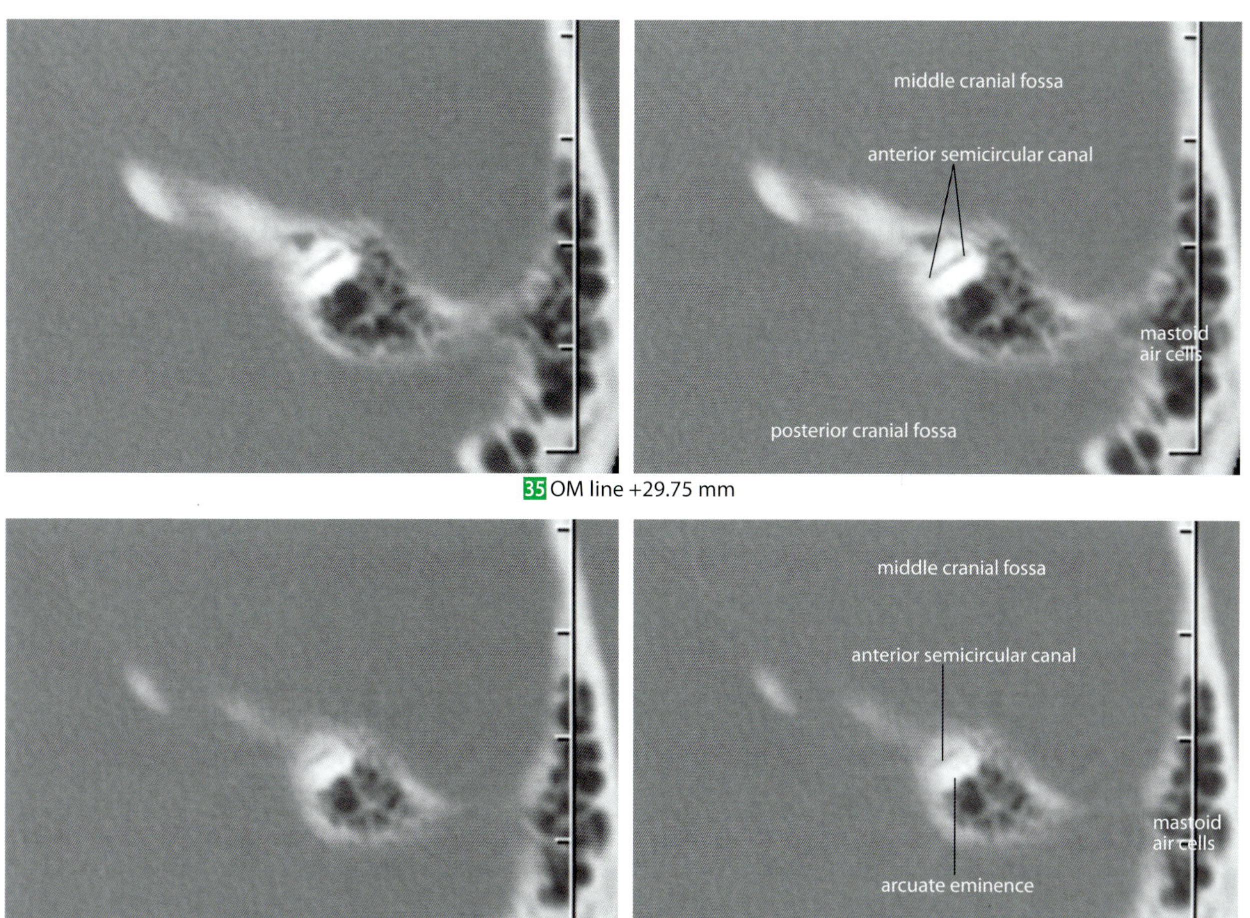

35 OM line +29.75 mm

36 OM line +30.38 mm

Male, 16 years, 10 months old: left coronal section

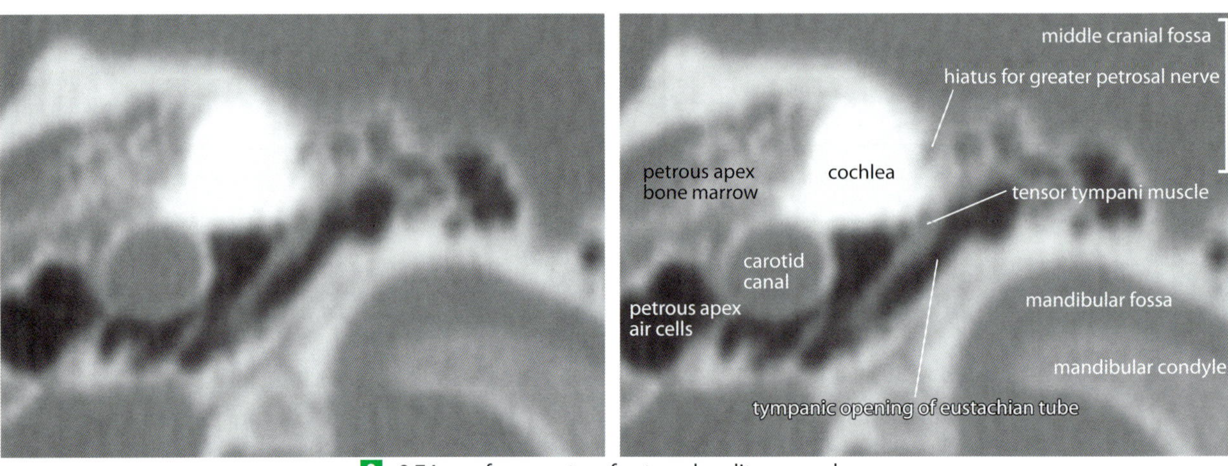

1 +10.39 mm from center of external auditory canal

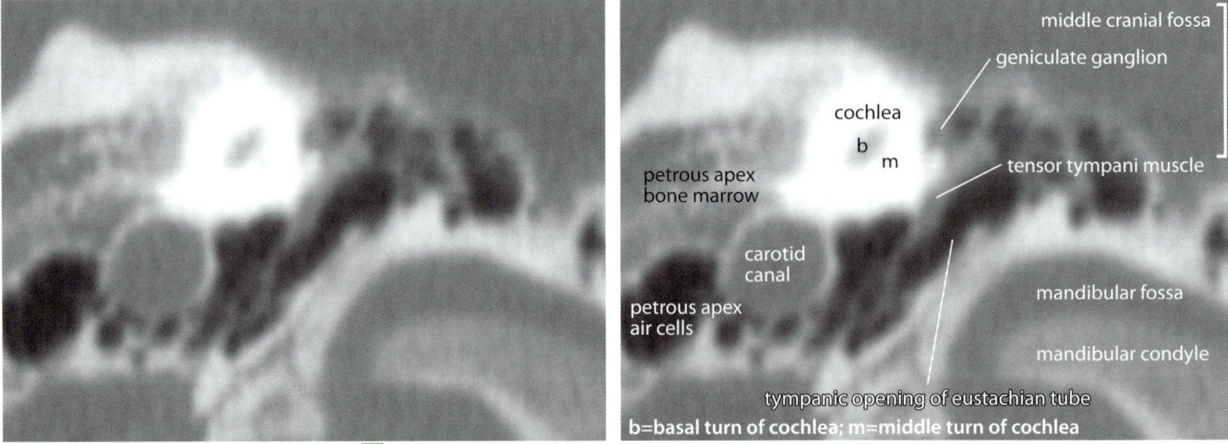

2 +9.74 mm from center of external auditory canal

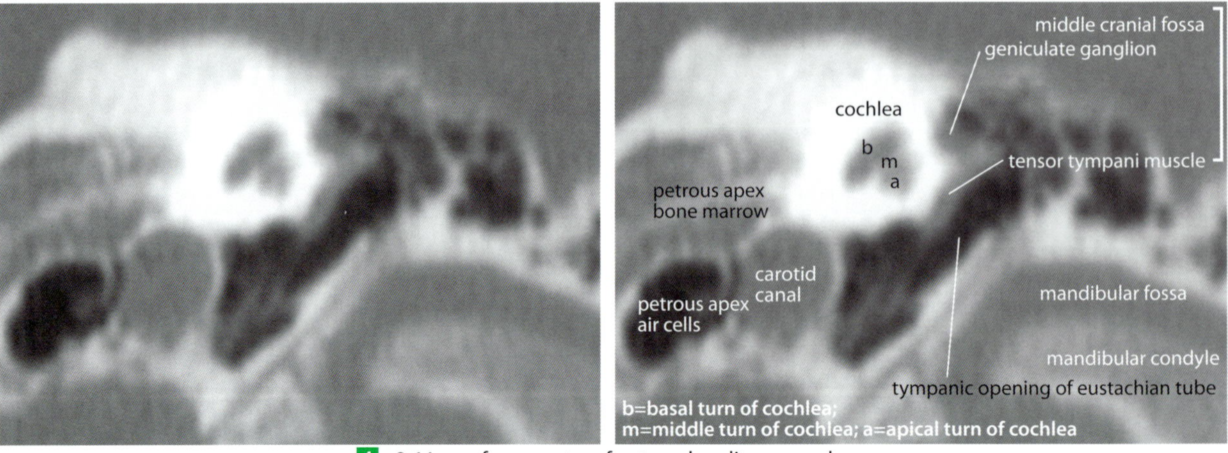

3 +9.09 mm from center of external auditory canal

4 +8.44 mm from center of external auditory canal

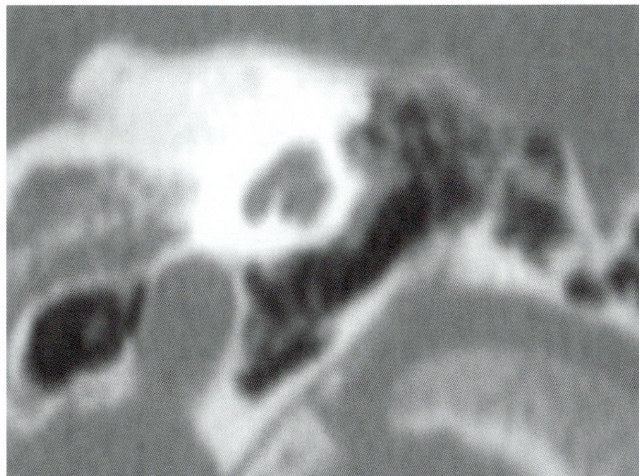

5 +7.79 mm from center of external auditory canal

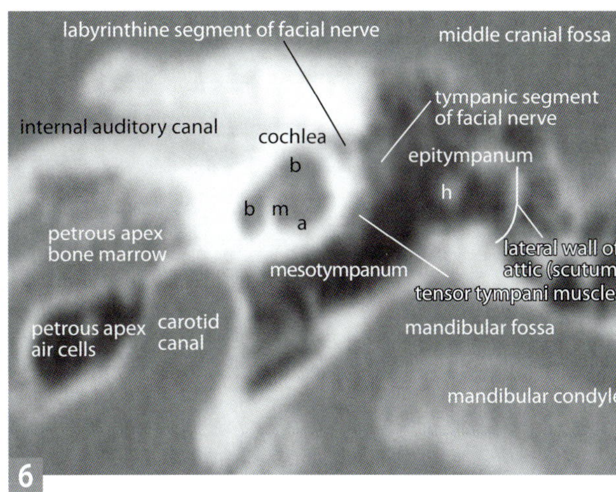

6

b=basal turn of cochlea; **m**=middle turn of cochlea;
a=apical turn of cochlea; **h**=head of malleus

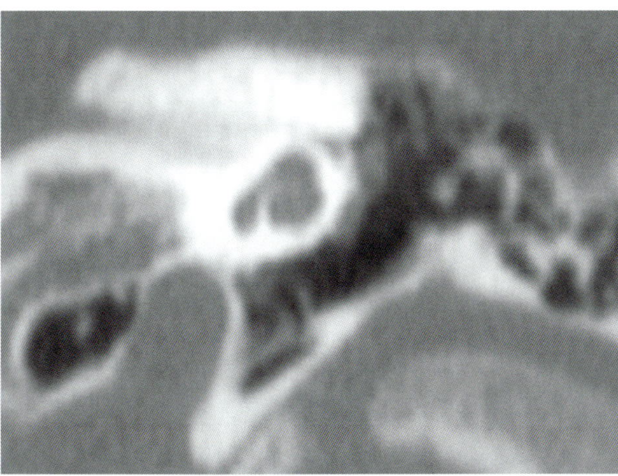

6 +7.14 mm from center of external auditory canal

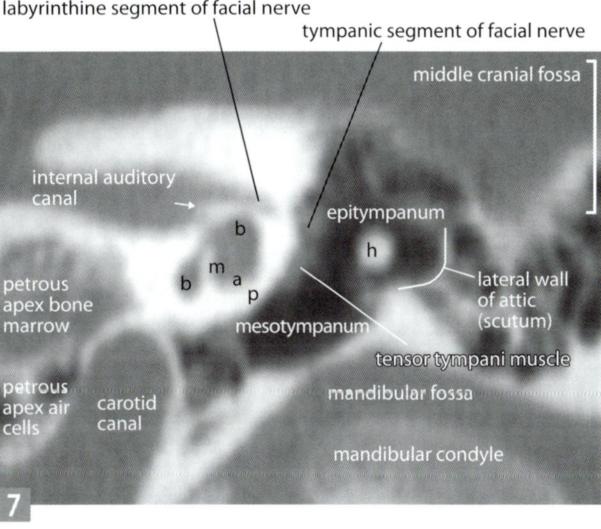

7

b=basal turn of cochlea; **m**=middle turn of cochlea;
a=apical turn of cochlea; **p**=promontory; =transverse crest;
h=head of malleus

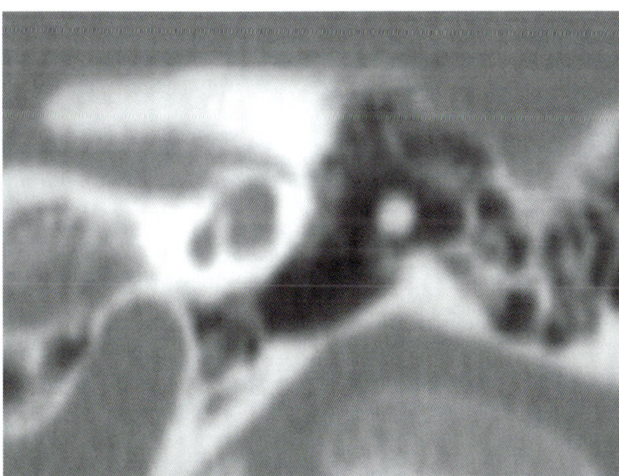

7 +6.48 mm from center of external auditory canal

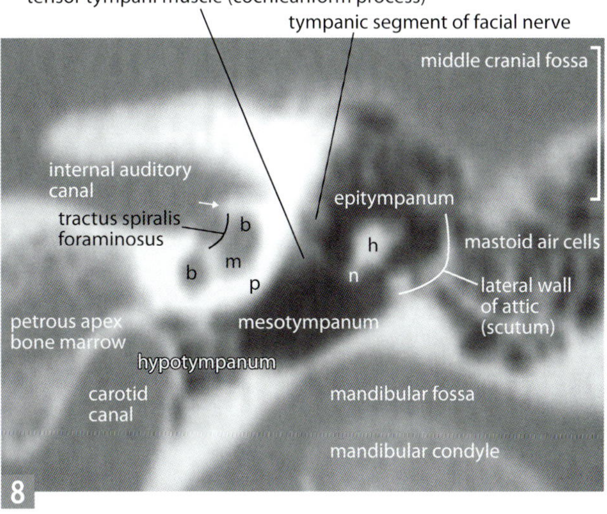

8

b=basal turn of cochlea; **m**=middle turn of cochlea;
p=promontory; =transverse crest; **h**=head of malleus;
n=neck of malleus

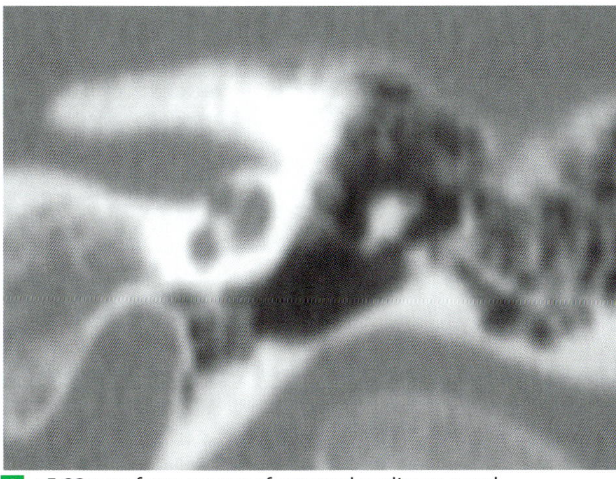

8 +5.83 mm from center of external auditory canal

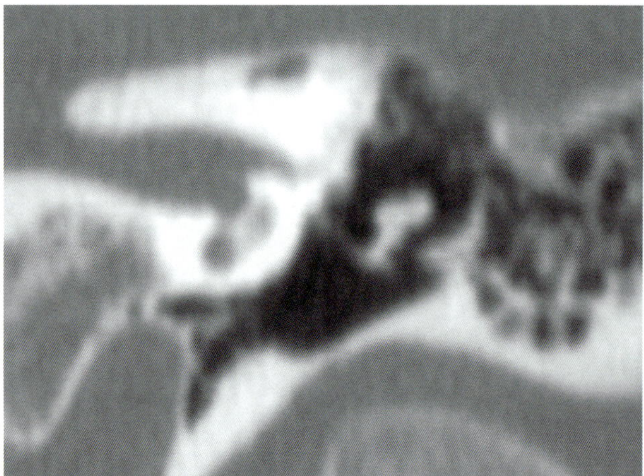

9 +5.18 mm from center of external auditory canal

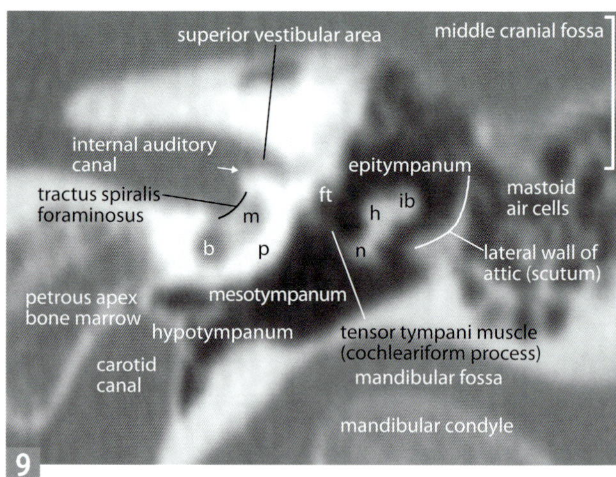

ft=tympanic segment of facial nerve; **b**=basal turn of cochlea; **m**=middle turn of cochlea; **p**=promontory; =transverse crest; **ib**=body of incus; **h**=head of malleus; **n**=neck of malleus

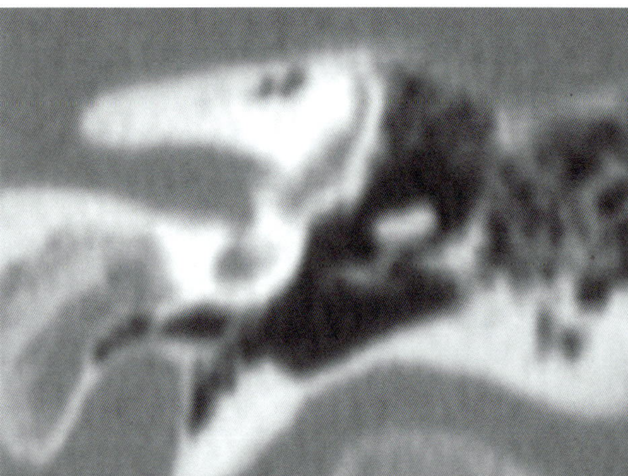

10 +4.53 mm from center of external auditory canal

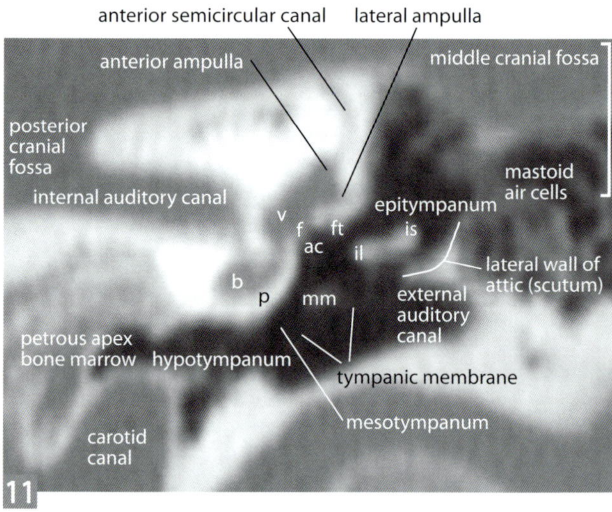

ft=tympanic segment of facial nerve; **v**=vestibule; **b**=basal turn of cochlea; **p**=promontory; **is**=short process of incus; **il**=long process of incus; **mm**=manubrium of malleus; **ac**=anterior crus of stapes; **f**=footplate of stapes

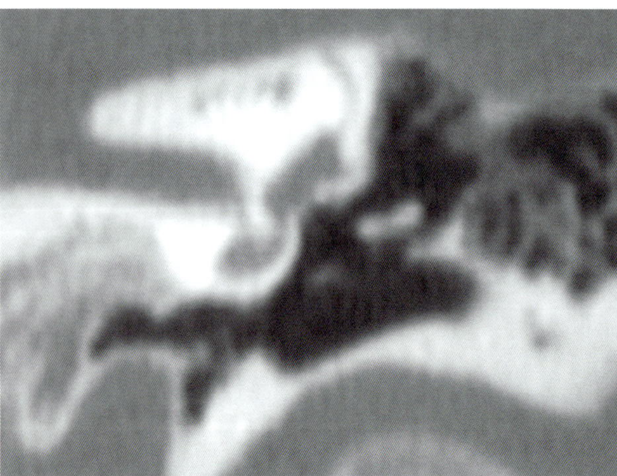

11 +3.88 mm from center of external auditory canal

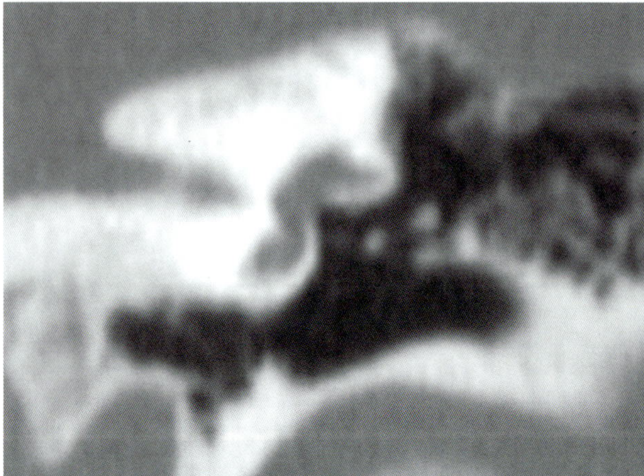

12 +3.23 mm from center of external auditory canal

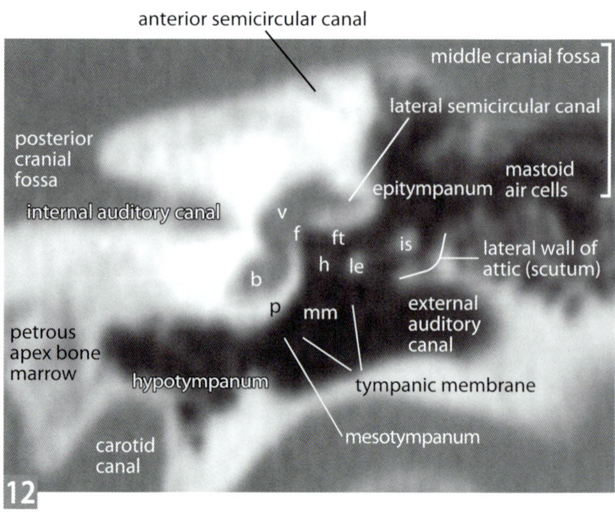

ft=tympanic segment of facial nerve; **v**=vestibule; **b**=basal turn of cochlea; **p**=promontory; **is**=short process of incus; **le**=lenticular process of incus; **h**=head of stapes; **f**=footplate of stapes; **mm**=manubrium of malleus

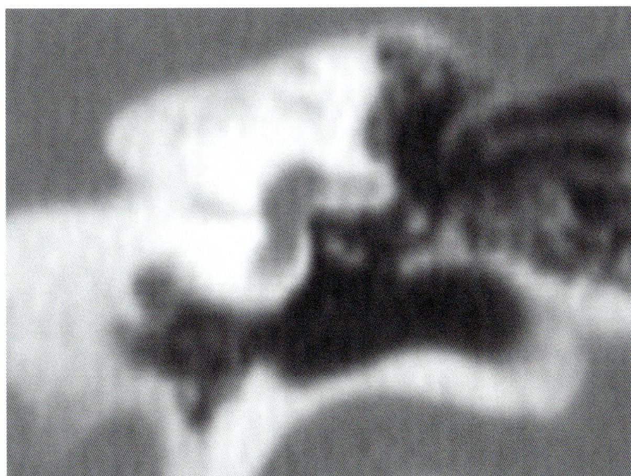

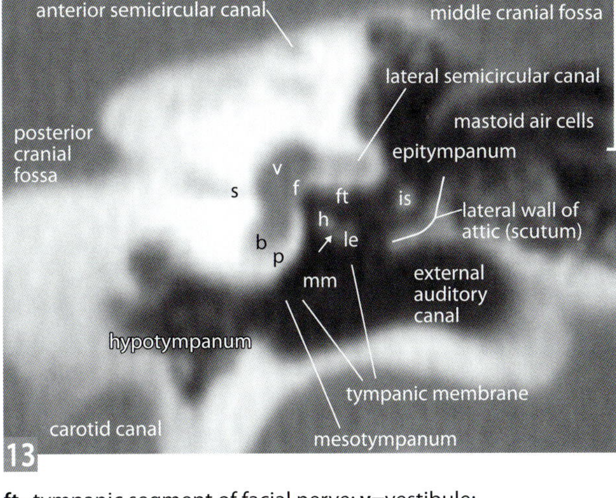

13 +2.58 mm from center of external auditory canal

ft=tympanic segment of facial nerve; **v**=vestibule;
b=basal turn of cochlea; **p**=promontory; **s**=singlar canal;
is=short process of incus; **le**=lenticular process of incus;
↗=incudostapedial joint; **h**=head of stapes; **f**=footplate of stapes;
mm=manubrium of malleus

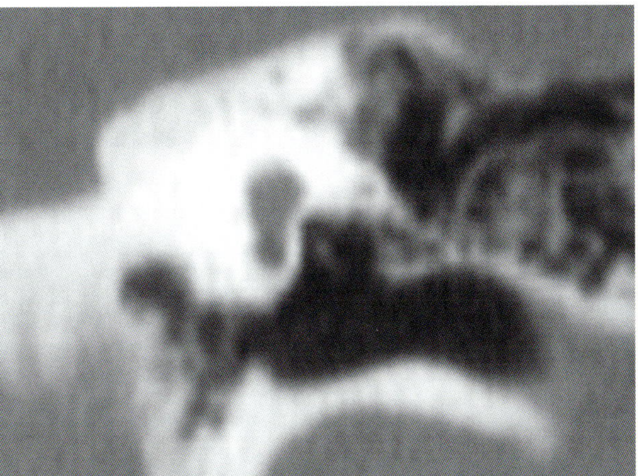

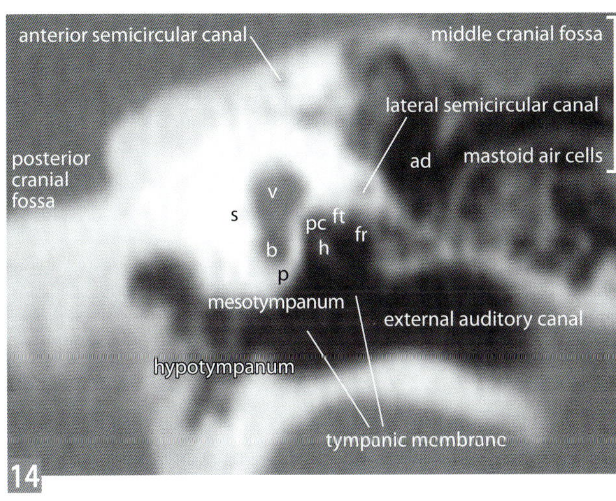

14 +1.92 mm from center of external auditory canal

ft=tympanic segment of facial nerve; **v**=vestibule;
b=basal turn of cochlea; **p**=promontory; **s**=singlar canal;
ad=aditus ad antrum; **h**=head of stapes;
pc=posterior crus of stapes; **fr**=facial recess

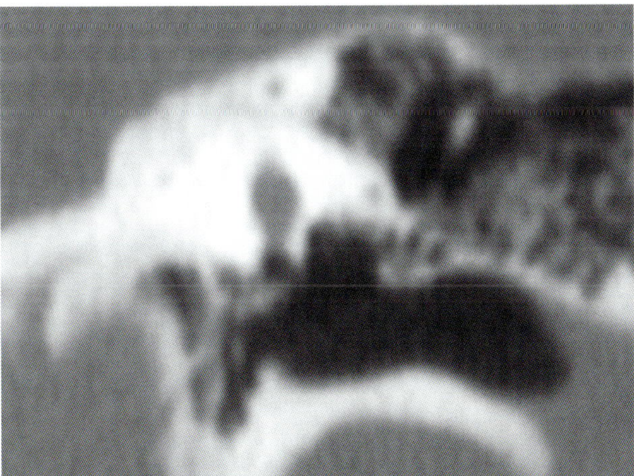

15 +1.27 mm from center of external auditory canal

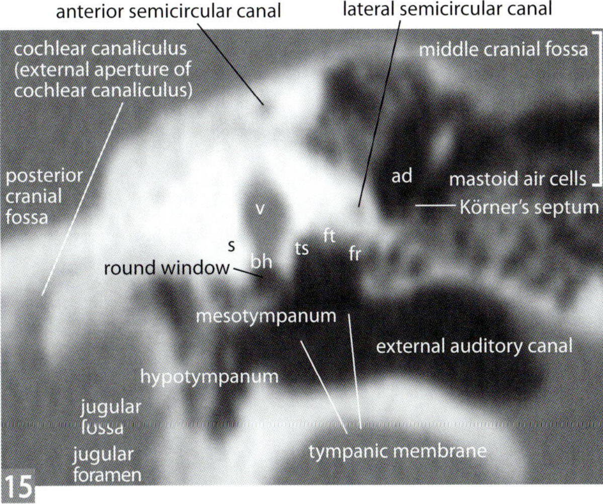

ft=tympanic segment of facial nerve; **v**=vestibule;
bh=basal turn of cochlea (hook portion); **s**=singlar canal;
ad=aditus ad antrum; **fr**=facial recess; **ts**=tympanic sinus

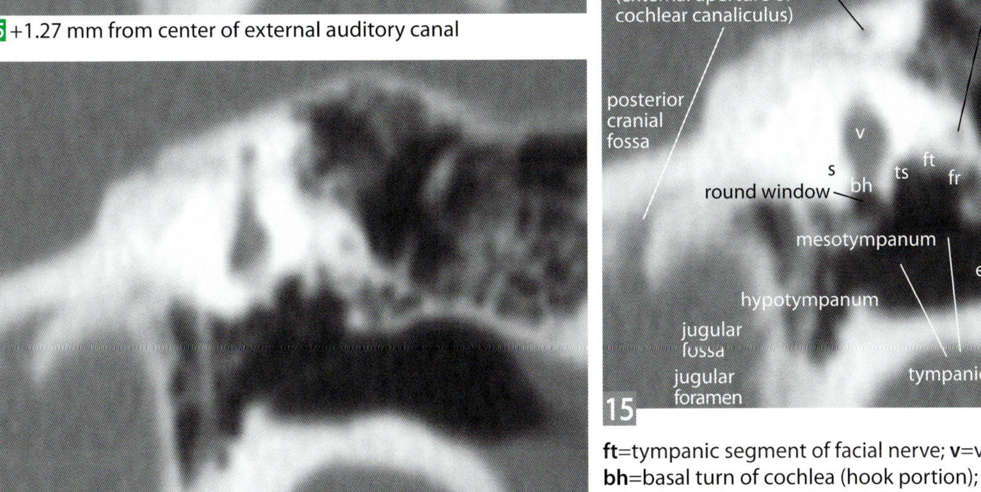

16 +0.62 mm from center of external auditory canal

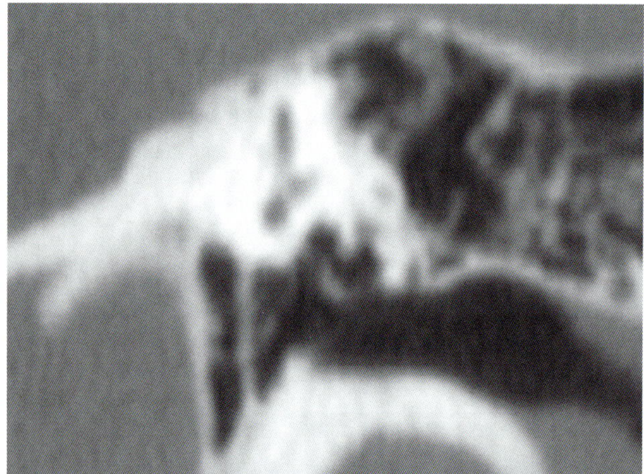

17 −0.03 mm from center of external auditory canal

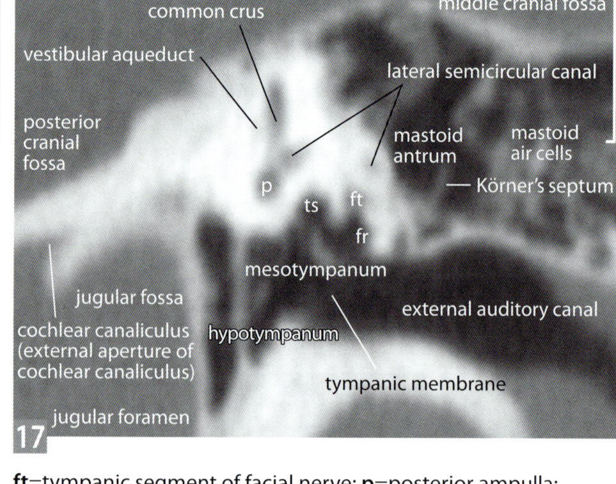

ft=tympanic segment of facial nerve; **p**=posterior ampulla;
fr=facial recess; **ts**=tympanic sinus

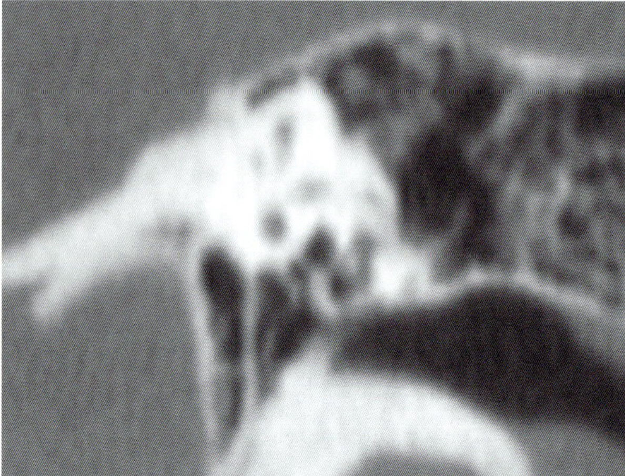

18 −0.68 mm from center of external auditory canal

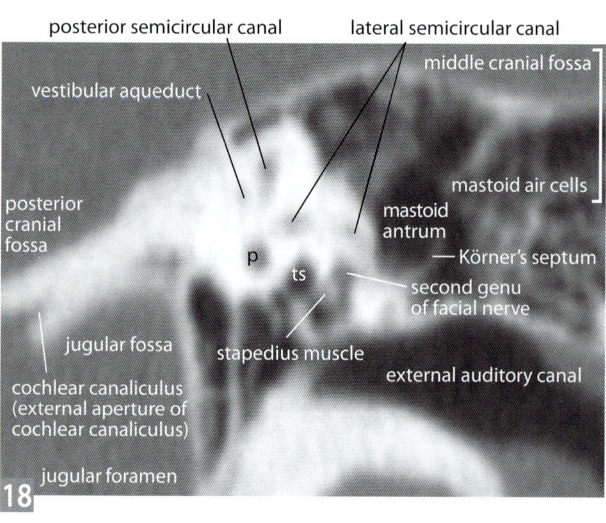

p=posterior ampulla; **ts**=tympanic sinus

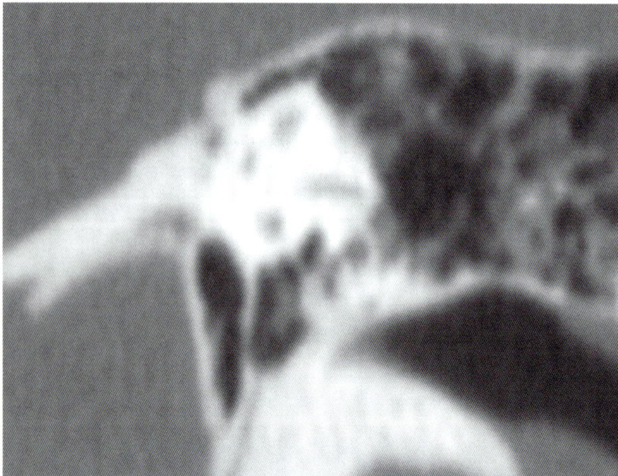

19 −1.34 mm from center of external auditory canal

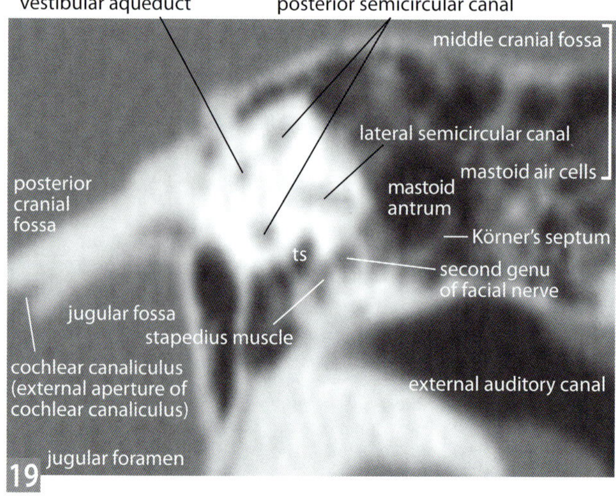

ts=tympanic sinus

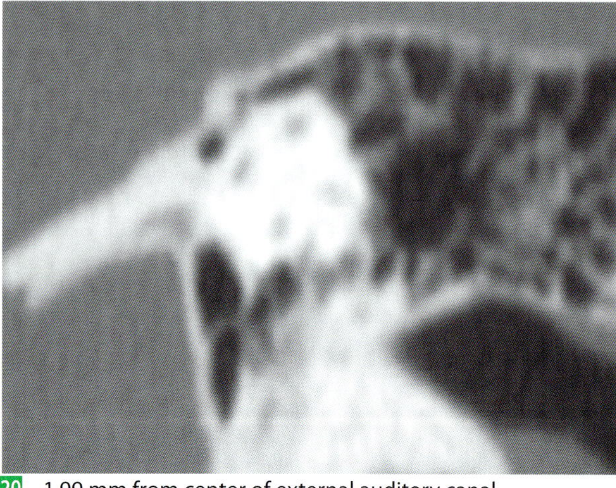

20 −1.99 mm from center of external auditory canal

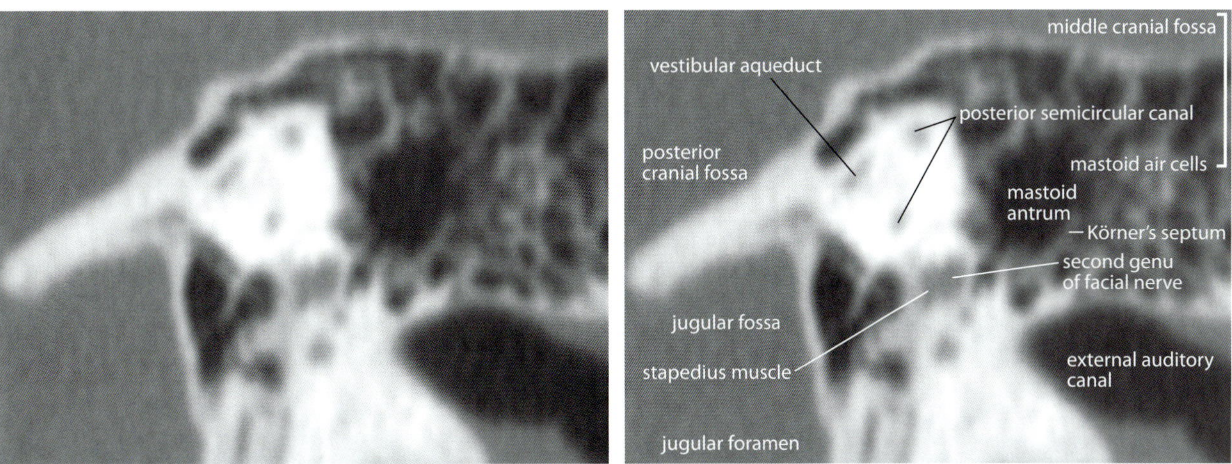

21 −2.64 mm from center of external auditory canal

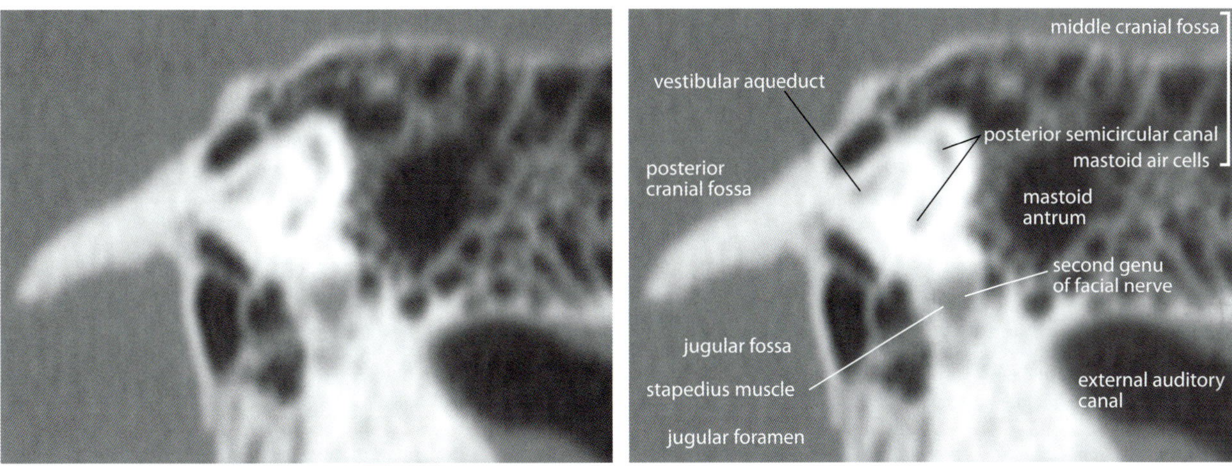

22 −3.29 mm from center of external auditory canal

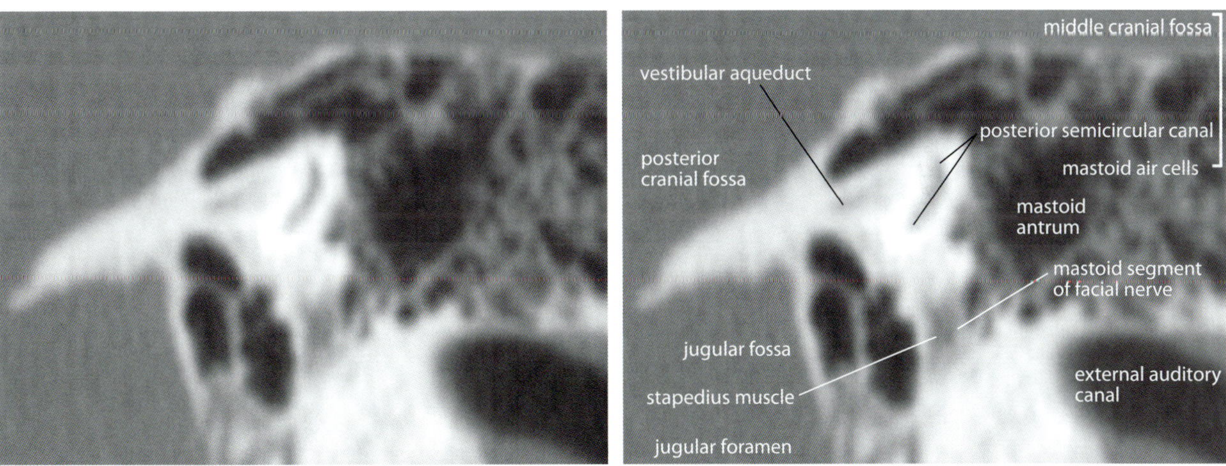

23 −3.94 mm from center of external auditory canal

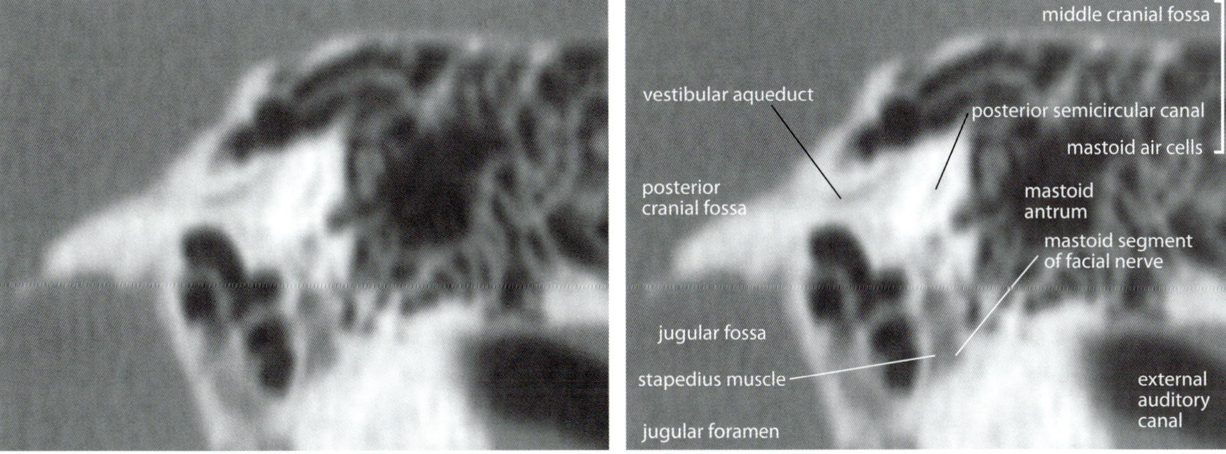

24 −4.59 mm from center of external auditory canal

Pediatric Ear Diseases
Diagnostic Imaging Atlas and Case Reports

Postnatal Growth of the Temporal Bone

Some parts of the temporal bone are fully formed at birth and undergo no postnatal change, while other parts undergo changes in size and shape that accompany postnatal growth. This forms the basis for the clinical understanding that since, for example, the cochlea, vestibule, and other components of the inner ear and auditory ossicles are fully formed at birth, the length and thickness of an electrode for a cochlear implant will be the same for an infant as for an adult, or that bone malformations of the inner ear and auditory ossicles undergo no postnatal changes. On the other hand, the external auditory canal, mastoid air cells, internal auditory canal, vestibular aqueduct, and other components exhibit changes in shape that accompany postnatal growth. Also, because postnatal development of the mastoid air cells is impaired by recurrent otitis media in infancy and childhood, their form may vary widely due not only to age, but also to diseases of the middle ear. A proper understanding of the temporal bone's normal structure with respect to age is important for accurate temporal bone imaging diagnosis and appropriate surgical intervention. In this chapter, we will examine CT images of each section of the temporal bone in children at different ages and explain how the various structures develop and change with age.

In this chapter, images taken from children at four months, one year, three years one month, and sixteen years ten months are used as representative examples, however these images are taken from different individuals and are not the product of an ongoing examination of a single child over time. Although the subjects all received CT exams for hearing loss or other reasons, samples were chosen from those who displayed no clear abnormalities in their CT images.

Chapter **2**

1 External Auditory Canal
2 Mastoid Air Cells
3 Internal Auditory Canal
4 Vestibular Aqueduct

❶ External Auditory Canal

At birth, the bony framework of the external auditory canal consists of the annular tympanic bone alone, with lateral structures composed almost entirely of cartilage. As shown in the image taken at four months after birth, only the superior half of the bony external auditory canal exists, namely the floor (1b: ⇐) of the tegmental air cells (❀) and the medial portion of the posterior wall of the mandibular fossa (1a: ⇐); the inferior half is still almost completely unformed (1b: ⇑). In both the axial and the coronal sections, the bony external auditory canal is not so much a bony canal as a trumpet-shaped hollow in the base of the skull that spreads out laterally from the tympanic cavity (1a: ✎, 1b: ⇐). On the other hand, the lumen of the external auditory canal is cylindrical, with a thick layer of soft tissue between the auditory canal's skin and bone surfaces. The diameter of the external auditory canal's lumen in an infant of this age is approximately half that of an older child, and in clinical settings the external auditory canals of newborns and infants are so narrow that it is frequently difficult to observe the entire tympanic membrane, even with a magnifying otoscope.

Examination of the image taken at one year shows that the external auditory canal is both larger in diameter and longer than that of the 4-month-old infant. As can be seen in the axial section image, both the anterior wall (2a: ⇐) and posterior wall (2a: ✎) of the bony external auditory canal have grown laterally. In the coronal section image, the lateral margin of the external auditory canal's superior wall (2b: ⇐) has moved laterally and slightly inferiorly, with the inferior portion of the bony wall growing laterally (2b: ⇑), causing the external auditory canal to form a cylindrical shape overall. However, the external auditory canal is still trumpet-shaped (2a: ✎). Infants in this age range frequently require cochlear implantations, but direct observation of the round window niche while performing mastoidectomy and posterior tympanotomy is often impaired by the lateral portion of the bony external auditory canal wall. In order to obtain satisfactory operating field of vision of the round window niche and to further perform cochlear fenestration procedures, it is necessary to either remove a portion of the bony part of the external auditory canal or thin out the bony wall and temporarily fracture it to permit viewing from a more anterior position.

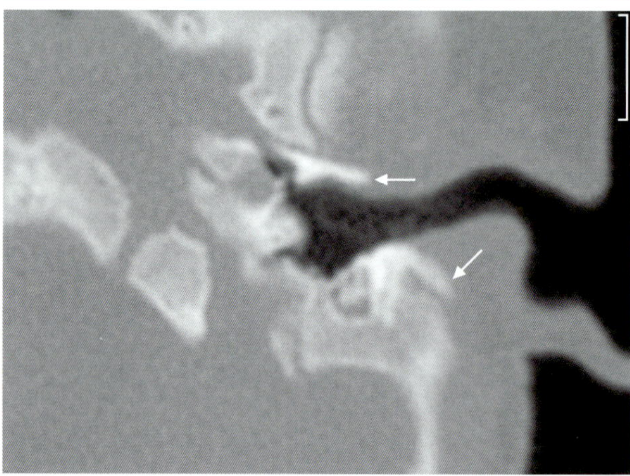

1a: 4 months old

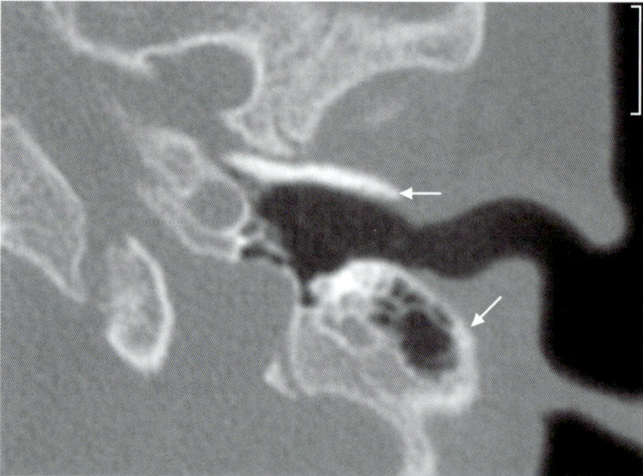

2a: 1 year old

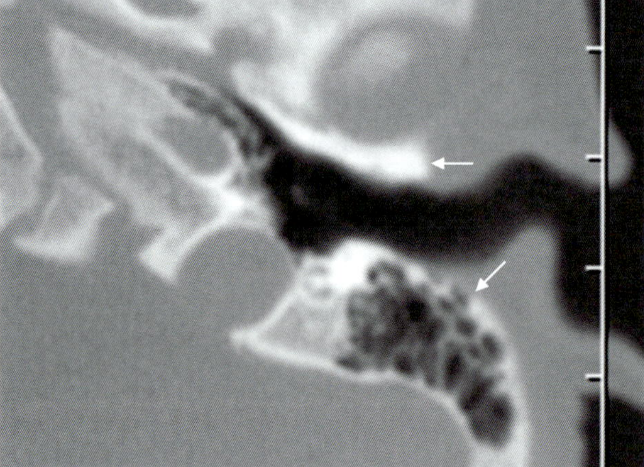

3a: 3 years, 1 month old

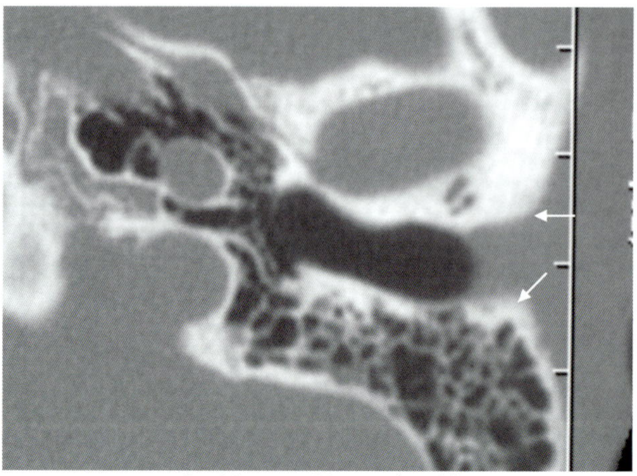

4a: 16 years, 10 months old

Coronal Section Images

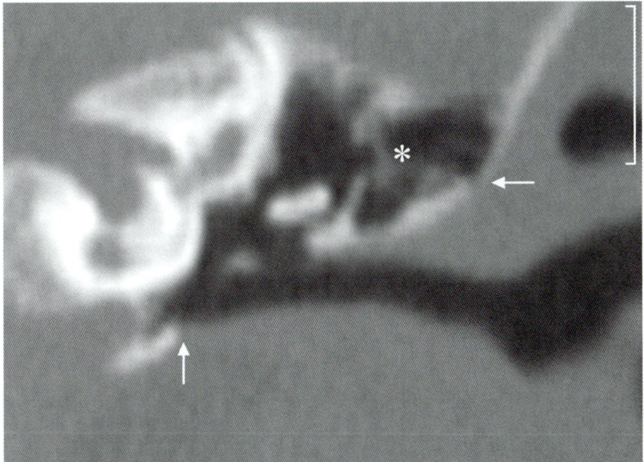

1b: 4 months old

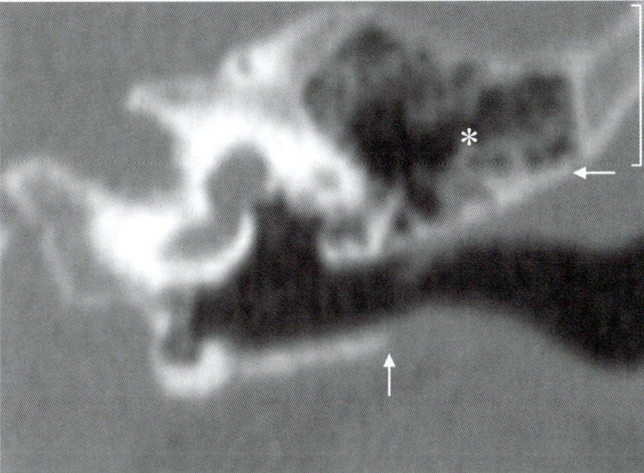

2b: 1 year old

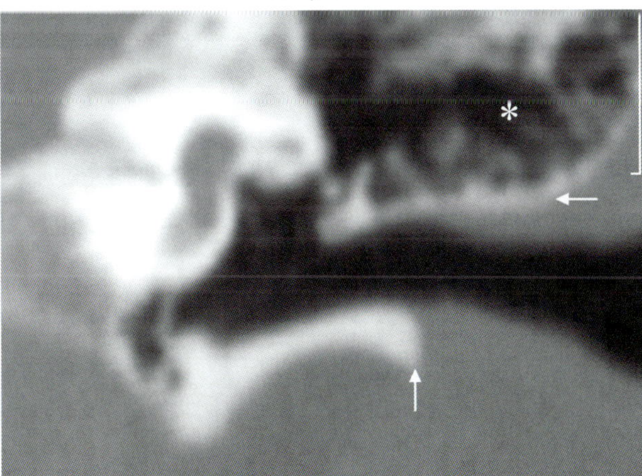

3b: 3 years, 1 month old

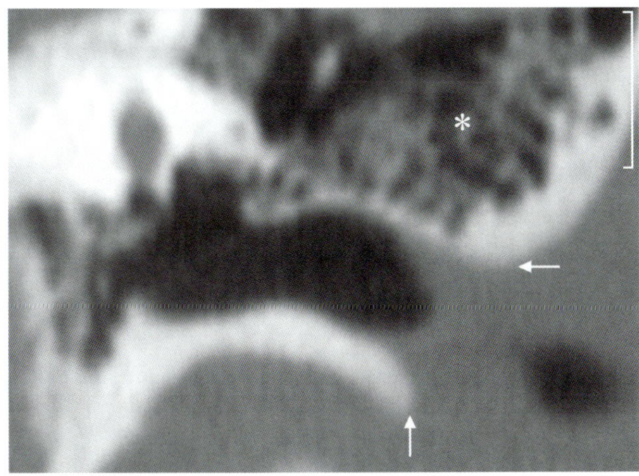

4b: 16 years, 10 months old

In the image taken at three years old, we observe that the bony external auditory canal has expanded and elongated. Accompanying this growth, the lateral margin of the external auditory canal's posterior wall has moved anteriorly (3a: ✎) and the lateral edge of the superior wall inferiorly (3b: ⇐), with the entire structure gradually forming into a tunnel shape of constant diameter. The bone of the anterior and inferior walls has thickened and extended laterally (3a: ⇐, 3b: ⇑).

The images from a child at 16 years old are essentially the same as for an adult. Little change is expected to occur in the size of the temporal bone or the skull overall, limited to a slight thickening of cortical bone. The lateral margin of the external auditory canal has further extended laterally and has formed a complete tunnel shape (4a: ⇐ ✎). The superior wall of the entrance to the external auditory canal is lower (4b: ⇐) and the inferior wall has further thickened and grown laterally (4b: ⇑). (Scale shown in images indicates 1 cm)

② Mastoid Air Cells

■ Mastoid Air Cell Development—Axial Section

The temporal bone is small at birth. The inner ear and auditory ossicles remain essentially unchanged, but the surrounding mastoid air cells expand with age, the external auditory canal grows, the internal auditory canal lengthens, and the petrous apex becomes extended. In newborns, the mastoid process is almost completely unformed and the temporal bone is positioned lower in the skull than in an adult, with its surface facing slightly inferior. After birth, the bony external auditory canal lengthens and the mastoid process becomes extended. The remarkable difference in temporal bone formation between an infant and an older child is mainly due to the different degrees of development of the mastoid air cells. Development of the mastoid air cells causes the lateral surface of the temporal bone to approach perpendicular, while the surface of the tympanic membrane gradually rises from its initial pronounced, downward-facing position [1].

Here, in order to examine the development of the temporal bone overall, and in particular the changes to the mastoid air cells, we present axial section images showing cross sections taken at the level of the inferior margin of the external auditory canal (1a–4a) and at the level of the malleus head and incus body in the middle area of the epitympanum (attic) (1b–4b).

First, we examine the development of the temporal bone in the axial section at the level of the inferior margin of the external auditory canal (1a–4a). In the image taken at four months, the temporal bone is not visible except for the inferior margin of the external auditory canal and the stylomastoid foramen (1a: ⇑) in the vicinity of the tympanic annulus. In other words, very little development of the mastoid process, hypotympanum, and other components of the inferior temporal bone has taken place between birth and this age. The facial nerve also exits the temporal bone at this level. At one year, the air cells of the hypotympanum become visible, and a slight amount of bone formation can be observed at the medial margin of the external auditory canal and the mastoid process. The facial nerve is clearly contained in a bony canal (mastoid segment of facial nerve, 2a: ⇑). At three years, development of the mastoid air cells is remarkable and extends to the sigmoid sinus posteriorly, and to the carotid canal anteriorly. However, the area around the facial canal (3a: ⇑) has not yet undergone pneumatization. At sixteen years old, air cell development is nearly complete, with pneumatization extending to the petrous apex, hypotympanum, mastoid tip, and to the lateral region of the sigmoid sinus and posterior. The area surrounding the mastoid segment of the facial nerve is also pneumatized (4a: ⇑).

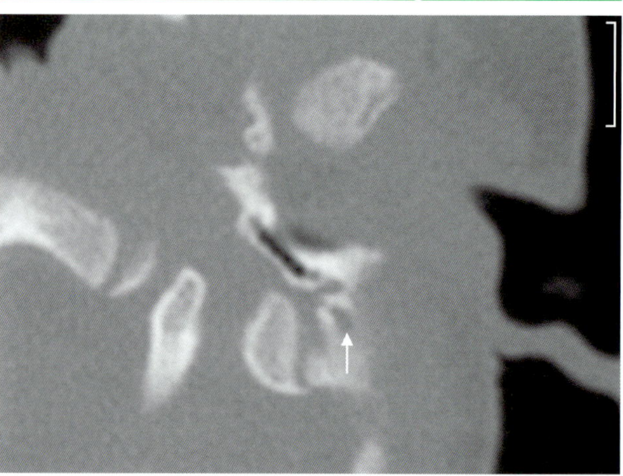

1a: 4 months old

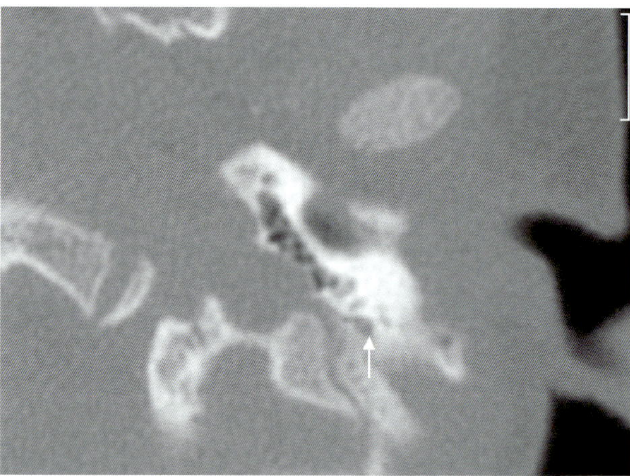

2a: 1 year old

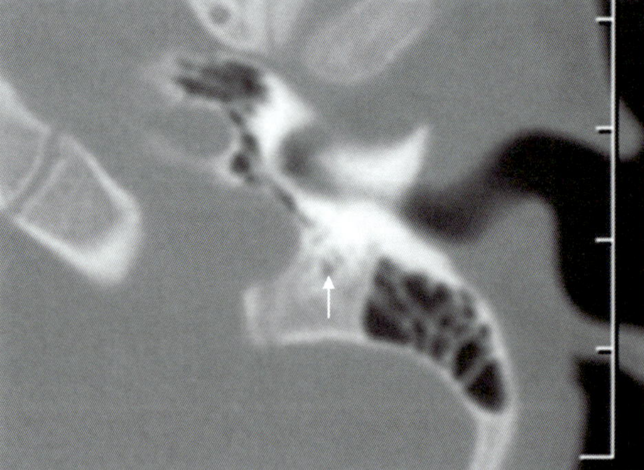

3a: 3 years, 1 month old

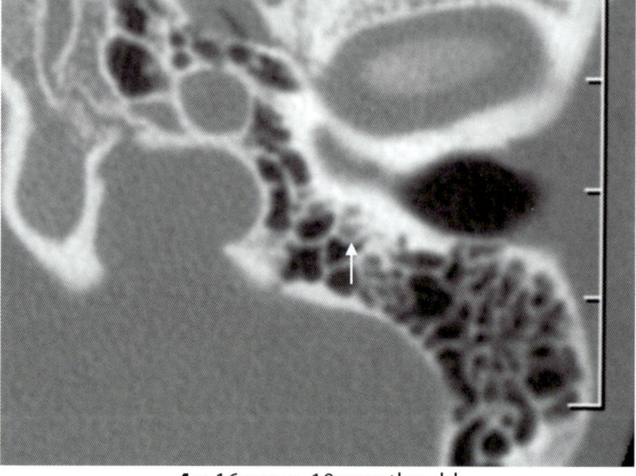

4a: 16 years, 10 months old

Axial Section Images

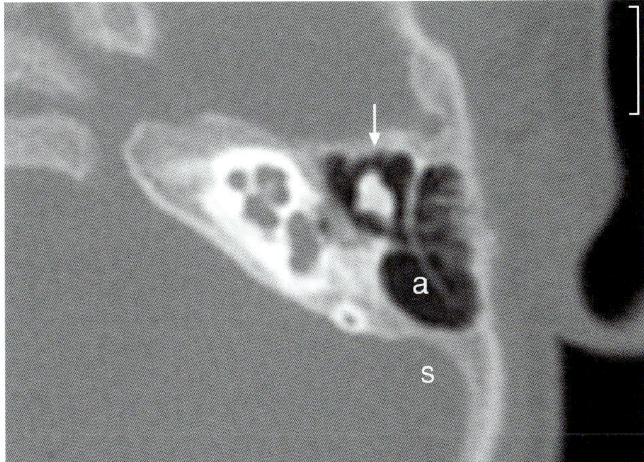

1b: 4 months old

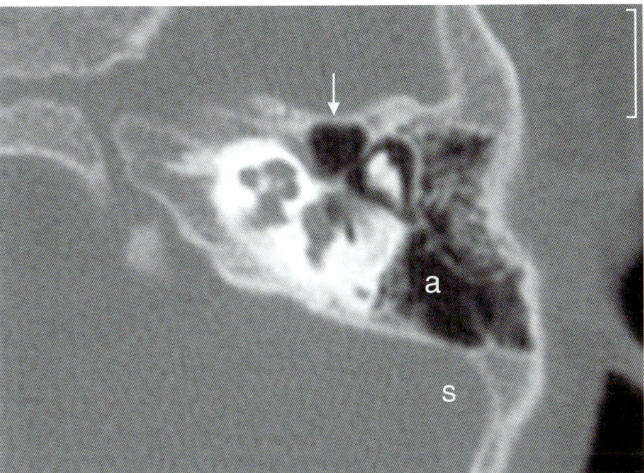

2b: 1 year old

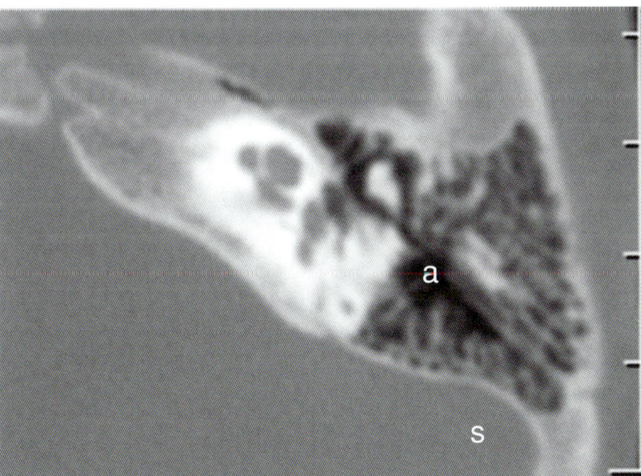

3b: 3 years, 1 month old

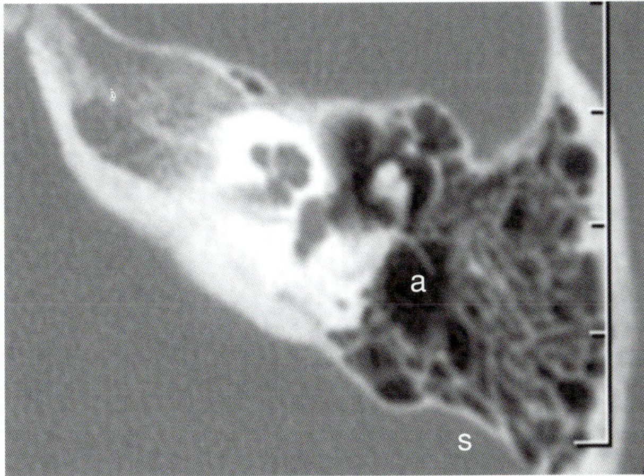

4b: 16 years, 10 months old

Next we examine the image taken at the level of the attic (1b–4b). In the image, "**a**" marks the mastoid antrum and "**s**" marks the sigmoid sinus. At zero years, pneumatic cavities are limited to the attic (1b: ⇓) and its lateral area, and to the mastoid antrum. The area between the sigmoid sinus and the mastoid antrum is still bone marrow, with no air cells. At one year, the formation of air cells is observed anterior to the attic in the supratubal recess (2b: ⇓), with pneumatization of the area lateral to the attic and in the periphery of the mastoid antrum progressing nearly to the sigmoid sinus. Observation of the image at three years (3b) clearly indicates that, along with overall air cell development, the temporal bone itself has become larger. The air cells extend from the mastoid antrum, reaching the sigmoid sinus. In the image at sixteen years (4b), the temporal bone has grown further and pneumatization extends to its borders. Posteriorly, the mastoid air cells extend lateral to the sigmoid sinus.

■ Mastoid Air Cell Development—Coronal Section

The coronal section images here show cross sections anteriorly in the malleoincudal joint region (1a–4a) and posteriorly in the central part of the mastoid antrum (1b–4b). First, we will examine the anterior images at the level of the malleoincudal joint region. The arrow mark (✐) in the images indicates the lateral wall of the attic.

At zero years, pneumatic cavities are visible not only in the attic, but also lateral to it. At this age, the inferior mastoid region (1a, previous page) showed no air cell development, but at the level of the attic, air cell development is present lateral to the lateral wall, indicating that air cell development in the temporal bone begins in the superior region of the temporal bone.

At one year, slight air cell development is visible immediately superior to the attic, while the temporal bone displays expansion and pneumatization in the area lateral to the attic's lateral wall (tegmental air cells). As seen on the previous page, development of the mastoid part begins with growth of the bone itself, followed by growth and expansion of air cells within, whereas at the attic level superior to the external auditory canal air cell growth can be observed from early infancy, with pneumatization and bone growth and expansion progressing simultaneously as the child grows older.

This process continues from three to around sixteen years old, with the temporal bone expanding laterally and thickening vertically. The tegmen portion of the attic has almost no air cells during infancy, with only a cavity continuing from the mastoid antrum, but later air cells develop in the tegmen portion, which is basically a cavity, and this area develops and enlarges. On the other hand, as in the case of adhesive otitis media and cholesteatoma samples shown in Chapter 4, "Inflammatory diseases of the middle ear," cases of recurrent otitis media are marked by impaired development of air cells lateral to the attic and a low-hanging middle cranial fossa floor. In such middle ear surgeries of the temporal bone, the low-hanging cranial base makes it difficult to secure sufficient field of view when approached laterally, necessitating an approach from inferior, which results in less working space. Therefore, it is important to examine air cell development of the tegmental air cells when determining whether middle ear surgery can be performed safely and securely. In observing the overall age-related lateral development of the temporal bone with respect to the medial and lateral portions of the attic's lateral wall, it is apparent that, whereas the width of the medial attic hardly changes (in other words, it is almost fully formed in infancy), the lateral portion continues to grow and widen.

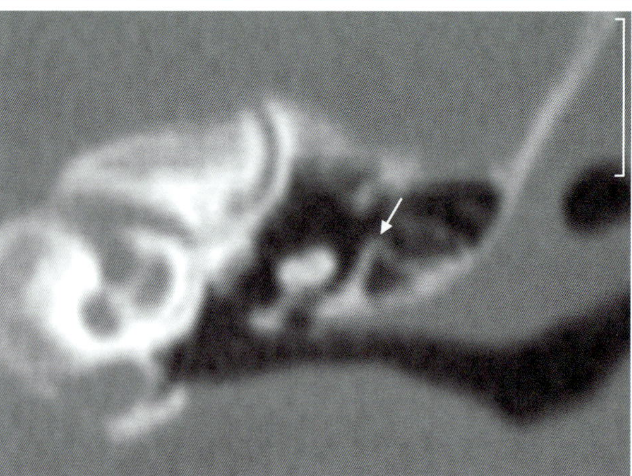

1a: 4 months old

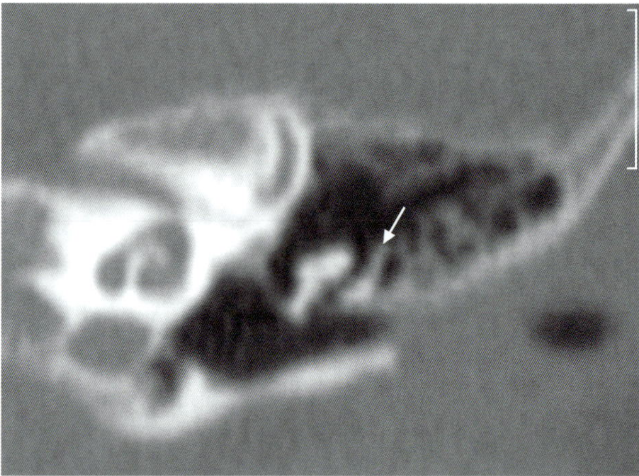

2a: 1 year old

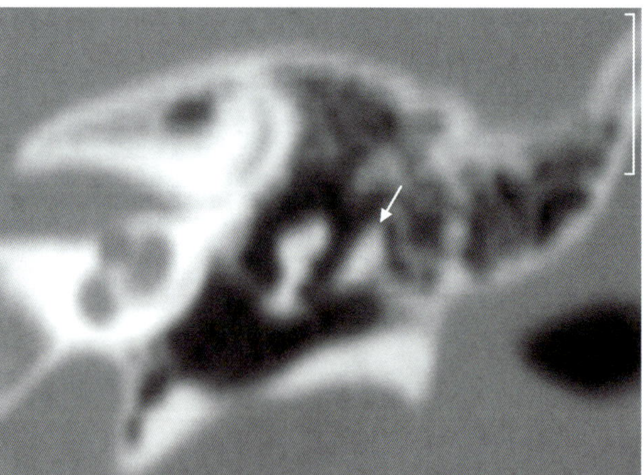

3a: 3 years, 1 month old

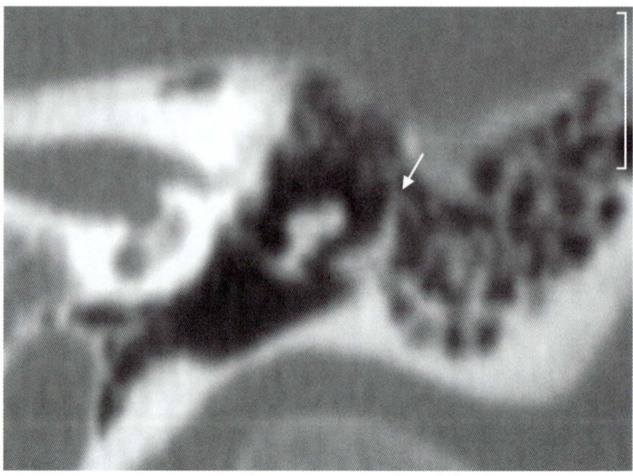

4a: 16 years, 10 months old

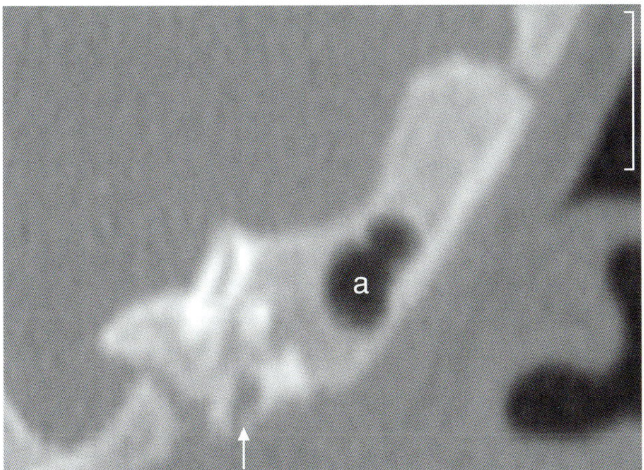

1b: 4 months old

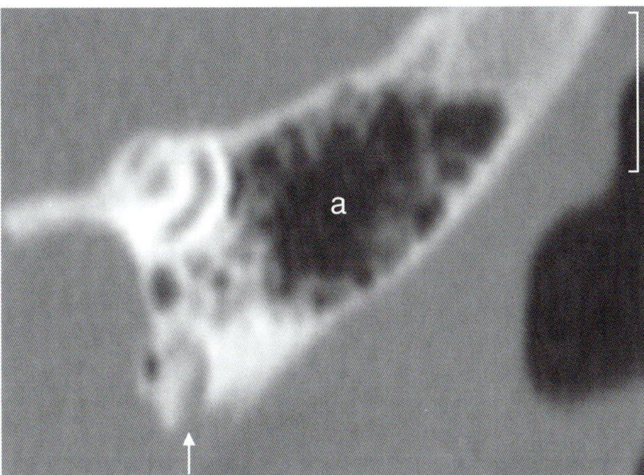

2b: 1 year old

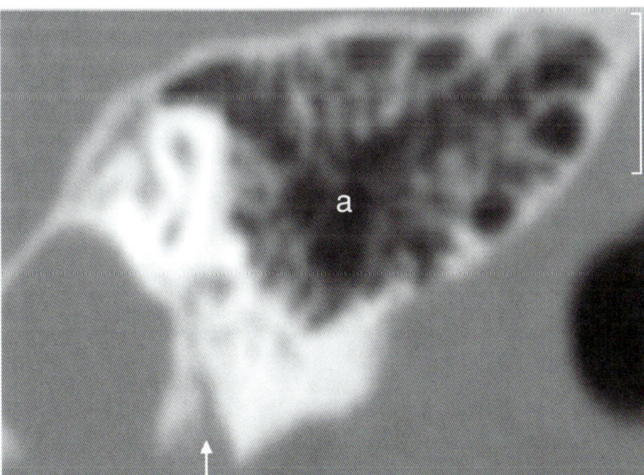

3b: 3 years, 1 month old

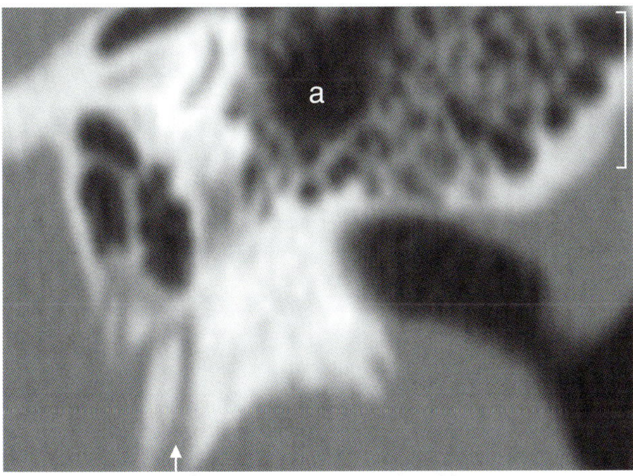

4b: 16 years, 10 months old

Next, we examine the cross section at the level of the mastoid antrum and the stylomastoid foramen (1b–4b). In the image, "**a**" indicates the mastoid antrum and "⇑" indicates the stylomastoid foramen. At zero years, the mastoid (1b) contains no pneumatic cavities other than the antrum, the rest being composed entirely of bone marrow. Later, pneumatization occurs centered on the mastoid antrum and spreading toward the periphery, until at 16 years, air cells have developed medially beyond the labyrinth. Note that the stylomastoid foramen, where the mastoid segment of the facial nerve exits (1b–4b: ⇑), has descended relative to the labyrinth with age. Also, with regard to the medial-lateral orientation, at zero years the stylomastoid foramen is almost exposed at the inferior margin of the temporal bone's lateral surface, whereas in older children it is located medial to the mastoid process, deeply medial to the temporal bone's lateral surface. When performing surgery on the infra-auricular region or inferior mastoid part in younger children, particularly infants, particular caution must be exercised in order to avoid damaging the facial nerve trunk.

(Scale shown in images indicates 1 cm)

References

1 Gulya AJ: Developmental anatomy of the ear. Glasscock ME III and Shambaugh GE Jr. eds Surgery of the ear. Saunders. Philadelphia, 1990:5–33.

❸ Internal Auditory Canal

The size of the inner ear does not change after birth, but the internal auditory canal continues to grow from birth to around puberty. Here we present a summary of normal development; for further details including examples of anomalies, please refer to Chapter 3, "Congenital anomalies: IAC stenosis." There are many reports showing measurements of the length and diameter of the internal auditory canal based on high-resolution CT findings, including cases in which hearing loss is both present and absent. According to the report by McClay [1], there is no significant difference in horizontal and vertical diameters of the internal auditory canal between groups with and without sensorineural hearing loss. However, in cases with inner ear malformation, the incidence of sensorineural hearing loss was higher when the diameter of the internal auditory canal was 2 mm or less.

While there is no universal standard established for abnormal enlargement of the internal auditory canal, the above-mentioned report by McClay et al [1] defines enlargement as a horizontal or vertical diameter of 8 mm or greater. However, enlargement of the internal auditory canal is generally considered to be unrelated to hearing loss.

Concerning age-related changes to the length of the internal auditory canal, Lang [2] states that it grows from around 5–7 mm at birth to 10–15 mm in adulthood. Measurements using 3-dimensional computer reconstructions based on histopathological specimens of the temporal bone [3] also show that, while the internal auditory canal's diameter increases very little with age, it does lengthen. In measurements taken according to McClay's method in temporal bone CT images shown here (1a,b–4a,b), the length of the internal auditory canal was 5.8 mm at four months, 7.7 mm at one year, 10.6 mm at three years, and 12.9 mm at sixteen years, indicating that it lengthens with age. The diameter of the internal auditory canal varies considerably between individuals, but does not show the same clear trend toward enlargement as for length. Consequently, the growth pattern for the internal auditory canal is best understood as a steady lengthening with little change in diameter.

The development of the internal auditory canal includes changes in direction as well as length. In the coronal section images, we see that the medial end of the internal auditory canal is elevated and its path slightly angled in infants, with an approach toward horizontal accompanying growth (1b–4b). In the axial section images, the medial end appears to be facing slightly posteriorly in early years, whereas in older children it faces almost directly medially. These spacial changes to the direction of the internal auditory canal may reflect relative growth differences between the temporal bone and the cerebellum, brain stem, and 7th and 8th cranial nerves in the posterior cranial fossa.

(Scale shown in images indicates 1 cm)

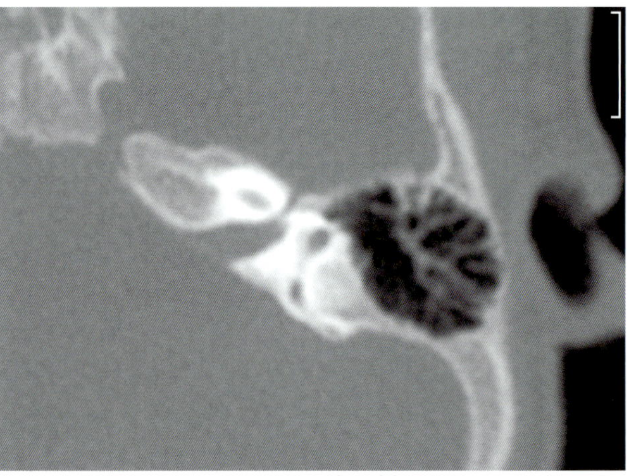

1a: 4 months old

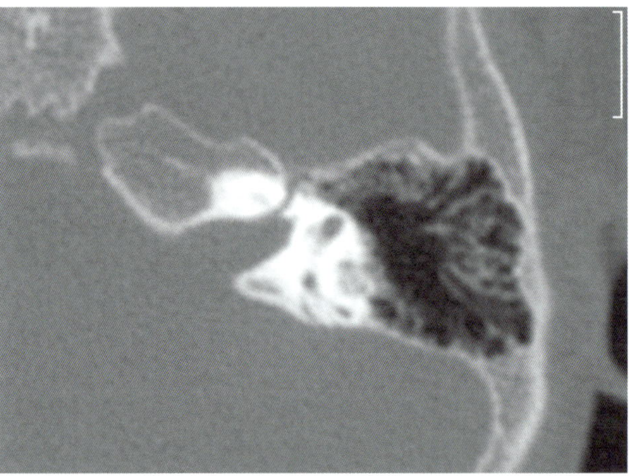

2a: 1 year old

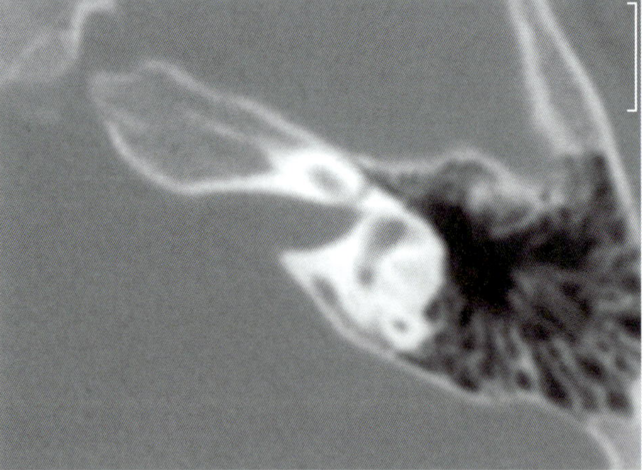

3a: 3 years, 1 month old

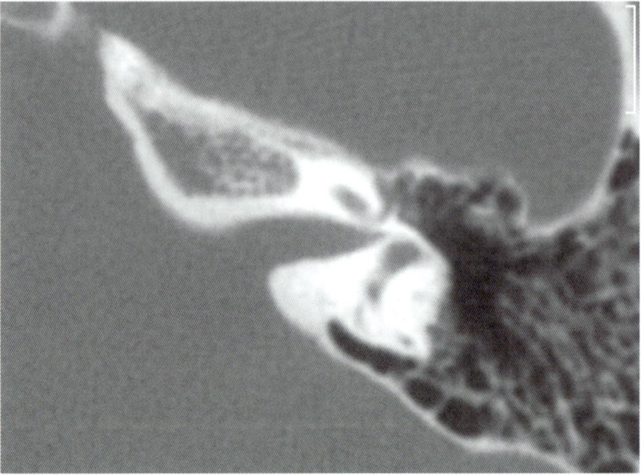

4a: 16 years, 10 months old

Axial Section Images

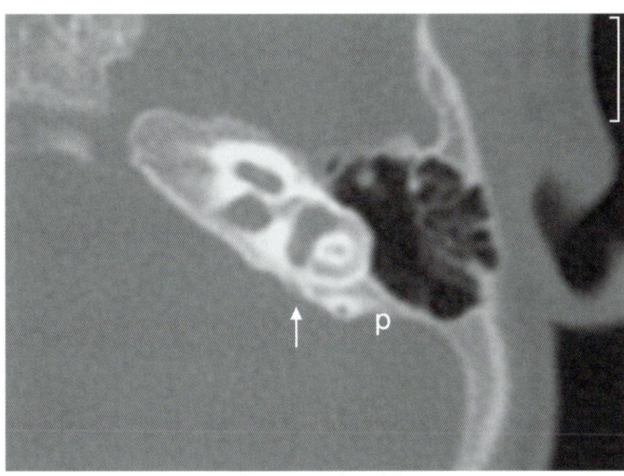

1b: 4 months old

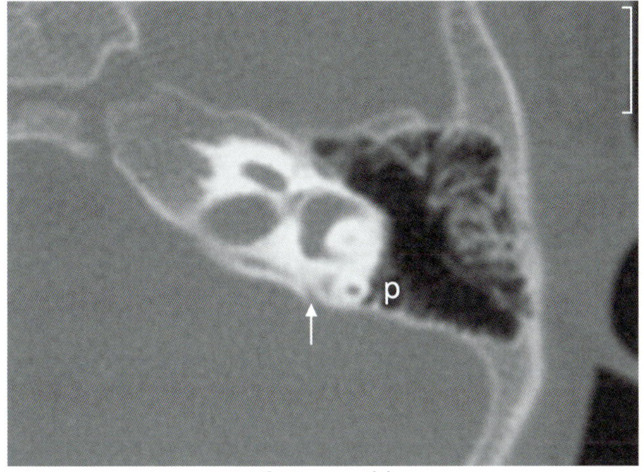

2b: 1 year old

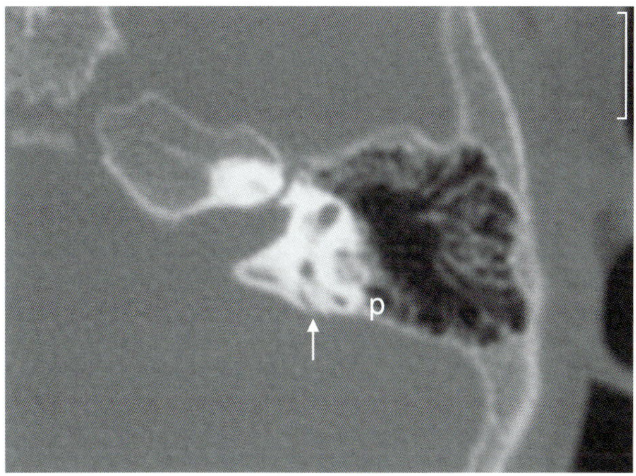

2c: 1 year old

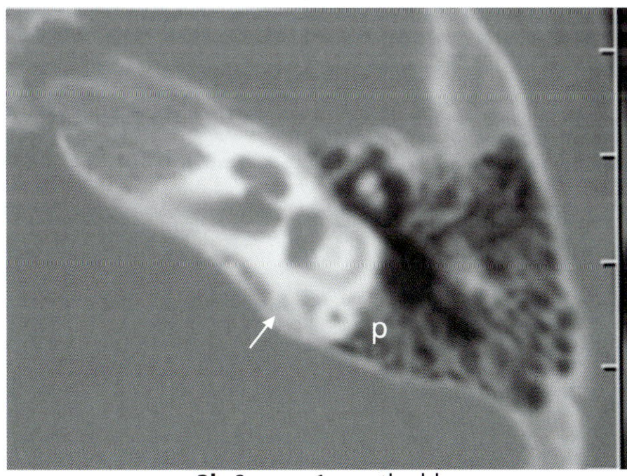

3b: 3 years, 1 month old

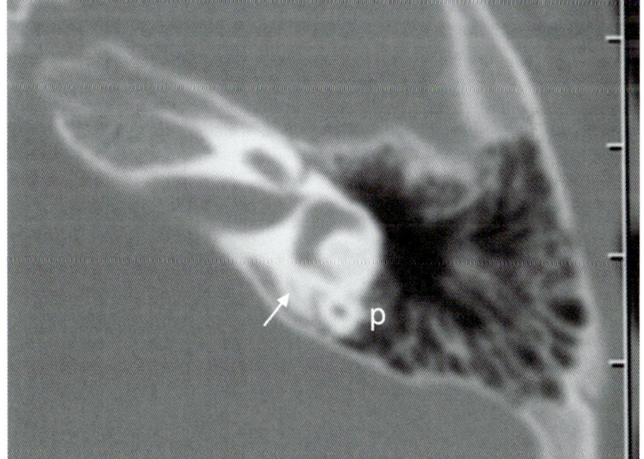

3c: 3 years, 1 month old

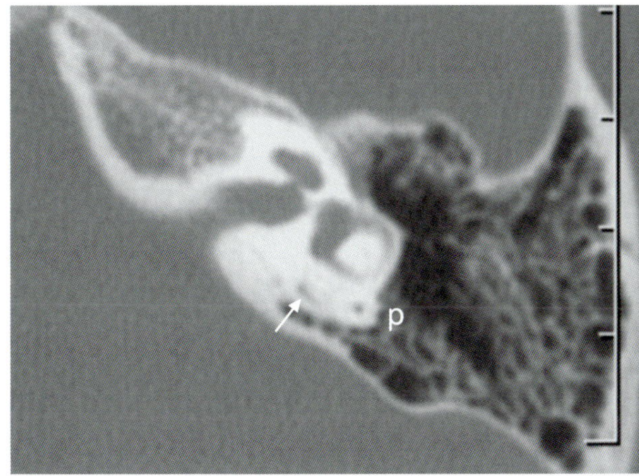

4b: 16 years, 10 months old

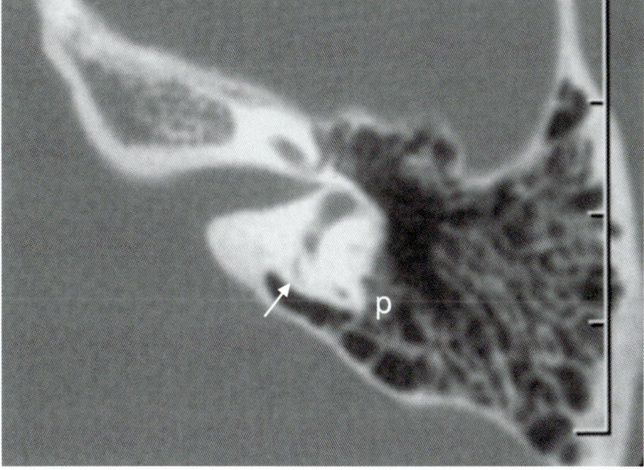

4c: 16 years, 10 months old

shows a slight depression.

Ménière's disease is not necessarily limited to a single cause and is considered to be a product of compound factors. Although, as previously stated, Ménière's disease patients have hypoplastic vestibular aqueducts and suppressed development of the temporal bone posterior to the posterior semicircular canal, mastoid air cell development in other areas is basically satisfactory and differs from the uniform inhibition of air cell development within the temporal bone seen in chronic otitis media. I have experienced cases of adult patients with typical bilateral Ménière's disease in whom CT images indicate that their posterior semicircular canals protrude into the posterior cranial fossa, from which one may postulate that Ménière's disease may be attributable to some form of congenital or genetic factor inhibiting temporal bone growth posterior to the posterior semicircular canal. (Scale shown in images indicates 1 cm)

References

1 Krombach GA, van den Boom M, Di Martino E, et al: Computed tomography of the inner ear: size of anatomical structures in the normal temporal bone and in the temporal bone of patients with Menière's disease. Eur Radiol 2005;15:1505–1513.

2 Yazawa Y, Kitahara M: Computed tomographic findings around the vestibular aqueduct in Ménière's disease. Acta Otolaryngol Suppl 1991;481:88–90.

3 Nidecker A, Pfaltz CR, Matefi L, Benz UF: Computed tomographic findings in Meniere's disease. ORL J Otorhinolaryngol Relat Spec 1985;47:66–75.

4 Fujita S, Sando I: Three-dimensional course of the vestibular aqueduct. Eur Arch Otorhinolaryngol 1996;253:122–125.

Pediatric Ear Diseases
Diagnostic Imaging Atlas and Case Reports

Congenital Anomalies

In congenital anomalies in children, and particularly in infants, as a rule the patients themselves do not complain of their symptoms. This is partly because they are too young to express their disability in words, but also because it is difficult for them to recognize their condition as a disability, as they have lived with it since birth. Consequently, except in cases such as microtia in which the anomaly is externally visible, hearing loss due to defects not externally apparent may remain undetected unless either the parents notice or it is picked up in a physical exam or screening test.

Furthermore, even when hearing loss is confirmed, if there is no finding of abnormality in the tympanic membrane the patient is sometimes diagnosed as "hearing loss of unknown origin" with no further pursuit of the etiology, whereupon a hearing aid is fitted and the road to an accurate diagnosis abandoned. In such cases, even when the cause was previously thought to be unknown, CT or MRI examination of the temporal bone can reveal valuable information. For example, if malformation of the inner ear is discovered, the cause of hearing loss can be explained to the parents, and if conductive system abnormalities are detected they may be ameliorated through surgery. Congenital anomalies in children can have a profound effect on the futures of both patient and family.

It is important to conduct sufficient testing, arrive at an accurate diagnosis at an early stage, and determine an appropriate treatment strategy. Imaging diagnosis has an important role to play in this process.

Chapter **3**

❶ External Auditory Canal
❷ Auditory Ossicles and Middle Ear
❸ Inner Ear
❹ Internal Auditory Canal

❶ External Auditory Canal

EAC Atresia and Stenosis

The external auditory canal (EAC) arises from the first external branchial cleft; the auricle from the first and second branchial arches; the auditory ossicles from the first branchial arch (head of malleus, body of incus) and the second branchial arch (handle of malleus, long process of incus, superstructure of stapes); the tympanic cavity from the first pharyngeal pouch; and the tympanic membrane from the first external branchial cleft and pharyngeal pouch. The first branchial cleft is located between the first and second branchial arches. Considering these embryological origins, it is understandable how malformations of the external and middle ear combine in a variety of forms. The inner ear, on the other hand, originates in the otic vesicle, which is dorsal to the branchial cleft and branchial arch. In other words, the inner and middle ear have different origins, and therefore their malformations can arise separately, although in actuality there are cases in which the two combine, so in imaging diagnosis of pediatric hearing loss it is necessary to examine both the inner and the middle ear.

Congenital EAC atresia occurs with a frequency of approx. one case in 10,000 births, frequently with combined malformation of the auricle and middle ear, and occurs bilaterally in 15–25% of cases [1–3]. It is more common in boys and, when unilateral, occurs more frequently on the right side [1–3]. Taking influence on language development into consideration, in bilateral cases a hearing acuity assessment should be performed as early as possible and the patient directed to wear a bone conduction hearing aid. At the same time, imaging should be used to obtain a detailed grasp of the condition of the malformation and meatotympanoplasty performed on at least one side. Formation of the external auditory canal occurs in conjunction with that of the auricle, so as a rule an auriculoplasty is performed prior to meatoplasty. A bone conduction hearing aid is used until the meatotympanoplasty is performed, but the bone conduction hearing aid must be a plate-spring type device that straddles the head and holds the bone-conduction vibrator tightly against the temporal bone. Special care must be taken to fix it in place, as it can easily be dislodged during activity and many children do not like wearing it. However, even in cases of bilateral EAC atresia not accompanied by inner ear malformation, hearing loss is around 65 dB [4], so one cannot expect healthy language development without the use of a hearing aid. Conversely, where there is no inner ear dysfunction the cause of hearing loss is conductive and therefore one can expect the use of a hearing aid to be highly effective. In cases in which the external auditory canal can be formed without repositioning the auricle, meatoplasty can be performed at an early stage. Even if hearing improvement is insufficient, sufficient otoacoustic effect for spoken language acquisition may be obtained from an air conduction hearing aid. In cases of external or middle ear malformation, examination of 3-dimensional reconstructed surface rendering image of the ear in addition to temporal bone CT images facilitates an accurate grasp of the relationship between the middle ear conduction mechanism and the auricle located on the surface, which is helpful in surgical planning [5].

In malformations of the external auditory canal and middle ear, many variations are possible with respect to the degree and location of the morphological defect, making discussion of the propriety or efficacy of surgery difficult for any given case. The Jahrsdoerfer score is used to organize and assign point values for each defect to permit a numerical evaluation of the malformation's overall condition. This score adds one point for the existence of each anatomical structure, assigning two points for the stapes only, for a total of ten points (table 1) [6]. The score correlates with post-operative hearing improvement, and it has been reported that significantly beneficial results can be obtained with a score of seven or higher [7].

In cases of atresia of the bony and cartilaginous portions of the external auditory canal, the tympanic segment of the facial nerve frequently follows a lower path than normal, making ossicular chain reconstruction difficult if it overhangs the oval window. The mastoid section normally diverts posterior to the external auditory canal and descends to the stylomastoid foramen, but if there is no external auditory canal there is no constraint on this portion of the nerve's path, so in many cases it descends anterior to normal [8].

In recent years, rather than using meatotympanoplasty to treat EAC atresia, it has become increasingly common policy to secure hearing through the use of a Bone Anchored Hearing Aid (BAHA) [9], Vibrant Soundbridge [10], or other implantable hearing devices. However, because in infants development of the temporal bone is incomplete, a BAHA device cannot be anchored directly to it. The method employed instead involves pressing the BAHA oscillator against the head with an elastic belt. Reports indicate that favorable language development can be obtained with this method [11], so we can expect its use to become more widespread in cases where early-stage surgery is difficult.

In cases of unilateral EAC atresia where hearing in the healthy side is good, auriculoplasty is strongly recommended, but physicians are divided as to whether or not to perform meatoplasty or reconstructive surgery on the conductive system. This is because if the abnormality is unilateral then as a rule there is no worry of delayed language development, while one must consider the possibility of complications such as post-operative infection or tympanic membrane lateralization, or the risk of surgical damage to the facial nerve due to abnormalities in the facial nerve path within the temporal bone.

Table 1. Grading system of candidacy for surgery of congenital aural atresia

Parameter	Points
Stapes present	2
Oval window open	1
Middle ear space	1
Facial nerve	1
Malleus/incus complex	1
Mastoid pneumatized	1
Incus-stapes connection	1
Round window	1
Appearance external ear	1
Total available points	10

From Jahrsdoerfer et al [6]

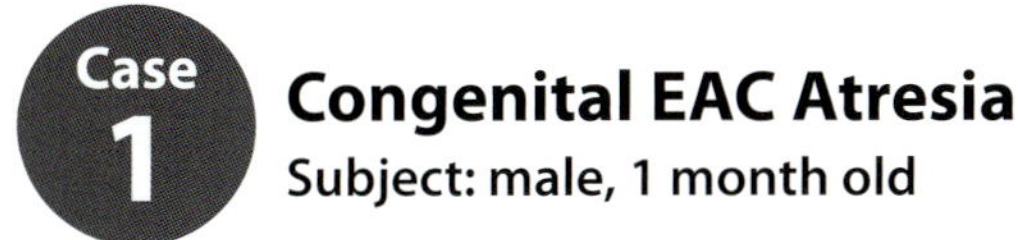

Case 1

Congenital EAC Atresia

Subject: male, 1 month old

■ History and Clinical Findings

Bilateral microtia and EAC atresia were confirmed immediately after birth. Further examination at a pediatric hospital revealed no combined anomalies elsewhere on the body. At three weeks after birth, the ABR V-wave threshold was 80 dB in both ears. The subject was referred to our department to consider a treatment strategy. ASSR (air conduction) thresholds were about 90 dB in the right ear and 110 dB in the left ear. A bone conduction ASSR test revealed threshold values of 10 dB in the mid-to-low frequency ranges and 40 dB in the high frequency range (4,000 Hz), resulting in a diagnosis of near normal bone conduction hearing. The right ear auricle was a lobule type, in which only the lobule exists, and the left ear a concha type, in which the concha exists with the upper half mostly absent [5].

■ Patient CT Findings

The CT images are of the left temporal bone. The bone completely occludes the external auditory canal (fig. 1:1) in the area where it would normally be located (fig. 1:n1). The development of the mastoid air cells is limited, but is considerable for a newborn, and there is no soft tissue density. In the ossicular chain, a portion of the body of the incus approaches the lateral epitympanum (attic) wall nearly to the point of contact (fig. 1:1). The anterior and posterior crus (fig. 1:2) and footplate (fig. 1:3) of the stapes are all visible. The facial nerve is almost normal in the labyrinthine segment, but the tympanic segment slightly overhangs the oval window (fig. 1:3) and the mastoid segment descends slightly more anterior than normal (fig. 1:1). All corresponding structures are indicated with arrows in the normal images (fig. 1:n1–n3) for comparison.

The coronal images reveal absence of the inferolateral portion of the temporal bone, with clear indication that the area where the external auditory canal would normally be located is replaced by skull-base soft tissue in this patient (fig. 2:1–3). Also, the head of the malleus and the body of the incus are in close proximity to the lateral attic wall, with almost no space between them (fig. 2:1). The incudostapedial joint is visible (fig. 2:3), with no apparent differences from the normal control (fig. 2:n3).

In the left ear, the mastoid and the epitympanum are located immediately medial to the post-tragus region, which is where the external auditory canal would normally have been located, making it possible to create the external auditory canal without moving the auricle. A meatotympanoplasty was performed at one year of age. The Jahrsdoerfer score for this case was nine, which predicts a favorable prognosis.

■ Surgical Findings

A mastoidectomy was performed as usual via postauricular incision and the atretic plate carefully removed to expose the ossicular chain. The handle of malleus was hypoplastic, with the head adhered to the atretic plate, which was surgically removed. A portion of the body of the incus also contacted the surrounding bone, limiting mobility, but was freed by removing the surrounding bone. The lenticular process of the incus was somewhat hypoplastic, but continuity of the incudostapedial joint was intact and the mobility of the stapes was normal. The tympanic membrane was formed using the temporalis fascia and a type II tympanoplasty performed, a pedicled connective tissue flap laid down on the mastoid segment, and the external auditory canal formed using a split thickness skin graft from the inguinal region. COR (conditioned orientation response audiometry) at six months after birth exhibited 40 to 55 dB unaided hearing levels, and everyday sound recognition, response, and vocalization improved.

Patient CT Findings	**Normal Control CT Findings**

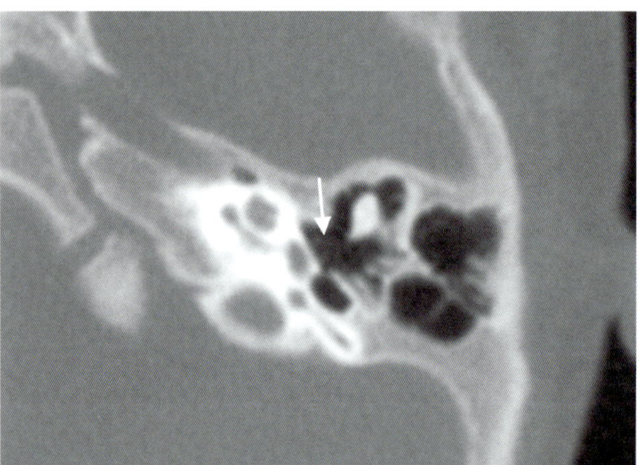

1. axial image

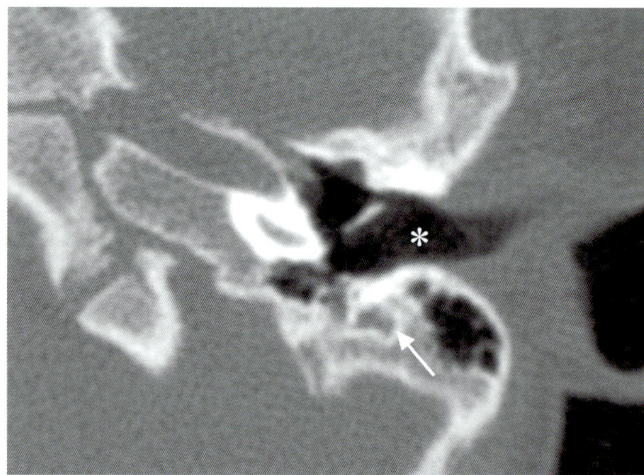

n1. axial image

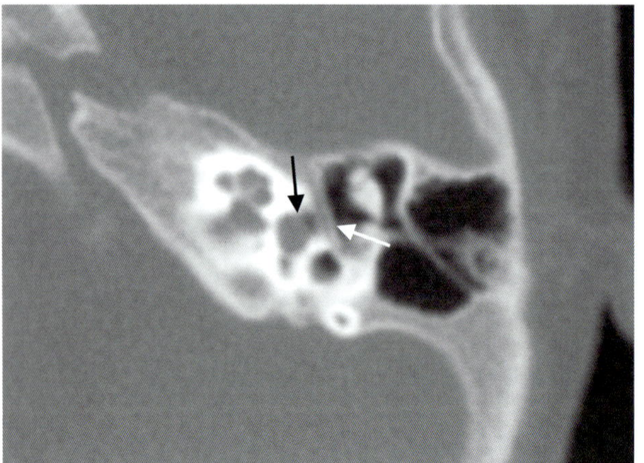

2. axial image

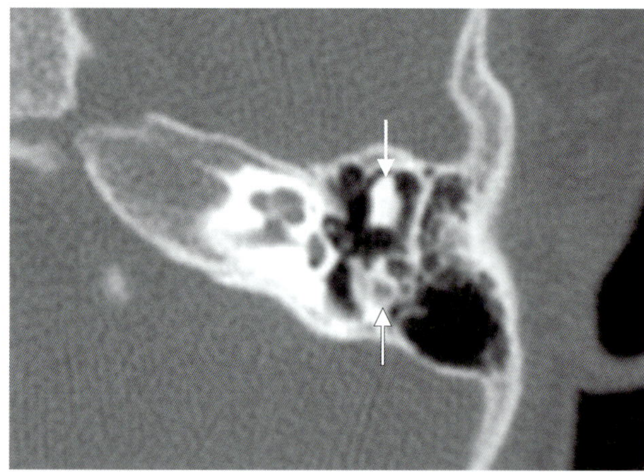

n2. axial image

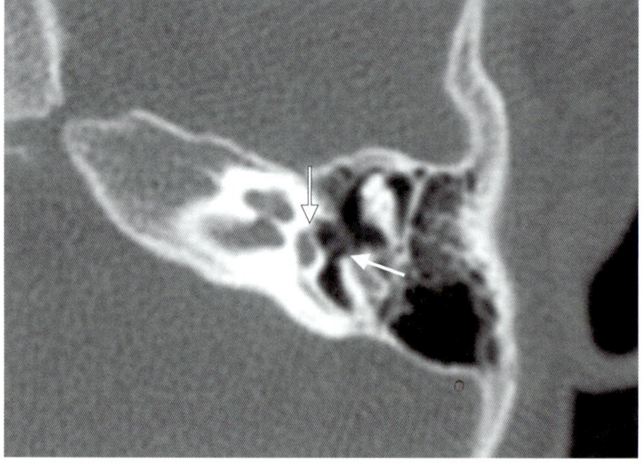

3. axial image

n3. axial image

Fig. 1. (Case 1) Left ear CT: preoperative

[Patient CT Findings]

《Normal Control CT Findings》

Patient CT Findings

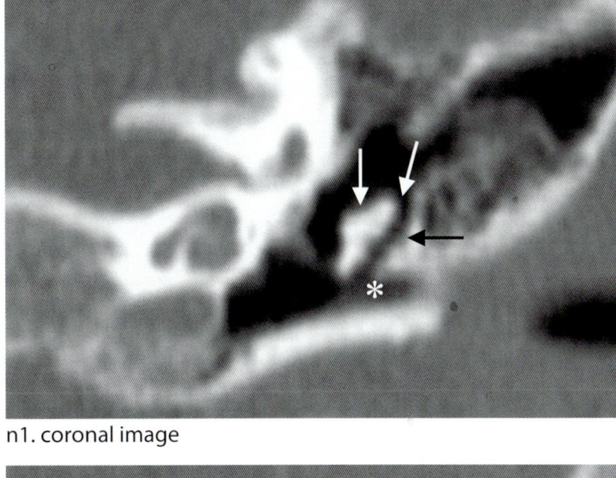

1. coronal image

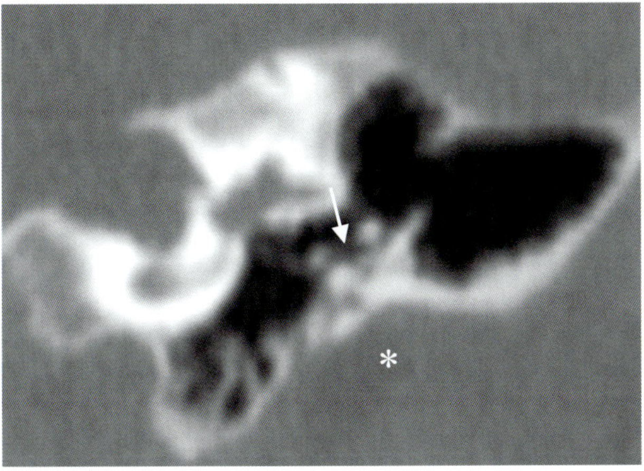

2. coronal image

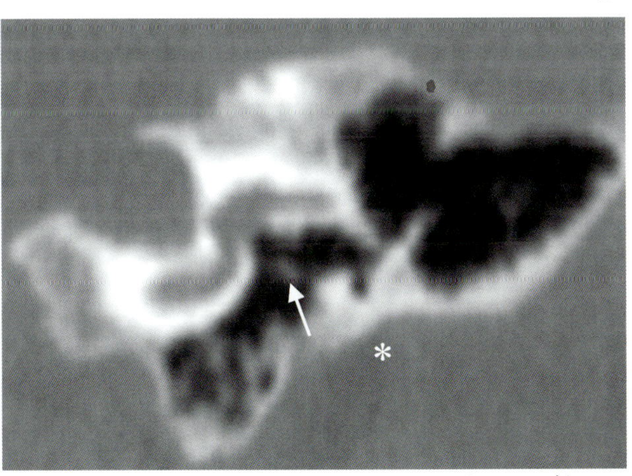

3. coronal image

Normal Control CT Findings

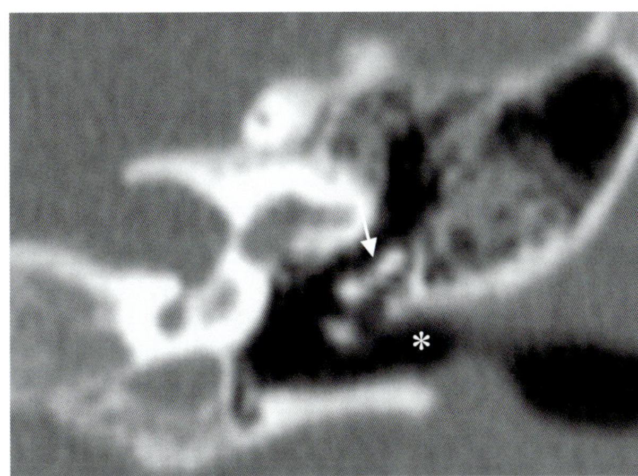

n1. coronal image

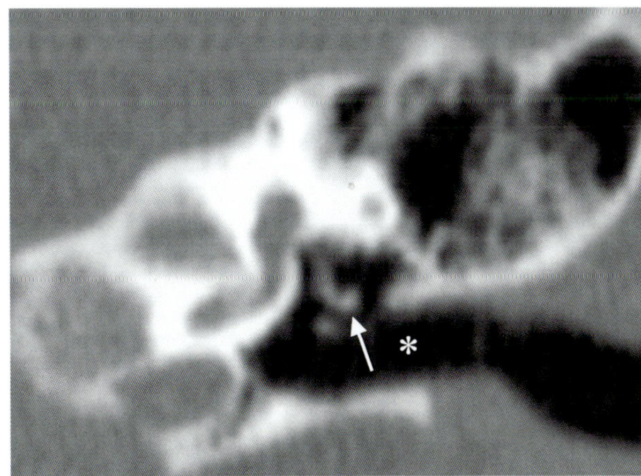

n2. coronal image

n3. coronal image

Fig. 2. (Case 1) Left ear CT: preoperative

[Patient CT Findings]

The inferolateral portion of the temporal bone is absent, with clear indication that the area where the external auditory canal would normally be located is replaced by skull-base soft tissue in this patient (1–3: ✿). Also, the head of the malleus and the body of the incus are in close proximity to the lateral attic wall (1: ⟵), with almost no space between them (1: ⌀). Slightly posterior, the ossicular chain (2: ⌀) can be observed contacting the lateral attic wall and atretic plate. In a cross-section posterior to this, the incudostapedial joint can be identified (3: ⌀).

⟪Normal Control CT Findings⟫

n1: A space (⌀) is visible between the malleus/body of the incus (⌀) and the lateral attic wall (⟵). ✿ indicates the external auditory canal. n2: There is no contact between the ossicular chain (⌀) and the lateral attic wall. ✿ indicates the external auditory canal. n3: ⌀ incudostapedial joint; ✿ external auditory canal.

Case 2 Congenital EAC Stenosis with Cholesteatoma
Subject: female, 1 year, 8 months

■ History and Clinical Findings
EAC stenosis was present in the left ear, with no malformation of the auricle. In the right ear, there were no abnormalities in the external auditory canal or tympanic membrane. Since one month previously the subject became upset if her left ear was touched, and since 20 days previously she exhibited swelling and redness in her left postauricular region. Two weeks previously the subject underwent incision and drainage of a postauricular abscess at her regular pediatric hospital. She received an antibiotic IV drip, but the left postauricular abscess returned and the subject was referred to our department for radical treatment. The left external auditory canal was extremely narrow and the periphery swollen, making observation of the lumen impossible. In an ASSR test conducted by the previous physician, air conduction threshold values averaged 98 dB, while the bone conduction ASSR threshold values averaged 28 dB.

■ Preoperative History and Patient CT Findings
The previous physician conducted a CT exam of the temporal bone at four months after birth. Even in findings at this time the external auditory canal cavity could not be confirmed due to EAC stenosis (fig. 3:1), but the image showed no osteolytic lesions, pneumatization in the middle ear was satisfactory, and there were no soft

<table><tr><td>

Patient CT Findings

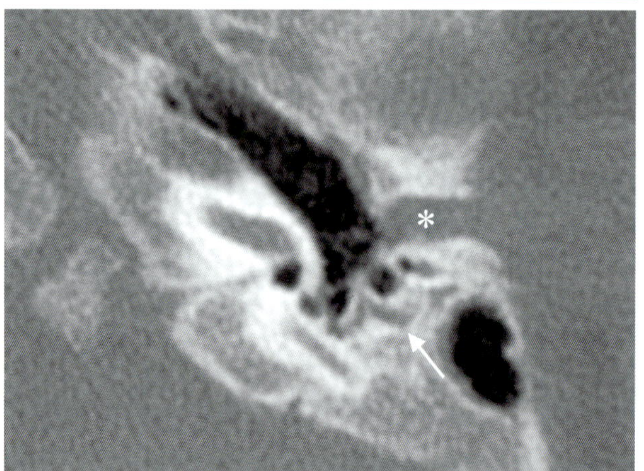

1. axial image

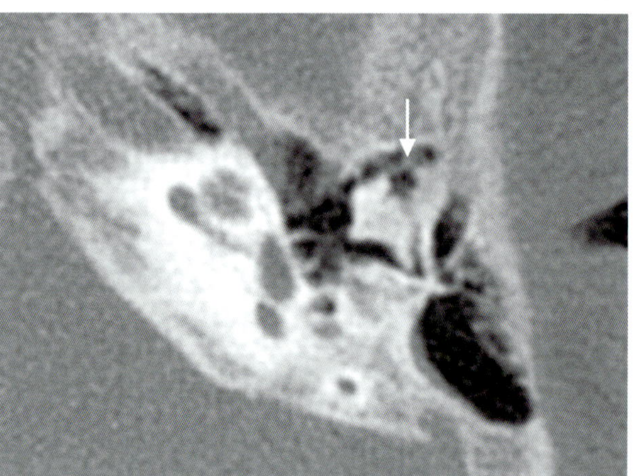

2. axial image

</td><td>

Normal Control CT Findings

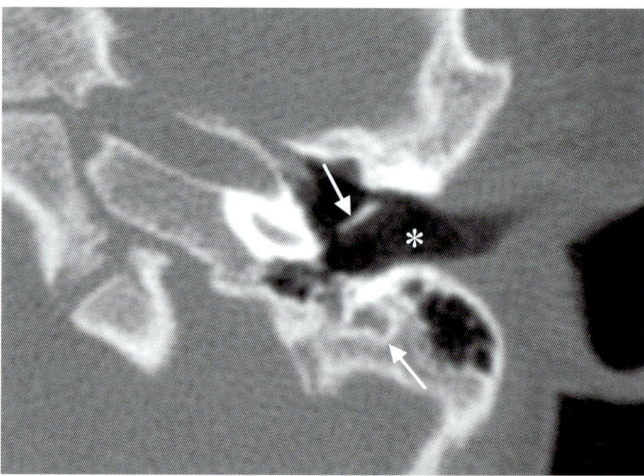

n1. axial image

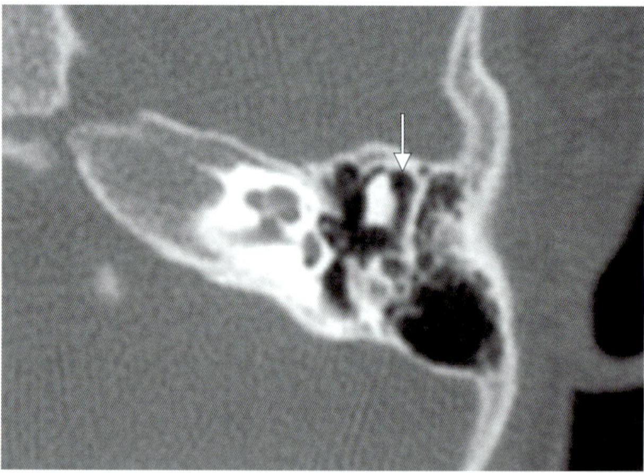

n2. axial image

</td></tr></table>

Fig. 3. (Case 2) Left ear CT: preoperative (4 months old)

[Patient CT Findings]
The external auditory canal cavity cannot be confirmed due to EAC stenosis (1: ✿), but the image shows no osteolytic lesions. Pneumatization in the middle ear is good and there are no soft tissue densities to suggest inflammation or cholesteatoma (1, 2). The mastoid segment of the facial nerve descends slightly anterior to normal (1: ✎). The bony external auditory canal in this case is narrower than the normal control (1, n1: ✿). Slightly posterior at the attic level, overall morphological abnormalities are almost imperceptible, but the space lateral to the malleus head and incus body is narrow (2: ⇣).

《Normal Control CT Findings》
n1: ✎ handle of malleus; ✿ external auditory canal; ✎ mastoid segment of facial nerve. n2: A space (⇣) exists between the ossicular chain and the lateral attic wall.

tissue densities to suggest inflammation or cholesteatoma (fig. 3:1, 2). The mastoid segment of the facial nerve descended slightly anterior (fig. 3:1) to normal (fig. 3:n1). At the level of the external auditory canal, the bony EAC in this case was clearly narrower (fig. 3:1, n1), as would be expected, but slightly posterior at the epitympanum level overall morphological abnormalities were almost imperceptible. However, the space lateral to the malleus head and incus body was narrower (fig. 3:2) than in the normal control (fig. 3:n2).

However, the temporal bone CT image taken at one year seven months (fig. 4) showed a soft tissue density mass spreading from the left external auditory canal to the tympanic cavity and a clear widening of the external auditory canal accompanying osteolysis (fig. 4:1–4), resulting in a diagnosis of external auditory canal cholesteatoma due to EAC stenosis. Figure 4, images 1 and 2 show axial sections, while 3 and 4 show coronal sections.

■ Surgical Findings

Five days after our initial examination, we performed surgery on the left external auditory canal to remove the cholesteatoma and provisionally widen the entrance. During surgery, continuous facial nerve monitoring was carried out to avoid damaging it. The bony external auditory canal entrance on the temporal bone's external surface was extremely small at 2–3 mm, but expanded medially due to osteolysis caused by the cholesteatoma. The cholesteatoma matrix contacted the medial wall of the tympanic cavity and extended posteriorly to the aditus ad antrum. The shape of the malleus was almost normal, but the long process of the incus was absent and the incudostapedial joint disrupted. The cholesteatoma had exerted pressure on the stapes, causing it to slant toward the promontory. The cholesteatoma was removed, a tympanic membrane formed using the temporalis fascia, a small piece of the auricle excised at the entrance to the external auditory canal, and the mastoid segment provisionally covered with a Palva

Patient CT Findings

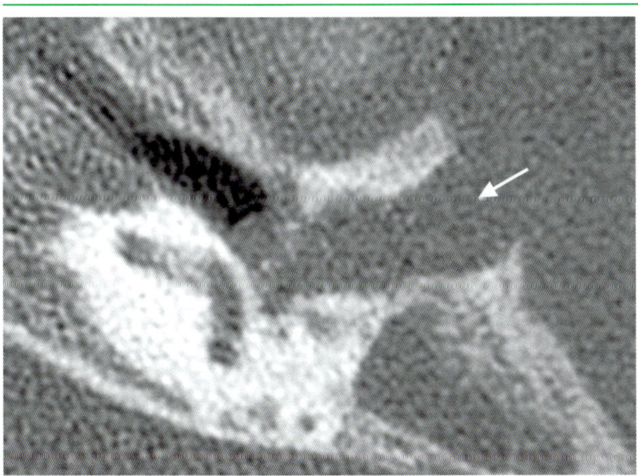

1. axial image

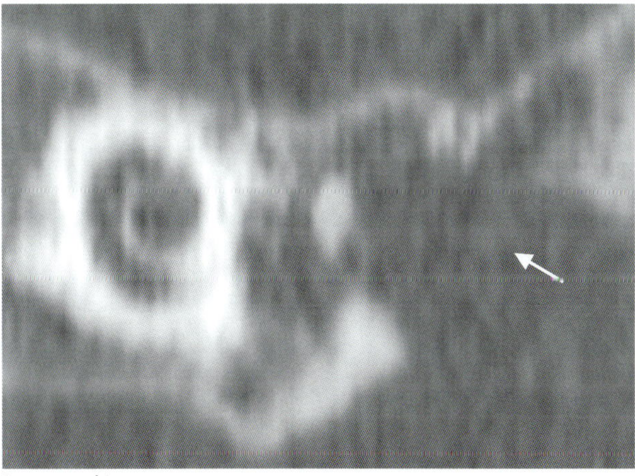

3. coronal image

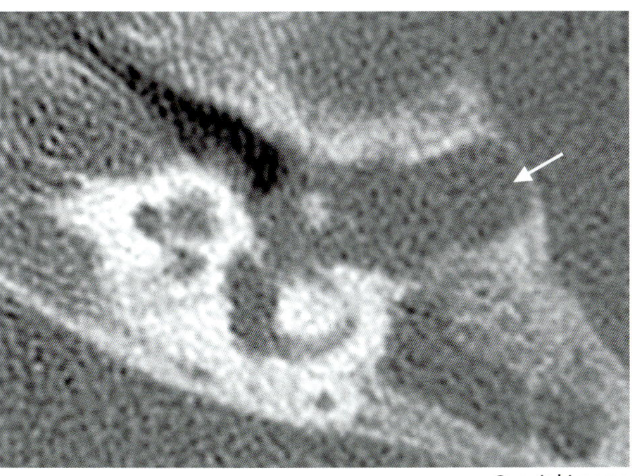

2. axial image

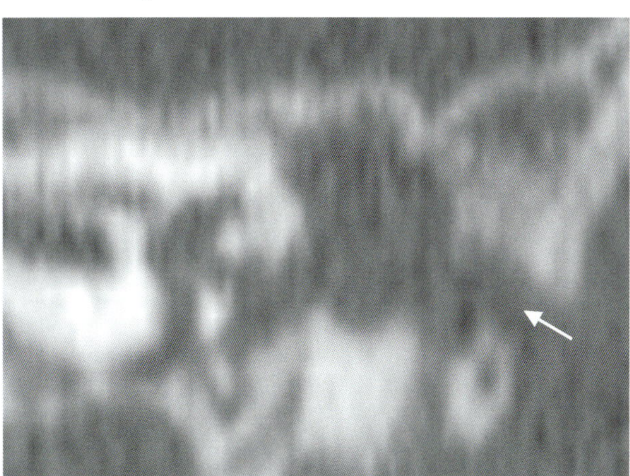

4. coronal image

Fig. 4. (Case 2) Left ear CT: preoperative (1 year 7 months old)

[Patient CT Findings]

This CT is of the left temporal bone at 1 year 7 months old. Note the soft tissue density mass spreading from the external auditory canal to the tympanic cavity and a clear widening of the external auditory canal accompanying osteolysis (1–4: ✎, ✎). Images 1 and 2 are axial; images 3 and 4 are coronal.

Patient CT Findings

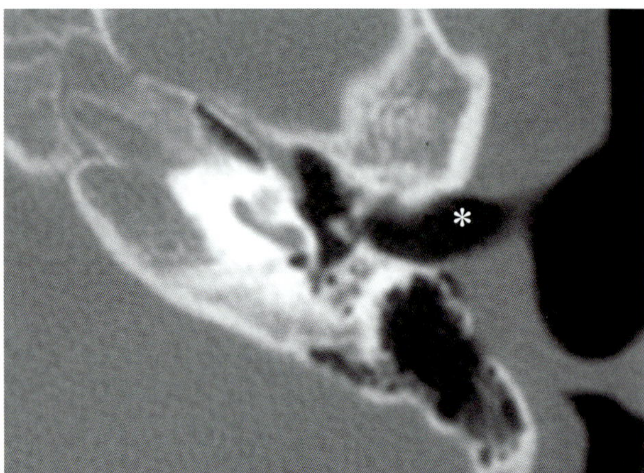

1. axial image

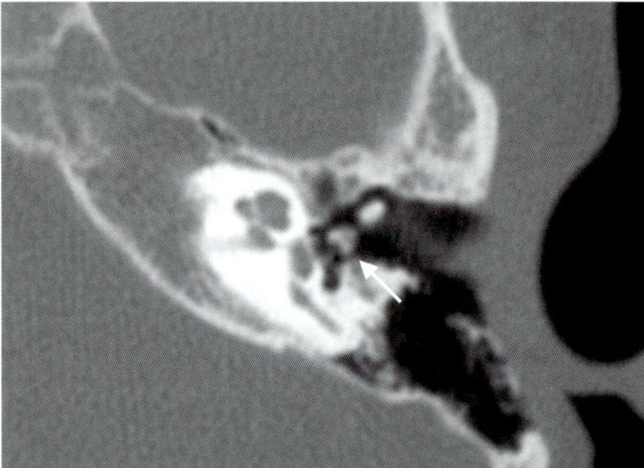

2. axial image

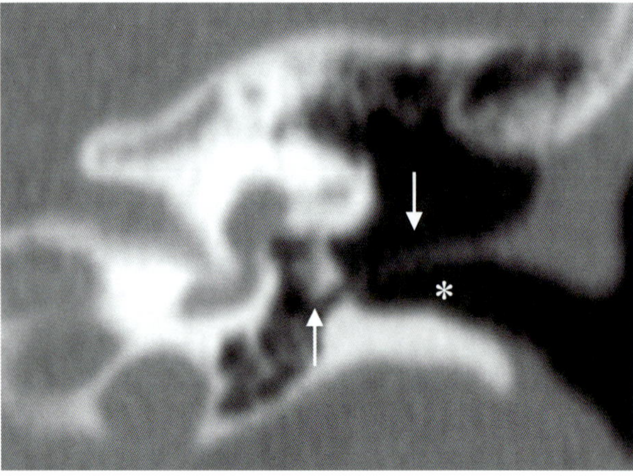

3. coronal image

Fig. 5. (Case 2) Left ear CT: 1 year 5 months postoperative (4 years 9 months old)

[Patient CT Findings]

The external auditory canal is wide (1, 3: ✳) and there are no findings of inflammation in the mastoid. The columella is in proper position (2: ↖, 3: ⇑). The posterosuperior wall of the external auditory canal (3: ⇓) is reconstructed of soft tissue, but pneumatization of the mastoid segment is favorable and there is no observable retraction or enlargement of the external auditory canal wall.

flap. Approx. one year later, after waiting for complete recovery from infection and inflammation, a meatotympanoplasty was performed. The external auditory canal was formed using a split thickness skin graft from the inguinal region and a type III tympanoplasty was performed using a sculpted incus as a minor columella. (Please see p.141 for tympanoplasty classifications)

■ Postoperative Course and Patient CT Findings

The postoperative course went favorably, with left average air conduction hearing improving to 30.0 dB, the external auditory canal wide (fig. 5:1, 3) as shown in the follow-up temporal bone CT (axial images: fig. 5:1, 2; coronal image: fig. 5:3), and no findings of inflammation in the mastoid. It is apparent that the columella is in proper position (fig. 5:2, 3). For the external auditory canal, a canal wall down tympanoplasty with soft wall reconstruction was performed. Pneumatization of the mastoid is good and there is no retraction or enlargement of the external auditory canal wall (fig. 5:3).

■ Examination and Treatment of Congenital EAC Atresia and Stenosis

Schuknecht classified congenital EAC atresia into four groups [12, 13]. Type A (meatal) atresia is limited to the fibrocartilagenous part of the external auditory canal. Type B (partial) shows narrowing of the cartilaginous and bony external auditory canal. Type C (total) includes cases of totally atretic ear canal with a well-pneumatized tympanic cavity. The ossicles are fused and most probably not connected to a malformed stapes. Type D (hypopneumatic total) atresia is a total atresia with poor pneumatization, which are poor surgical candidates for hearing improvement.

In examples of (A) and (B) with stenosis in the cartilaginous part, keratinized waste products from the skin is obstructed and an external auditory canal cholesteatoma forms, sometimes progressing toward the tympanic cavity and damaging the ossicular chain. Some reports suggest that congenital EAC stenosis gives rise to external auditory canal cholesteatoma in around 10% of cases [14]. In EAC stenosis in infants, full observation of the tympanic membrane is often impossible even with using a small diameter fiberscope. In such cases, a CT exam is essential at time of initial visit and every one to several years thereafter. In cases of (B) involving stenosis of both the bony and cartilaginous parts, the tympanic membrane is present but of small diameter, with frequent malleus malformation and fixation to the lateral attic wall. Conductive hearing loss is basically common among all cases (B) to (D), but pure tone audiometry cannot be carried out until around five years of age, so it is difficult in newborns and infants to differentiate between sensorineural hearing loss and conductive hearing loss using pure-tone audiometry. In actuality, as seen both in this case and in Case 1, the anomalies in the conduction system must be determined as a result of comprehensive diagnosis of all findings, including temporal bone CT images, air and bone conduction ASSR, ABR, stapedial reflex, and so on.

In cases of (C) and (D) involving complete atresia, aberrant courses of the facial nerve are commonly observed. In middle ear surgery that does not involve malformations, the prominence of the lateral semicircular canal and the short process of the incus form the referrence point for surgical site orientation. However, in cases involving EAC atresia and middle ear malformations, as was evident in the two cases presented here, this relative spatial relationship changes, and in order to avoid damaging the facial nerve it is necessary to use CT images to confirm the facial nerve path and spatial relationships of the ossicles and lateral semicircular canal for each case. It is also essential to use facial nerve monitoring during surgery.

References

1 Roberson JB Jr, Reinisch J, Colen TY, Lewin S: Atresia repair before microtia reconstruction: comparison of early with standard surgical timing. Otol Neurotol 2009;30:771–776.

2 Chandrasekhar SS, De la Cruz A, Garrido E: Surgery of congenital aural atresia. Am J Otol 1995;16:713–717.

3 El-Begermy MA, Mansour OI, El-Makhzangy AM, El-Gindy TS: Congenital auditory meatal atresia: a numerical review. Eur Arch Otorhinolaryngol 2009;266:501–506.

4 Ishimoto S, Ito K, Karino S, et al: Hearing levels in patients with microtia: correlation with temporal bone malformation. Laryngoscope 2007;117:461–465.

5 Asato H, Kaga K: Shojisho•gaijidoheisasho nitaisuru kino to keitai no saiken. (Microtia & atresia combined approach by plastic and otologic Surgery) Kanehara & Co., Ltd. Tokyo, 2009. (in Japanese.)

6 Jahrsdoerfer RA, Yeakley JW, Aguilar EA, et al: Grading system for the selection of patients with congenital aural atresia. Am J Otol 1992;13:6–12.

7 Shonka DC Jr, Livingston WJ 3rd, Kesser BW: The Jahrsdoerfer grading scale in surgery to repair congenital aural atresia. Arch Otolaryngol Head Neck Surg 2008;134:873–877.

8 Yu Z, Han D, Gong S, Wang Z, et al: Facial nerve course in congenital aural atresia -identified by preoperative CT scanning and surgical findings. Acta Otolaryngol 2008;128:1375–1380.

9 Béjar-Solar I, Rosete M, de Jesus Madrazo M, Baltierra C: Percutaneous bone-anchored hearing aids at a pediatric institution. Otolaryngol Head Neck Surg 2000;122:887–891.

10 Frenzel H, Hanke F, Beltrame M: Application of the Vibrant Soundbridge in bilateral congenital atresia in toddlers. Acta Otolaryngol 2010;130:966-970.

11 Verhagen CVM, Hol MKS: Coppens-Schellekens W, Snik AFM, Cremers CWRJ. The Baha Softband: A new treatment for young children with bilateral congenital aural atresia. Int J Pediatr Otorhinolaryngol 2008;72:1455–1459.

12 Schuknecht HF: Congenital aural atresia. Laryngoscope 1989;99: 908–917.

13 De la Cruz A, Fayad JN: Congenital aural atresia. In Nadol JB, Jr, McKenna MJ, eds. Surgery of the ear and temporal bone. Philadelphia, Lippincott Williams & Wilkins, 2005:3325-3335.

14 Yellon RF: Congenital external auditory canal stenosis and partial atretic plate. Int J Pediatr Otorhinolaryngol 2009;73:1545–1549.

Points

❶ Congenital EAC atresia occurs with a frequency of approx. one in 10,000; 15–25% of cases are bilateral.

❷ Microtia often accompanies EAC atresia and stenosis.

❸ The embryological origins of the external/middle ear and the inner ear are different, but combined malformations sometimes occur.

❹ Auditory, language development, and other functional testing is required along with visual, imaging, and other morphological examination.

❺ A diagnosis of conductive hearing loss is facilitated by temporal bone CT imaging, bone conduction ABR, bone conduction ASSR, stapedial reflex, and other testing.

❻ In cases of cartilaginous part stenosis, temporal bone CT examination is essential as external auditory canal cholesteatoma often occurs.

❼ Cases of EAC atresia and stenosis are often accompanied by fixation of the ossicles to the bony wall of the attic and the atretic plate.

❽ In cases of EAC atresia, facial nerve anomalies also occur, with the nerve's path running inferior (tympanic segment) and anterior (mastoid segment) to normal.

❾ In determining the surgical indication, overall consideration must be given to such factors as location of the malformation, complications, whether the malformation is bilateral or unilateral, and other factors.

❿ The Jahrsdoerfer score, which provides a numerical evaluation of the condition of EAC atresia, is useful in estimating the effectiveness of surgery.

❷ Auditory Ossicles and Middle Ear

Congenital Ossicular Malformation

Congenital ossicular malformation may accompany EAC atresia or stenosis, or it may occur independently. Here we will examine cases in which there are no anomalies of the external auditory canal, as cases accompanying EAC atresia and stenosis were already covered in the previous section. Approx. 30% of cases of ossicular malformation are bilateral [1], with some reports finding no sex difference [2] and others finding it slightly more common in females [1]. Ossicular anomalies are diverse, with possible malformation and partial defects in each of the three auditory ossicles, along with resulting joint disruption (primarily the incudostapedial joint) and fusion/fixation either among the auditory ossicles or with the surrounding bone.

Classifications of ossicular malformation have been attempted from the standpoints of morphology, embryology, and treatment, but here as one example we will present the classification system advocated by Cremers et al [3], which is based on the type of surgery required (table 2). According to this classification, Class 1 is when there is fixation of the stapes but no other anomalies; Class 2 is when, in addition to fixation of the stapes, there are anomalies in other auditory ossicles; Class 3 is when the stapes is mobile and there are anomalies in other auditory ossicles; and Class 4 is when there is atresia of the labyrinthine window. In terms of surgical intervention, Class 1 indicates that standard stapes surgery is sufficient; Class 2 indicates that, in addition to stapes surgery, surgical procedures on other auditory ossicles will be required; Class 3 indicates the anomaly can be dealt with through ossicular chain reconstruction involving procedures on auditory ossicles other than the stapes; and Class 4 indicates the need for new fenestration to the inner ear. Following this classification system, Cases 1 and 2 presented here are Class 2, Case 3 is Class 3, and Case 4 is Class 4 (accompanied by drooping of the facial nerve). Of these cases, only Case 4 failed to obtain hearing improvement. A survey of the literature indicates that the record of postoperative hearing improvement for Class 4 cases is less favorable than in other classes [2, 3], indicating that prudence is required when considering surgical indication.

Fixation of the footplate of the stapes occurs in 69% of overall cases according to a report by Teunissen and Cremers [3], in 59% according to Park et al [2], and 26% according to Kojima et al [1]. Despite the variation, a high incidence rate is indicated in all samples. Kojima's report also indicates a frequency of over 46% for incudostapedial joint discontinuity. Fixation of the footplate of the stapes cannot be diagnosed through imaging, and even supposing there is no stapedial reflex this may also be due to discontinuity or fixation of the malleus or incus, making it impossible to determine in advance whether or not the stapes is fixed in cases of ossicular malformation. Consequently, diagnosis of ossicular malformation frequently requires an exploratory tympanotomy in addition to physiological and imaging tests. If anomalies of the ossicular chain are confirmed during the exploratory tympanotomy, the surgeon can then proceed to perform conduction reconstructive surgery in accordance with the findings obtained. However it is necessary to formulate a surgical plan in advance that includes the possibility of stapes surgery, and also to obtain the informed consent of the patient.

As mentioned in the section on otosclerosis, even in children there are cases of stapes fixation due to otosclerosis [4] or bone metabolism disorders that are difficult to differentiate from stapes fixation as a result of congenital malformation. Findings that indicate otosclerosis include decalcification in the anterior end of the oval window and gradual progression of hearing loss, but decalcification is not observed in all CT images of otosclerosis and it takes time to confirm longterm hearing deterioration, so it would seem that in practical terms differential diagnosis is not always possible.

Stapes Surgery in Children

There has been much debate over whether or not to conduct stapes surgery for congenital stapes fixation and otosclerosis in children. The main points to consider are whether or not longterm, stable hearing improvements can be obtained, what risks are involved in surgery, whether or not otitis media affects the inner ear, and so on. House et al [5] started their article stating "Stapedectomy on a child? Never! But we believe there are indications.", and showed that their results of stapedectomy in children appear to be as satisfactory as results in adults. Ordinarily,

Table 2. Classification of congenital anomalies of middle ear

Class	Main Anomaly	Subclassification	No. of Ears
1	Congenital stapes ankylosis		44
2	Stapes ankylosis associated with another congenital ossicular chain anomaly		55
3	Congenital anomaly of ossicular chain but mobile stapes footplate	Discontinuity in ossicular chain	11
		Epitympanic fixation	20
4	Congenital aplasia or severe dysplasia of oval window or round window	Aplasia	10
		Dysplasia — Crossing facial nerve	3
		Persistent stapedial artery	1

From Teunissen and Cremers [3]

we can perform stapes surgeries safely in children and can obtain favorable results with no greater incidence of complication than in adults [4–6]. However, the youngest recipients of stapes surgery in these reports are around five years old. Taking into consideration the general age at which postoperative rest becomes substantially possible and the occurrence of otitis media is reduced, it would seem safer to wait until children reach school age or later to perform stapes surgery. Prior to that, during infancy, it is important to provide hearing aid appropriate to the level of hearing loss and take action to ensure that hearing and language development are not impaired. These cases essentially involve conductive hearing loss, so the effect to be gained from a hearing aid is substantial.

CT Diagnosis of Ossicular Malformation

In CT diagnosis of congenital ossicular malformation one observes the morphology of each auditory ossicle and whether or not there is space between it and the surrounding bone. In particular, fixation of the the head and neck of the malleus or the lateral process of the incus to the surrounding bone and discontinuity of the incudostapedial joint due to defects in the lenticular process of the long process of the incus or the head of the stapes are frequently observed. There are also many slight variations from normal in the shape and position of each of the auditory ossicles, necessitating a close comparison with the normal control images. The thickness of the anterior limb of the stapes is 0.5 mm or less and only occupies a small part in the CT image slab, so it is depicted in the CT image as grey rather than white and, if not properly captured in the cross-section, cannot be viewed in its entire form. Therefore when the stapes is poorly depicted in the CT image it is difficult to determine whether a finding is due to an anomaly in the stapes itself or to the partial volume effect in the image, and one must also consider functional test results such as hearing and the stapedial reflex. As mentioned above, in the end an exploratory tympanotomy is often required.

References

1 Kojima H, Miyazaki H, Tanaka Y, Moriyama H: Komaku seijo na jikotsukikei 72 ji no kento. (72 Cases of the auditory ossicle malformations but with normal findings in the tympanic membrane.) Nippon Jibiinkoka Gakkai Kaiho (Tokyo) 1998;101:1373–1379. (in Japanese with English abstract.)
2 Park K, Choung YH: Isolated congenital ossicular anomalies. Acta Otolaryngol 2009;129:419–422.
3 Teunissen EB, Cremers CWRJ: Classification of congenital middle ear anomalies: report on 144 ears. Ann Otol Rhinol Laryngol 1993; 102:606–612.
4 Lescanne E, Bakhos D, Metais JP, et al: Otosclerosis in children and adolescents: a clinical and CT-scan survey with review of the literature. Int J Pediatr Otorhinolaryngol 2008; 72:147–152.
5 House JW, Sheehy JL, Antunez JC: Stapedectomy in children, Laryngoscope 1980;15:1804–1809.
6 Millman B, Giddings NA, Cole JM: Long-term follow-up of stapedectomy in children and adolescents. Otolaryngol Head Neck Surg 1996; 115:78–81.

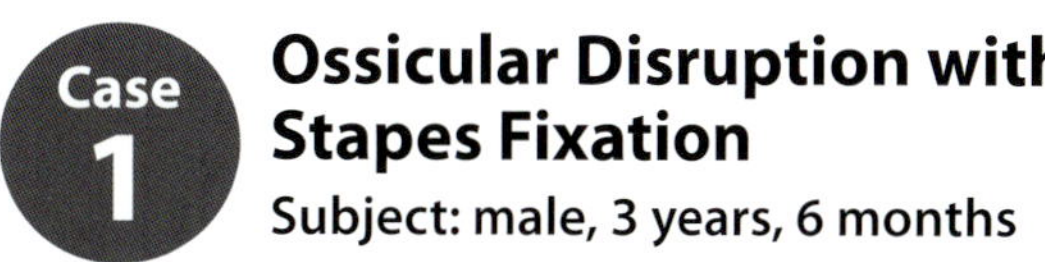

Case 1 — Ossicular Disruption with Stapes Fixation

Subject: male, 3 years, 6 months

■ History and Clinical Findings

The subject was born with auricular deformity and was placed under the observation of a plastic surgeon since soon after birth. At around one year old, his parents noticed that he spoke few words, but at his three-year health exam he was able to understand two-word sentences so observation continued as before. However, recently he frequently failed to react to whispers or answer even when called in a loud voice and so was referred to our department. The auricles on both sides were bent over— so-called lop ear—but there was no stenosis of the external auditory canal and no clear abnormal findings for the tympanic membrane. However, no stapedial reflex was observed despite a type A tympanogram for both ears (fig. 6). Static compliance (SC) for this case was 1.0 cc, slightly higher than the normal range of 0.2 to 0.9 cc, suggesting some form of excess mobility in the tympanic membrane or ossicular chain. ASSR (air conduction) test thresholds were elevated, with 100–110 dB in the low frequency range and 50–60 dB for the mid-to-high ranges. A bone conduction ASSR test revealed thresholds in the neighborhood of 30 dB for both ears, for a finding of conductive hearing loss (fig. 7).

■ Patient CT Findings

Here we discuss the left side, but the findings are essentially the same for both sides. Mastoid air cell development is normal and there is no soft tissue density to indicate inflammation. In observing the vicinity of the ossicular chain, first we note that the anatomical structures around the tip of the incus long process are not clearly depicted, so that the lenticular process is unobservable (fig. 8:1), and that the stapedius tendon appears to be inside the bony tube (fig. 8:1). Normally the stapes can be observed as an arch formed by the anterior and posterior crus, but in this case such an arch structure is not apparent (fig. 8:2). In the cross-section in which the base of the crus can be observed, in the normal control sample both the anterior and posterior crus are identified, but in this case there is only a thickening in one location at the center of the footplate (fig. 8:3), leading one to suspect a malformed stapes with just a single crus. Also, the tympanic segment of the facial nerve runs inferior to normal, so that the facial canal is thickly depicted immediately lateral to the footplate of the stapes in the same cross-section as the footplate (fig. 8:3).

■ Surgical Findings

Because conductive hearing loss is suspected in this case, we decided to first perform a left exploratory tympanotomy, with ossicular chain reconstruction if possible. Observing inside the tympanic cavity, the tip of the long process of the incus was gradually tapered, and the lenticular process was deficient and fixed to the head of the stapes by funicular soft tissue. Also the stapedius tendon was inside the bony tube and this tube was fused directly to the head of the stapes. The footplate of the stapes was a bluish color due to slight thinness and a single crus stood up from the center of the footplate. The footplate of the stapes was fixed to the surrounding bone, with no mobility whatsoever. The tympanic segment of the facial nerve was more inferior than normal and slightly overhung the oval window.

In this case, in order to carry out ossicular chain reconstruction, it was necessary to either extract the deformed upper structure of the stapes and perform a small fenestration slightly inferior to the oval window, or perform stapedectomy. Also, because the long process of the incus was hypoplastic, if a teflon wire piston was used the wire would need to be attached to the malleus. Since the child was still only three years old and there were various risks, it was decided not to perform stapes surgery but rather to close the incision as is and use a hearing aid. The parents were consulted and plans have been made to perform stapes surgery once the child reaches school age.

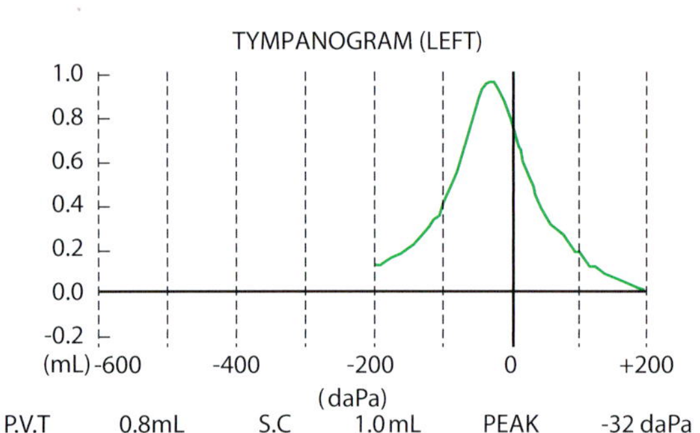

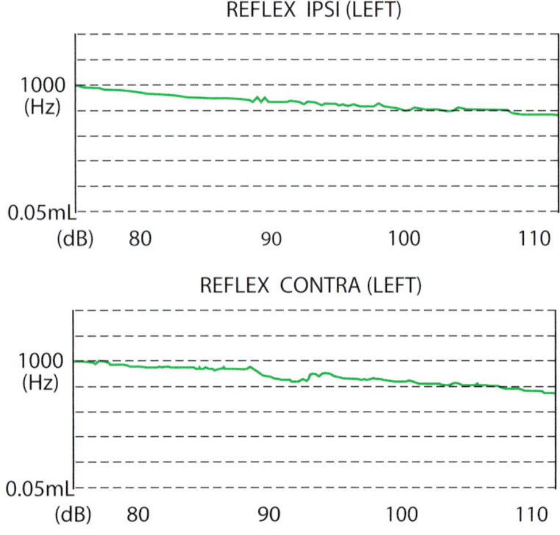

Fig. 6. (Case 1) Tympanogram and stapedial reflex test findings: preoperative.

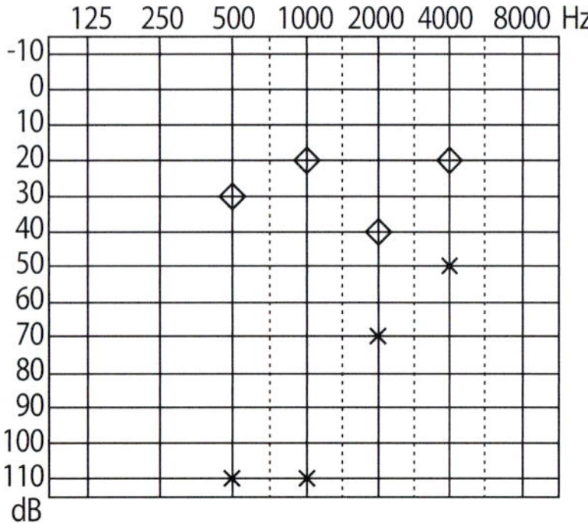

Fig. 7. (Case 1) ASSR findings; preoperative
(✕: air conduction threshold; ◇: bone conduction threshold)

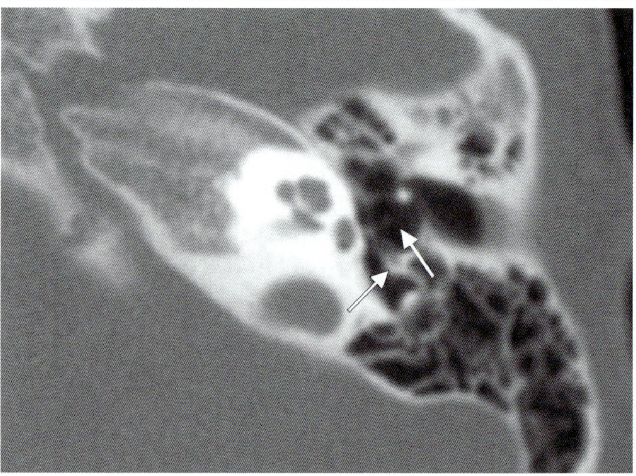
1. axial image

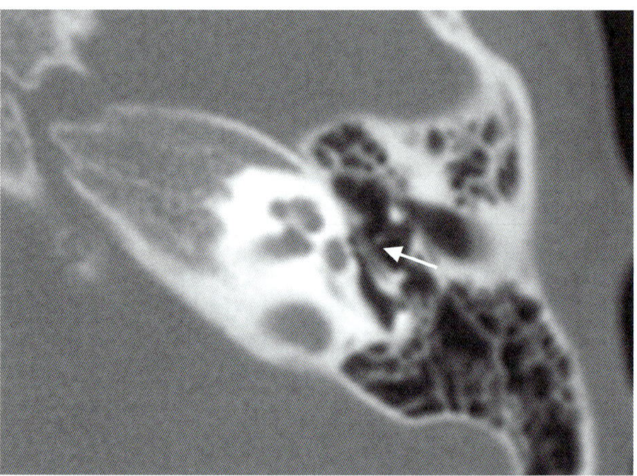
2. axial image

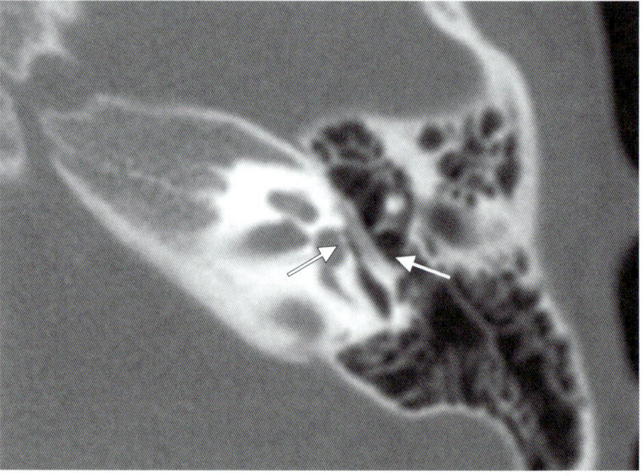
3. axial image

Fig. 8. (Case 1) Left ear CT: preoperative

[Patient CT Findings]

The anatomical structures around the tip of the incus long process are not clearly depicted, so the lenticular process is unobservable (1: ✎), and the stapedius tendon appears to be inside the bony tube (1: ↗). Normally the stapes can be observed as an arch formed by the anterior and posterior crus, but in this case such an arch structure is not apparent (2: ✎). In the cross-section in which the base of the crus can be observed, there is only a thickening in one location at the center of the footplate (3: ✎), leading one to suspect a malformed stapes with just a single crus. Also, the tympanic segment of the facial nerve runs inferior to normal, so that the facial canal is thickly depicted immediately lateral to the footplate of the stapes in the same cross-section as the footplate (3: ✎)

Normal Control CT Findings

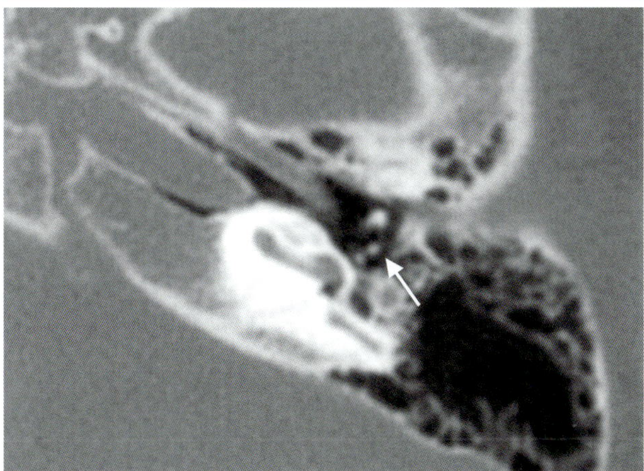

n1. axial image

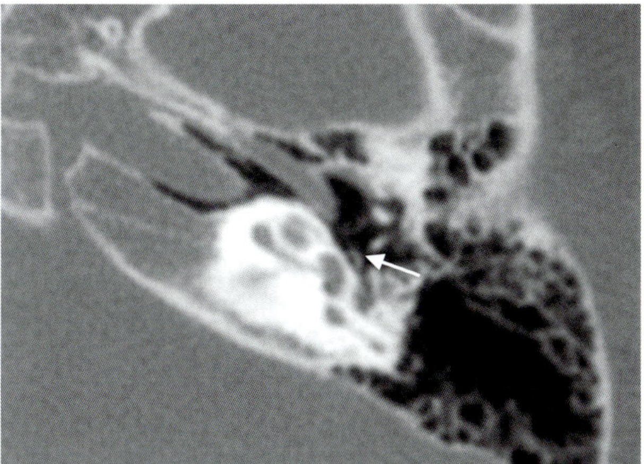

n2. axial image

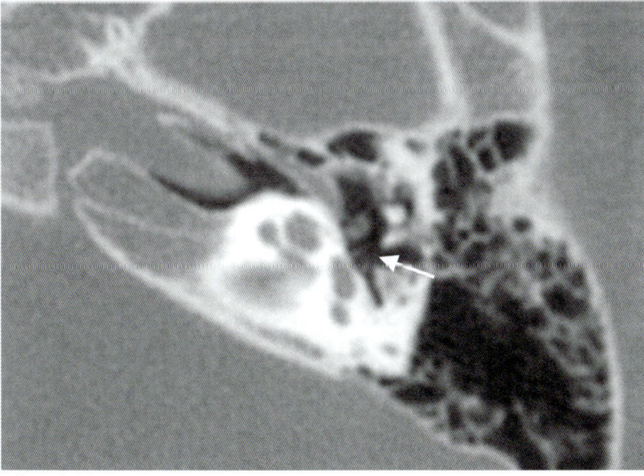

n3. axial image

《Normal Control CT Findings》

n1: ↖ lenticular process of incus; n2: ↙ arch of stapes;
n3: ↙ anterior and posterior crus of stapes

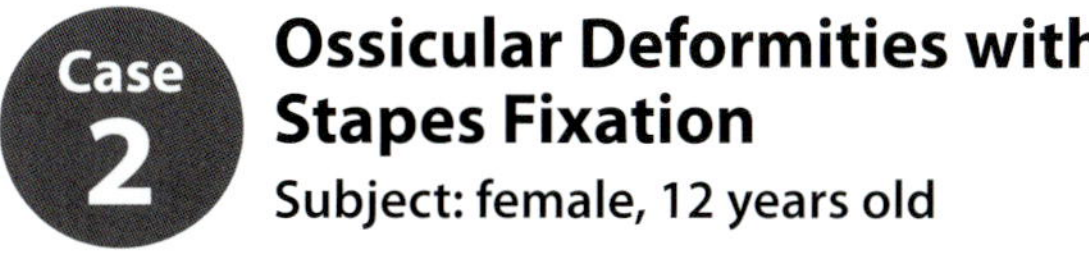

Ossicular Deformities with Stapes Fixation

Subject: female, 12 years old

■ History and Clinical Findings

The subject underwent plastic surgery at nine months old for a cleft palate. A family member noticed her hearing loss at around age five. Testing done at her regular pediatric hospital found bilateral mixed hearing loss between moderate and severe, and she was referred to our department to assess whether or not surgical intervention would be appropriate.

Pure tone audiometry conducted by us indicated mixed hearing loss with average hearing level of 50.0 dB right and 66.7 dB left (fig. 9). On initial inspection the tympanic membrane appeared almost normal, but further observation revealed that its diameter was slightly smaller and the handle of the malleus slightly shorter than normal. Surgery was performed on both sides, however here we will discuss only the left ear, in which hearing loss was worse.

■ Preoperative Patient CT Findings

Mastoid air cell development is deficient, but no effusion or other soft tissue density is apparent. The vicinity around the tip of the long process of the incus is unclear and the lenticular process is unrecognizable (fig. 10:1). This case does not include a cross-section in which the incudostapedial joint itself is displayed, and disruption is suspected. The superstructure of the stapes is slightly asymmetrical in form, but the head, anterior crus, and posterior crus of the stapes are all visible (fig. 10:1). The cross-section of the long process of the incus is flatter than normal (fig. 10:2) and the neck of the malleus contacts the anterolateral wall of the external auditory canal (fig. 10:2), with suspected fixation. Also, the space lateral to the body of the incus, which normally can be observed as quite wide, is narrow in this case (fig. 10:3). Fixation is probable here as well.

■ Surgical Findings

The posterosuperior wall of the bony segment of the external auditory canal and the lateral attic wall were carefully removed. With the ossicular chain clearly visible, it was apparent that the neck of the malleus contacted and was fixed to the anterior tympanic spine, and furthermore the short process of the incus was fixed to the surrounding bone, with no mobility in either. The long process of the incus was bent medially toward the tip, and the

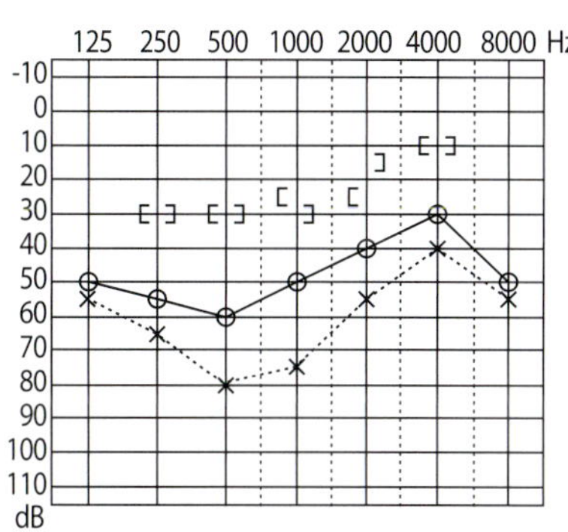

Fig. 9. (Case 2)
Audiogram: preoperative

Patient CT Findings

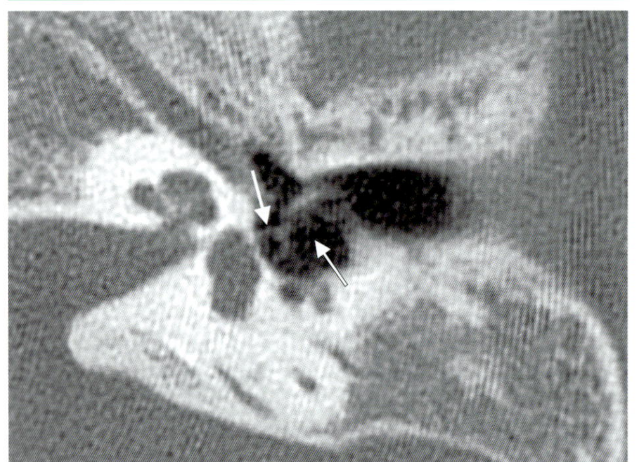

1. axial image

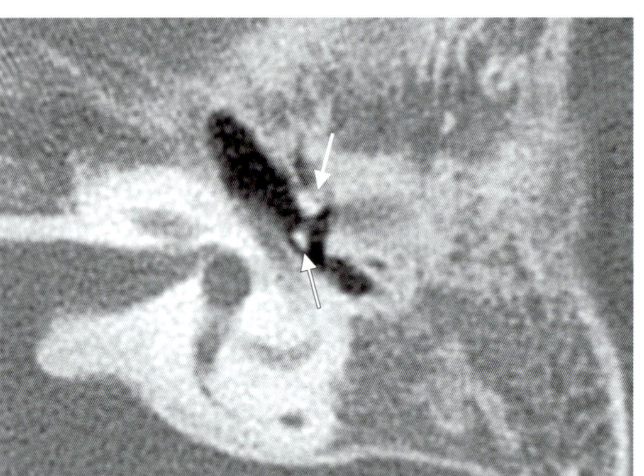

2. axial image

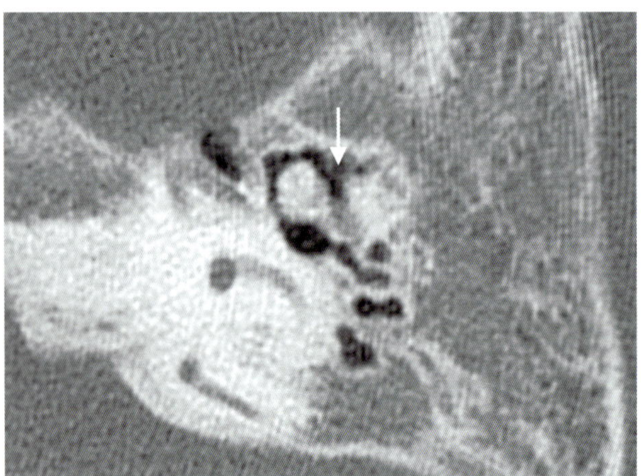

3. axial image

Normal Control CT Findings

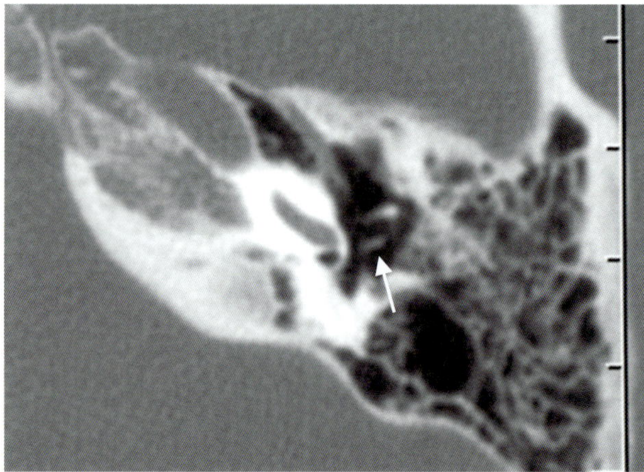

n1. axial image

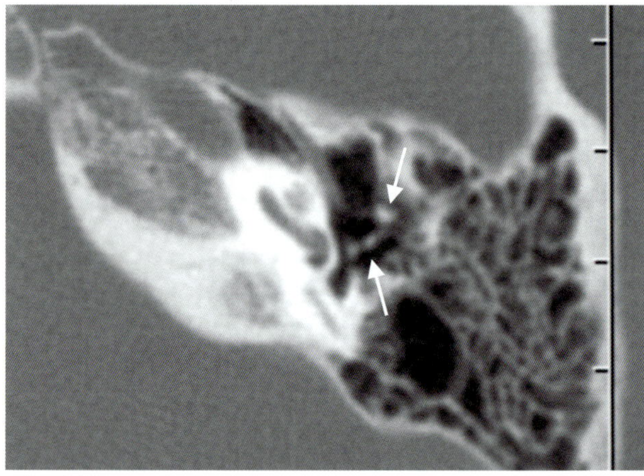

n2. axial image

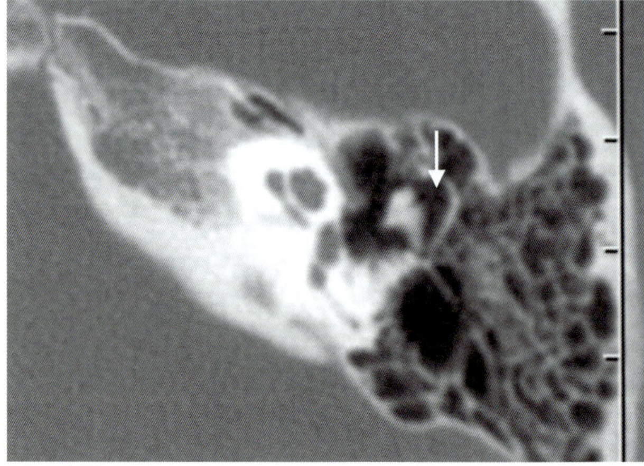

n3. axial image

Fig. 10. (Case 2) Left ear CT: preoperative

[Patient CT Findings]

The vicinity around the tip of the long process of the incus is unclear and the lenticular process is unrecognizable (1:). This case does not include a cross-section in which the incudosta-pedial joint itself is displayed, and disruption is suspected. The superstructure of the stapes is slightly asymmetrical in form, but the head, anterior crus, and posterior crus of the stapes are all visible (1:). The cross-section of the long process of the incus is flatter than normal (2:), and the neck of the malleus contacts the anterolateral wall of the external auditory canal (2:), with suspected fixation. Also, the space lateral to the malleus head and the body of the incus, which normally can be observed as quite wide, is narrow in this case (3:). Fixation is probable here as well.

《Normal Control CT Findings》

n1: incudostapedial joint. n2: neck of malleus; long process of incus and head of stapes. n3: Wide space ( ) between the head of malleus/body of incus and the lateral attic wall.

Patient CT Findings

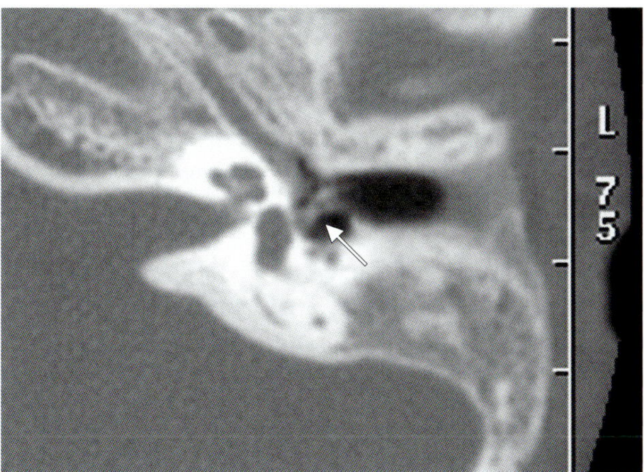

1. axial image

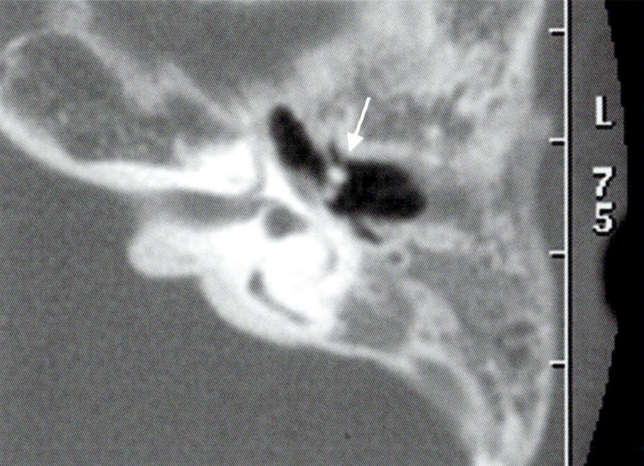

2. axial image

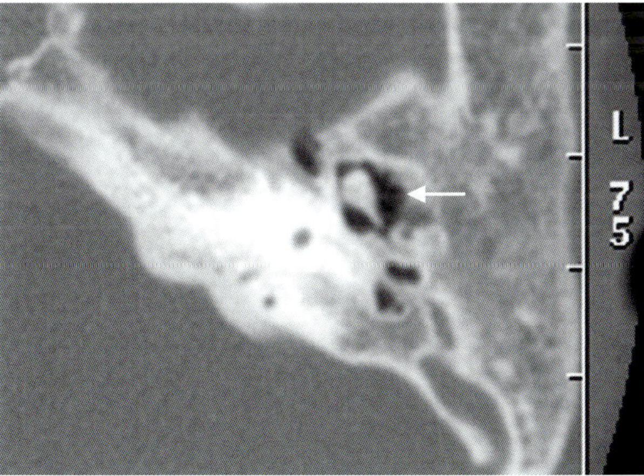

3. axial image

Fig. 11. (Case 2) Left ear CT: postoperative

lenticular process was absent and contact with the head of the stapes was only via funicular soft tissue. The head, anterior crus, and posterior crus of the stapes were present, but the footplate was fixed, with no apparent mobility.

The funicular soft tissue connecting the long process of the incus to the head of the stapes was severed and the bone in the vicinity of the malleus and incus adhesions carefully removed, freeing up the malleus and incus to move normally. It was decided that, as the long process of the incus was malformed, it would be difficult to perform standard stapes surgery by fastening the hook of the teflon wire piston to the long process, so a Rosen probe was used to carefully mobilize the stapes so that it slanted in the facial canal/promontory direction. The fixation between the stapes footplate and surrounding bone was released, resulting in a substantial gain in stapes mobility. Finally, type III tympanoplasty was performed by inserting a sliver of auricular cartilage into the space between the head of the stapes and the stump of the long process of the incus.

■ Postoperative Patient CT Findings and Postoperative Course

On examination of the postoperative CT image (fig. 11), first we notice that the incudostapedial joint is slightly enlarged and is connected via a tissue shadow with moderate density, which we may assume is the interpolating segment made from the sliver of auricular cartilage (fig. 11:1). Also note that, compared to the preoperative image, a new space has been created anterolateral to the neck of the malleus (fig. 11:2) and lateral to the body of the incus (fig. 11:3), due to the surgical removal of the superior wall of the bony segment of the external auditory canal and the lateral attic wall.

Postoperatively, hearing level in the left ear averaged 25.0 dB and the air-bone gap had improved to 3.3 dB (fig. 12). Currently, four years after the surgery, there is no change. Only mobilization of the stapes footplate was performed and there was concern that it would re-fixate, but currently it is progressing favorably. If the stapes footplate should re-fixate, we plan to perform stapes surgery. Also, a canal wall down tympanoplasty with soft wall reconstruction was performed in this case, with no bony reconstruction of the deep part of the bony segment of the external auditory canal that had been removed. This prevents fixation of the ossicular chain to the surrounding bone and vibrates from the tympanic membrane to the continuous external auditory canal wall, which is thought to contribute to acquisition and maintenance of favorable postoperative hearing.

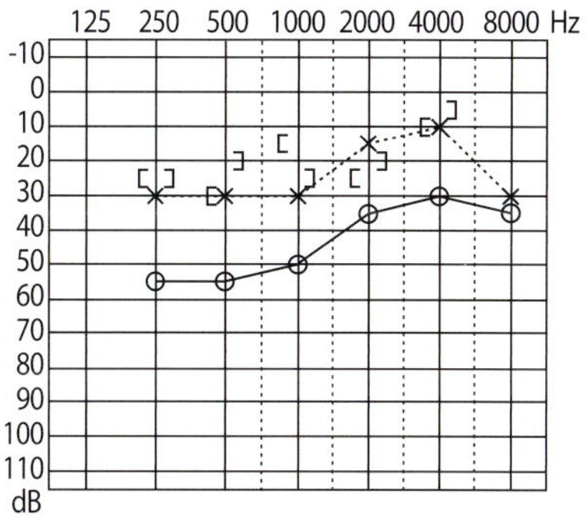

Fig. 12. (Case 2)
Audiogram: postoperative

Case 3 — **Ossicular Deformities**
Subject: female, 7 years old

■ History and Clinical Findings

Originally the subject was not aware of any abnormalities, nor had any been identified, but upon visiting ENT clinic due to a cold, an abnormality in her left tympanic membrane was identified and she was referred to our department. There were no abnormalities in the right ear. The left tympanic membrane showed no redness or retraction, but the handle of the malleus appeared slightly shorter and more vertical than normal. In pure tone audiometry the left ear had average air conduction hearing of 65.7 dB and bone conduction of 25.0 dB, with an air-bone gap of 40.7 dB (fig. 13a). The tympanogram was type As (fig. 13b), and no thickening or other qualitative abnormalities were observed in the tympanic membrane itself, so it was inferred that there must be some sort of mobility restriction in the ossicular chain. No stapedial reflex was present (fig. 13c). Basically it was conductive hearing loss, so an imaging examination was conducted to study the possibility of improving the subject's hearing through surgery.

■ Preoperative Patient CT Findings

Overall mastoid air cell development is satisfactory. There is no soft tissue density in the middle ear, negating the possibility of inflammatory disease. There is also no indication of anomalies in the inner ear or internal auditory canal. Observing the left ossicular chain, the malleus is slightly deformed and somewhat inferior to normal. There is no space where the anterior mallear ligament should normally be, and the neck of the malleus and the anterior tympanic spine are touching (fig. 14:1). In the normal control image, the handle of the malleus is pointing in the direction of the promontory and there is sufficient space between it and the anterior wall of the external auditory canal and other surrounding bone (fig. 14:n1, n2). There are no abnormalities in the stapes, but the tip of the long process of the incus cannot be clearly ascertained (fig. 14:2), nor can the joint between it and the stapes head (the incudostapedial joint) be confirmed. In the corresponding normal control image, the lenticular process of the incus is clearly depicted (fig. 14:n2). Viewing the cross-section of the central part of the incus, the head of the malleus (fig. 14:3) is depicted slightly smaller in this case than that of the normal control (fig. 14:n3). Also, as is often seen in cases of middle ear malformation, the space between the body of the incus and the lateral attic wall is narrow (fig. 14:3), in clear contrast to the normal control (fig. 14:n3).

In the coronal section as well, normally one can observe the corner at the tip of the long process of the incus where it bends at right angles from the lenticular process to reach the head of the stapes (fig. 15:n1), but in this case it cannot be identified (fig. 15:1). Also, the incus is adjacent to the lateral attic wall (fig. 15:1), and clearly lacks the usual space (fig. 15:n1).

Based on the above CT findings, we suspected fixation of the neck of the malleus and body of the incus to the surrounding bone, along with congenital disruption of the incudostapedial joint due to absence of the tip of the incus (lenticular process).

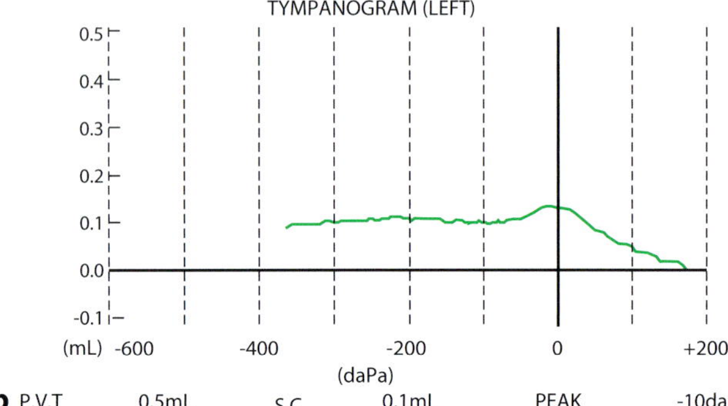

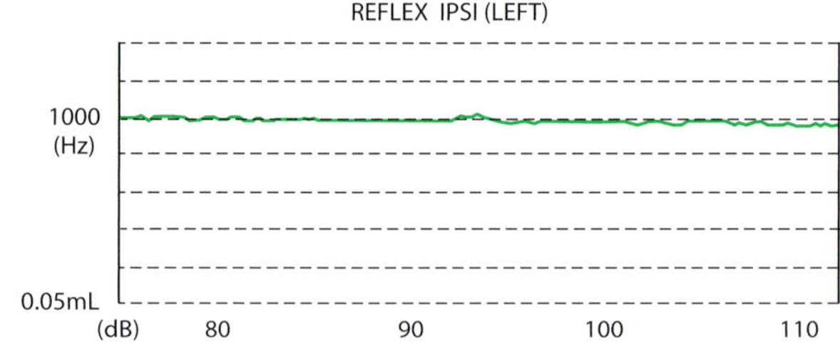

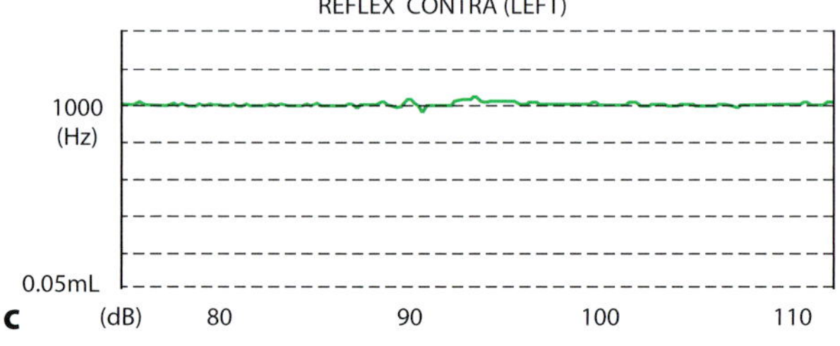

Fig. 13. (Case 3) Hearing test findings: preoperative. **a**= audiogram; **b**= tympanogram; **c**= left ear stapedial reflex

Patient CT Findings

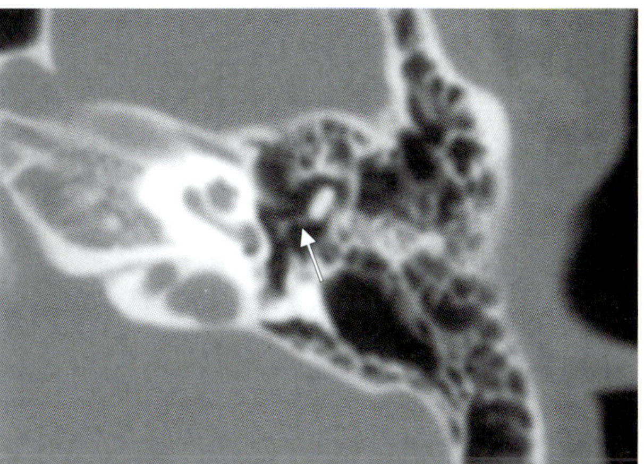

1. axial image

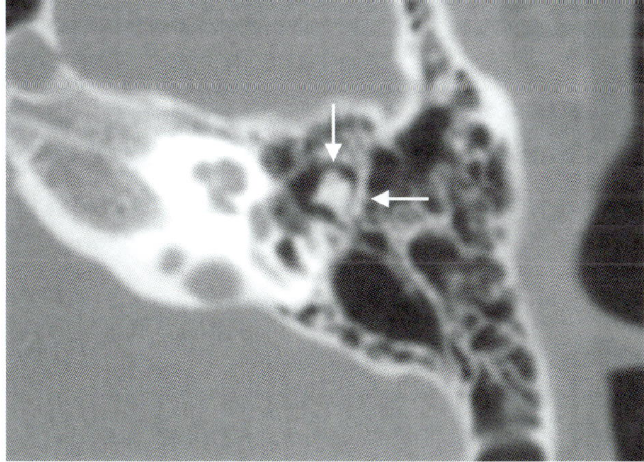

2. axial image

3. axial image

Normal Control CT Findings

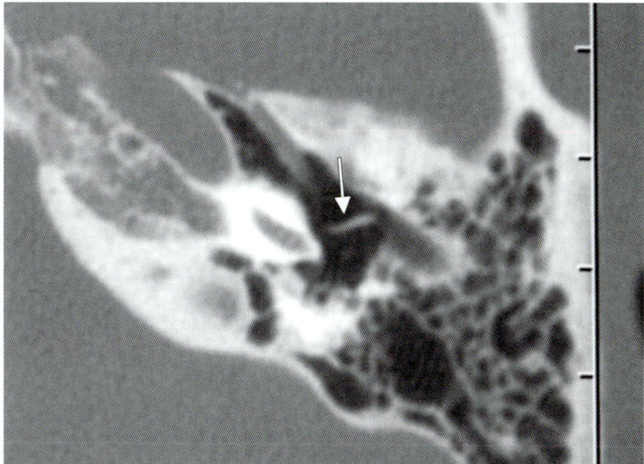

n1. axial image

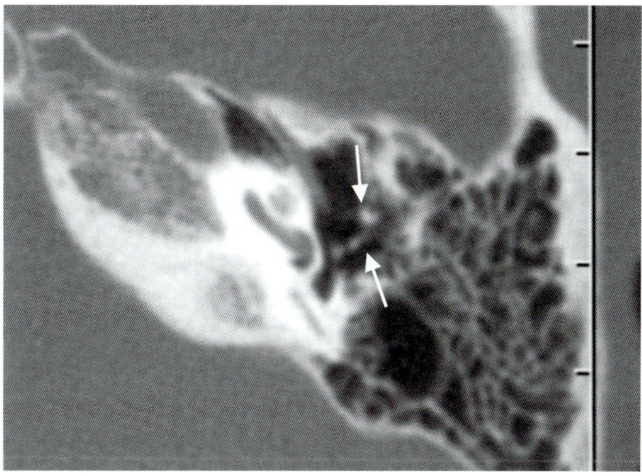

n2. axial image

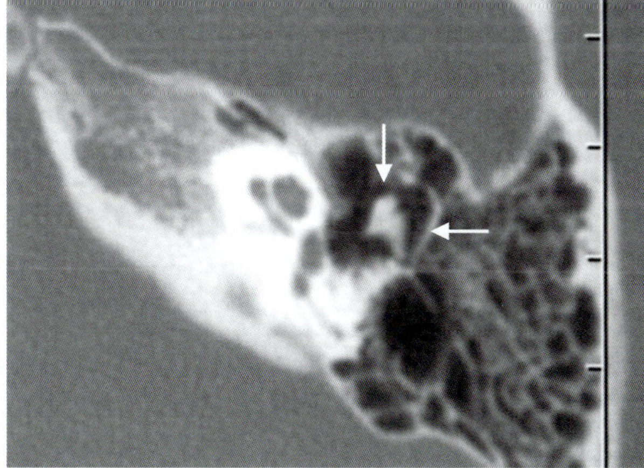

n3. axial image

Fig. 14. (Case 3) Left ear CT: preoperative

[Patient CT Findings]

The malleus is slightly deformed and somewhat inferior to normal and the neck of the malleus and the anterior tympanic spine are touching (1: ⇩). There are no abnormalities in the stapes, but the tip of the long process of the incus cannot be clearly ascertained (2: ⇧), nor can the joint between it and the stapes head (the incudostapedial joint) be confirmed. Viewing the cross-section of the central part of the incus, the head of the malleus in this case (3: ⇩) is depicted slightly smaller than that of the normal control (n3: ⇩). Also, as is often seen in cases of middle ear malformation, the space between the body of the incus and the lateral wall of the attic is narrow (⇐).

《Normal Control CT Findings》

n1: ⇩ handle of malleus. n2: ⇩ neck of malleus; ⇧ long process of incus and lenticular process. n3: ⇩ head of malleus; ⇐ lateral attic wall.

Patient CT Findings

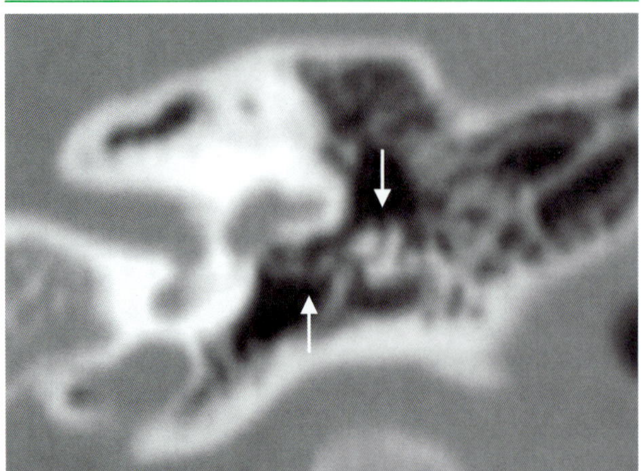

1. coronal image

Fig. 15. (Case 3) Left ear CT: preoperative

[Patient CT Findings]

The corner at the tip of the long process of the incus where it bends at right angles from the lenticular process to reach the head of the stapes cannot be identified (1: ⇑). Also, the body of the incus is adjacent to the lateral attic wall (1: ⇓)

Normal Control CT Findings

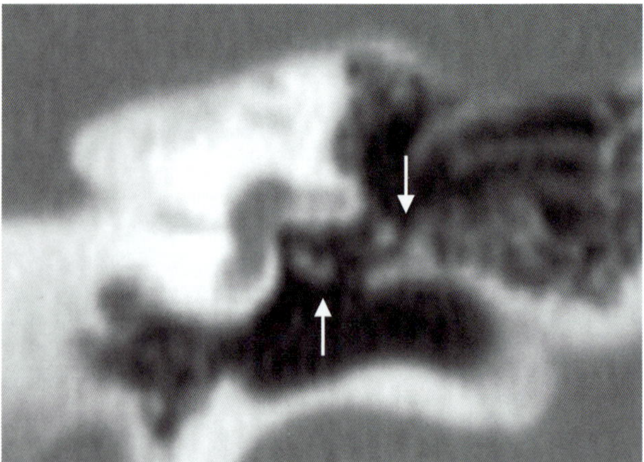

n1. coronal image

《Normal Control CT Findings》

n1: ⇑ area where the tip of the long process of the incus bends from the lenticular process to reach the head of the stapes; ⇓ space between the body of the incus and the lateral attic wall.

■ Surgical Findings

A left exploratory tympanotomy was performed. The neck and head of the malleus were malformed and fixed to the anterior tympanic spine and the lateral attic wall. The posterosuperior part of the bony segment of the external auditory canal was carefully removed to expose the incudostapedial joint, revealing that approx. ⅓ of the tip of the long process of the incus was extremely thin and curved gently to contact the head of the stapes. What appeared as a disruption in the CT image may have been due to the thinness of the tip of the long process of the incus and the lack of a bone mass corresponding to the lenticular process. Upon severing the incudostapedial joint, it was observed that the stapes displayed no abnormalities and its mobility was favorable. A portion of the lateral attic wall was removed and the incus that had been fixed to it extracted. It was also established that the head and handle of the malleus were separate in the vicinity of the neck, a finding that could not be confirmed in the preoperative CT image. The head of the malleus was severed and a type III ossiculoplasty was performed using the sculpted incus as a short columella to connect the stapes head and malleus handle.

Postoperative course was good, with left ear average hearing level of 23.3 dB eight months after surgery—a greater than 40 dB improvement over preoperative values—and the air-bone gap had virtually disappeared (fig. 16).

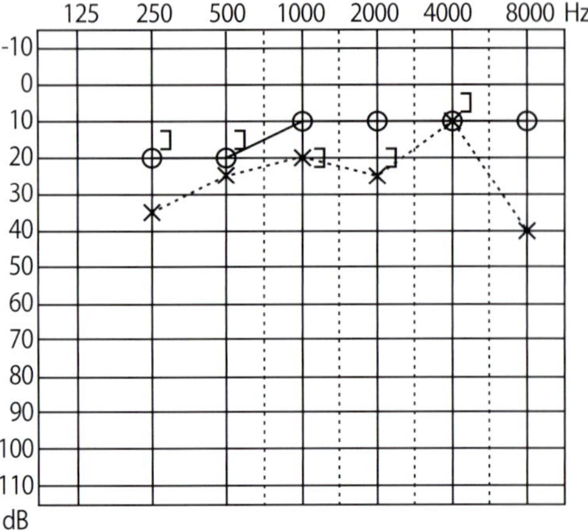

Fig. 16. (Case 3) Audiogram: 8 months postoperative

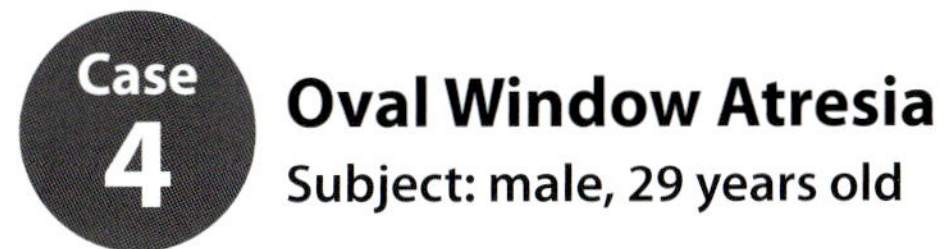

Case 4 — Oval Window Atresia
Subject: male, 29 years old

■ History and Clinical Findings

The subject had suffered from bilateral hearing loss since infancy and came to us with the hope of improving hearing in his right ear. He had mixed hearing loss, with average hearing level of 78 dB in the right ear and 59 dB in the left ear.

■ Patient CT Findings

The CT image is of the right temporal bone. Both mastoid air cell development and pneumatization are satisfactory. Observing the oval window in the axial section, it is apparent that it is obstructed by bone roughly 1 mm thick, though the central portion is slightly thinner (fig. 17:1). The thickness of the oval window atresia in this case is readily apparent when compared to the image of a normal stapes footplate (fig. 17: n1). The same finding can be made in the coronal section. In all of the cross-sections, including the coronal image, the oval window is obstructed by bone (fig. 17:2). The head of the malleus and body of the incus are normal (fig. 17:1), but the long process of the incus is unclear and the superstructure of the stapes cannot be identified. There are no clear abnormalities in the shape of the bony labyrinth.

Patient CT Findings	**Normal Control CT Findings**

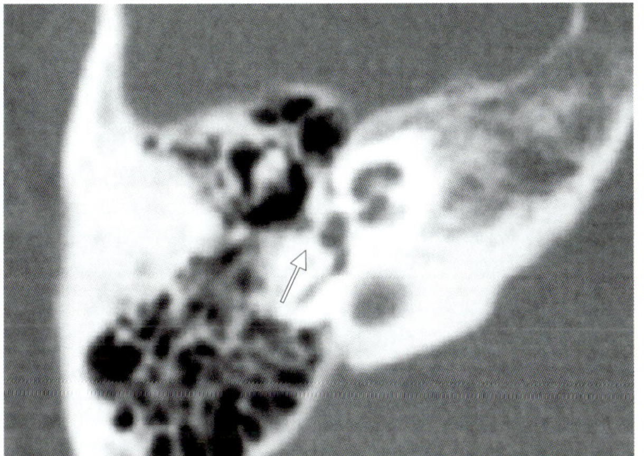

1. axial image

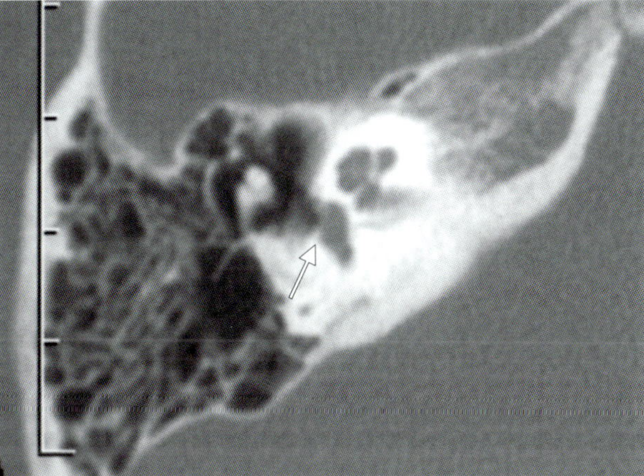

n1. axial image

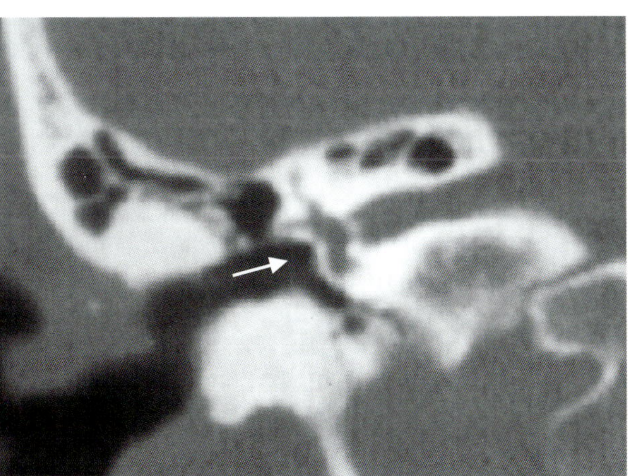

2. coronal image

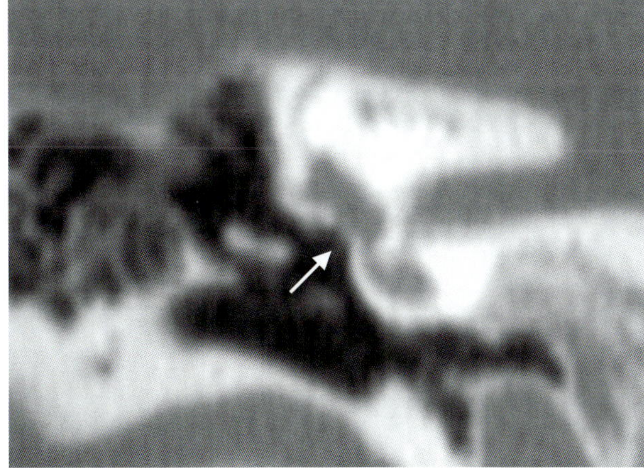

n2. coronal image

Fig. 17. (Case 4) Right ear CT: preoperative

[Patient CT Findings]
Both mastoid air cell development and pneumatization are satisfactory. The oval window is obstructed by bone roughly 1 mm thick, though the central portion is slightly thinner (1: ⇗). The same finding can be observed in the coronal section (2: ⇨). The head of the malleus and body of the incus are normal (1), but the long process of the incus is unclear and the superstructure of the stapes cannot be identified.

《Normal Control CT Findings》
n1: ⇗ footplate of stapes. n2: ⇗ oval window and footplate of stapes.

■ Surgical Findings

This was a difficult case with oval window atresia, but the possibility was pursued of improving hearing through an exploratory tympanotomy. A right exploratory tympanotomy was performed with prior explanation that stapes surgery may be carried out if circumstances warranted. During surgery it was observed that the stapes was missing and the oval window could not be identified. The tympanic segment of the facial nerve ran inferiorly to the area corresponding to the oval window. (In this case the resolution of the CT image was low, making it impossible to accurately confirm the path of the facial nerve.) The long process of the incus was malformed but present, so fenestration of the inner ear was carried out in the area corresponding to the oval window, a teflon wire piston inserted, and the wire attached to the long process of the incus. Hearing improved temporarily postoperatively, but later dropped to preoperative levels.

Points

❶ Diagnosis of ossicular malformation requires pure tone audiometry, a stapedial reflex test, and a temporal bone CT exam.

❷ In cases of hearing loss where mastoid air cell development and pneumatization are satisfactory, one should be mindful of the possibility of congenital malformation.

❸ In cases of unilateral hearing loss in children when the subject is only partially aware of the hearing loss, there is a high probability that it is congenital.

❹ The frequency of stapes footplate fixation is high, but confirmation through CT imaging is difficult.

❺ In cases where either the neck of the malleus, head of the malleus, body of the incus, or short process of the incus are in extremely close proximity to the lateral attic wall, there is a possibility of fixation.

❻ Ossicular chain disruption occurs frequently at the incudostapedial joint, making it important when examining the CT image to focus attention on whether the lenticular process of the incus and the head of the stapes are making contact.

Case 5

Skull Base Vascular Anomalies (CHARGE Syndrome)

Subject: male, 14 years old

■ History and Clinical Findings

The subject had responded poorly to sound since birth. He had other physical impairments, including partial choroid membrane deficiency (coloboma) of the eye, right nasal cavity stenosis (without choanal atresia), hypoplasia of the semicircular canals in the inner ear, right facial nerve paresis with dysphagia, underweight (growth hormone deficiency), middle ear malformation, patent ductus arteriosus, mild developmental retardation, and square face, which resulted in a diagnosis of CHARGE syndrome. The use of hearing aids was not effective. Due to the coexistence of multiple handicaps, the expected level of effectiveness from cochlear implants needed to be set lower than for hearing loss alone, but after consultation with the child's parents he underwent surgery at five years old, with the objective of achieving environmental sound recognition and partial recognition of spoken language.

In the child's preoperative CT exam, bilateral mastoid air cell development was found to be deficient and the middle ear space more or less limited to the tympanic cavity. Moreover, on the left side, the mastoid was occupied by a broadly meandering blood vessel. Existence of cranial nerve VIII was confirmed bilaterally via MRI. Because the left mastoid was occupied over a broad area by an aberrant blood vessel and there was a risk of macrovascular damage when preparing both the electrode insertion path and the well for embedding the receiver-stimulator unit, it was decided to perform the operation on the right side. Since, except for the sealed external auditory canal and the cochlear implantation area, the preoperative image is essentially the same as the postoperative image shown below, it is not shown here in order to avoid duplication.

■ Surgical Findings

The right mastoid air cells were completely undeveloped, so in order to insert the electrode via the external auditory canal a postauricular incision was made and all of the external auditory canal skin and tympanic membrane detached and extracted through the external auditory canal. Then a groove was created in the bone running posteriorly from the external auditory canal and a depression formed posterosuperiorly in the temporal bone to accommodate the receiver-stimulator unit. Transcanal confirmation of the round window niche was made, and fenestration of the cochlea's scala tympani performed anteriorly. The tip of the electrode array was fully inserted without problem, but the conducting wire at the base would not fit, so it was looped around once inside the external auditory canal. In order to prevent the cochlear implant's electrodes from being exposed to the external auditory canal, the cartilaginous segment of the external auditory canal was severed and sutured, and the inlet to the bony segment of the external auditory canal sealed with a bony plate.

Postoperatively a very gradual response to sound stimulation was obtained, and currently eight years later the average threshold with cochlear implant is 40 dB. The subject is unable to discern words through hearing alone,

Patient CT Findings

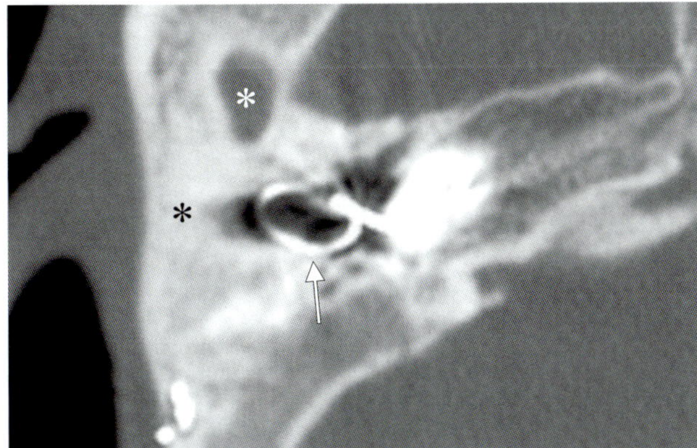

1. axial image

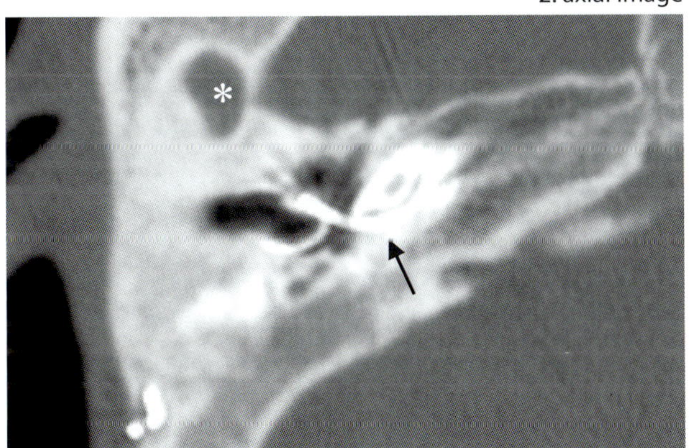

2. axial image

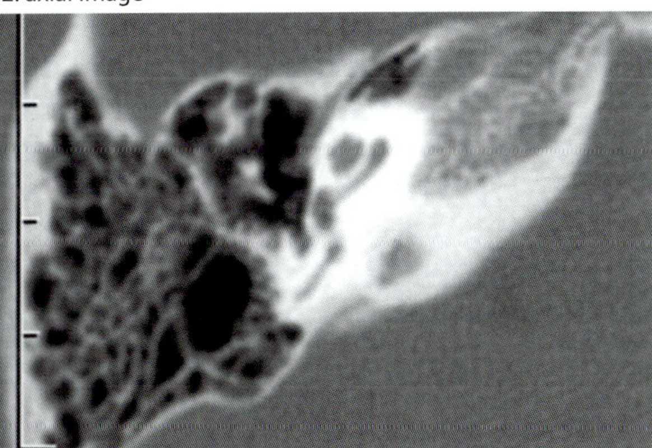

3. axial image

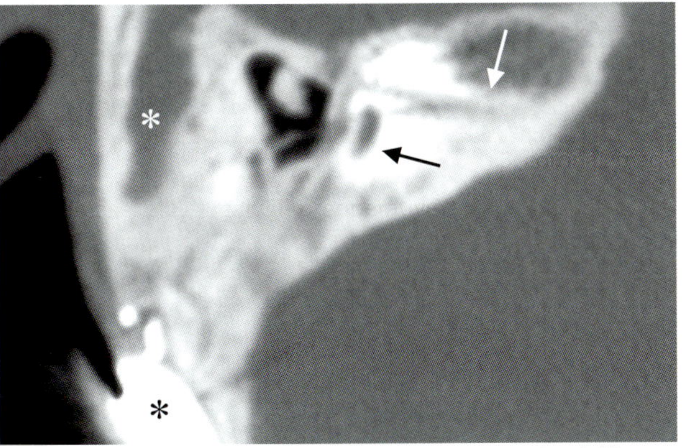

4. axial image

Normal Control CT Findings

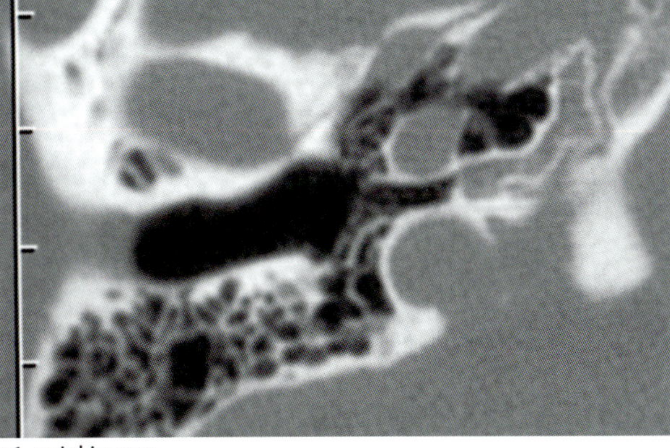

n1. axial image

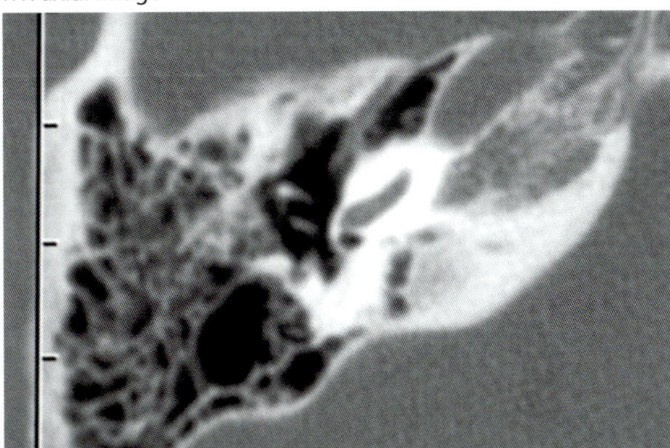

n2. axial image

n3. axial image

n4. axial image

Fig. 18. (Case 5) Right ear CT: 9 years postoperative (age 14)

[Patient CT Findings]

The external auditory canal shows thick bony occlusion (1: ✳, 2: ✱). The conducting wire of the cochlear implant passes through the temporal bone (1: ✎) and forms a loop in the lumen of the external auditory canal (2: ⇡) before entering the cochlea (3: ↖). In the vestibular system, the lateral semicircular canal is missing, forming only the vestibule (4: ↩), and the internal auditory canal is also narrow (4: ♪). The receiver-stimulator unit (4: ✱) is appropriately embedded in the lateral part of the skull. The structures marked "❀" are the PGF in figure 18:1 and the PSS in figures 18:2–4 (refer to text for explanation)

Patient CT Findings

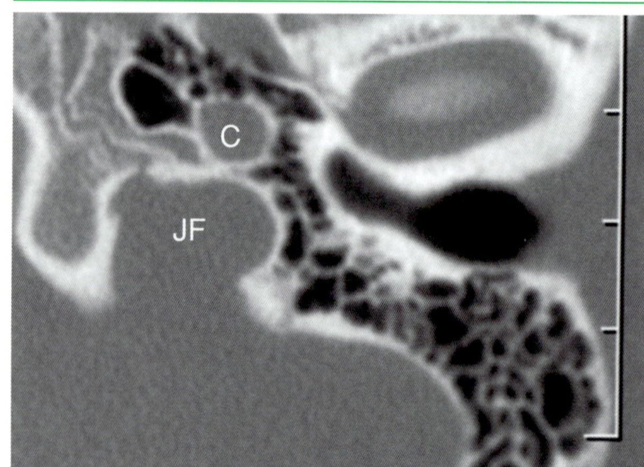

1. axial image

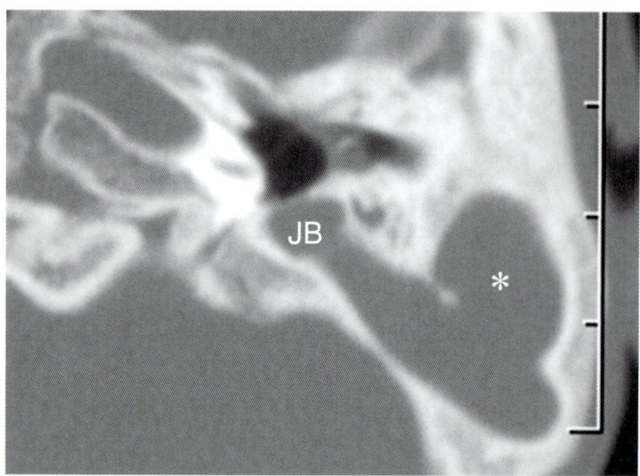

2. axial image

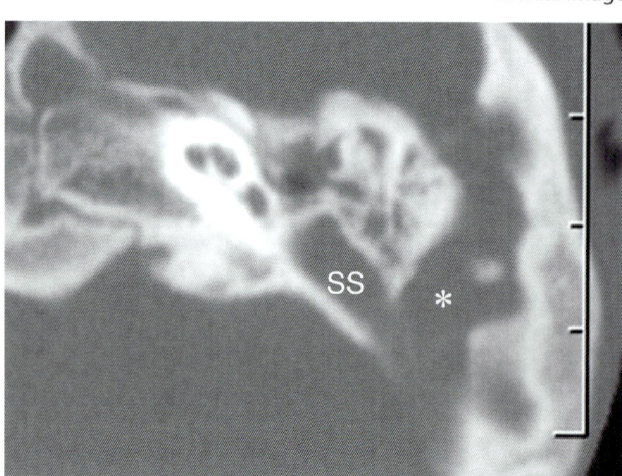

3. axial image

Normal Control CT Findings

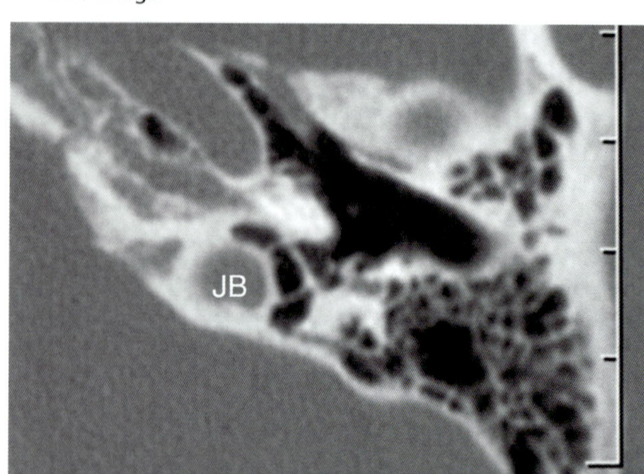

n1. axial image

n2. axial image

n3. axial image

Fig. 19. (Case 5) Left ear CT: 9 years postoperative (age 14)

[Patient CT Findings]

On the left side, the PSS (❋) is enlarged, bifurcating from the sigmoid sinus (3: **SS** and ❋) and running anteriorly (2: ❋), exiting the temporal bone at the upper external auditory canal (1: ✐). The internal carotid artery is of normal size (1: **C**), but the jugular foramen (1: **JF**) is clearly smaller than normal. Also, the position of the jugular bulb (2: **JB**) is located more laterally than normal.

《Normal Control CT Findings》

n1: **C**=internal carotid artery; **JF**=jugular foramen.
n2: **JB**=jugular bulb. n3: **SS**=sigmoid sinus.

but in combination with lip reading has 100% vowel recognition and can perceive simple words. Hearing, while auxiliary, plays a firm role in the subject's everyday life.

Postoperative CT Findings

The CT image shows the child at 14 years old, nine years after surgery. Mastoid air cell development is deficient, but there is no soft tissue density in the tympanic cavity, nor is there effusion retention or cholesteatoma due to remnant skin. The external auditory canal shows thick, bony occlusion (fig. 18:1, 2). The conducting wire of the cochlear implant, which is external to the cochlea, passes through the temporal bone and along the external auditory canal, forming a loop in the lumen of the external auditory canal (fig. 18:2) before entering the cochlea (fig. 18:3). In the vestibular system, the lateral semicircular canal is missing, forming only the vestibule (fig. 18:4), and the internal auditory canal is also narrow (fig. 18:4). The receiver-stimulator unit (fig. 18:4) is appropriately embedded in the lateral part of the skull, with no excessive protrusion or intracranial invagination observable. In the area of the border between the lateral margin of the pyramid and the pars squamosa there is a band of soft tissue density about 5 mm wide (fig. 18:4) which, if followed anteriorly, exits the temporal bone posterior to the temporomandibular joint (fig. 18:1–3). This structure, marked "�֍", which I will discuss later, is the petrosquamosal sinus (PSS) and its emissary the postglenoid foramen (PGF).

On the left side (fig. 19), the PSS is enlarged, bifurcating from the sigmoid sinus (fig. 19:3) and running anteriorly (fig. 19:2), exiting the temporal bone at the upper external auditory canal (fig. 19:1). The internal carotid artery is of normal size (fig. 19:1), but the jugular foramen (fig. 19:1) is clearly smaller than normal. Also, the position of the jugular bulb (fig. 19:2) is located more laterally than normal.

CHARGE Syndrome

Since CHARGE syndrome was first reported by Hall [1] in 1979, it has appeared in a comparatively large number of reports. It is thought to result from abnormal differentiation, setting, interaction, and migration of neural crest cells. A number of criteria for diagnosis of this disease have been proposed, but an updated diagnostic criteria recently proposed by Verloes [2] is as follows. He lists three major signs and five minor signs. The major signs are: 1) coloboma (iris or choroid, with or without microphthalmia); 2) atresia of choanae; 3) hypoplastic semicircular canals. The minor signs are: 1) rhombencephalic dysfunction (brainstem dysfunctions, cranial nerve VII to XII palsies and neurosensory deafness); 2) hypothalamo-hypophyseal dysfunction (including GH and gonadotrophin deficiencies); 3) abnormal middle or external ear; 4) malformation of mediastinal organs (heart, esophagus); 5) mental retardation. A patient with three major signs or two major signs and two or more minor signs is categorized as typical CHARGE syndrome; two major signs and one minor sign as partial/incomplete CHARGE syndrome; and fewer than that as atypical CHARGE syndrome. The case currently under consideration displays two major signs and all five minor signs, and so is classified as typical CHARGE syndrome.

Vascular Malformations of the Temporal Bone

Cerebral blood flow drains mainly through the internal jugular vein, but a portion drains through the external jugular vein. There are two routes that connect the two: one passes from the superficial and deep middle cerebral veins and through the cavernous sinus to the pterygoid plexus, and the other is via the emissary veins. Of the emissary veins, the one running from the sigmoid sinus to the mastoid foramen is observed frequently. However, the emissary route referred to as the petrosquamosal sinus (PSS), which runs from the anterior portion of the transverse sinus anteriorly along the petrosquamous suture and exits from the temporal bone through the postglenoid foramen (PGF) located anterior to the external auditory canal and posterior to the temporomandibular joint to arrive at the temporal fossa, ordinarily undergoes involution in the fetal or early postnatal stages, so it is rare to encounter it in a clinical setting [3]. The PGF can be observed in around 3.5% of humans, but in 40–50% of monkeys [4]. However, with advances in imaging diagnosis, the number of cases of skull base malformation in which the PSS can be confirmed is rising [5], and a case of CHARGE syndrome involving enlarged PSS has been reported [6]. The PSS normally either does not exist or is vestigial with no functional significance, however in cases of malformation such as the present one it has a large diameter and is believed to play an important role along with the internal jugular vein system in draining blood from the brain. This vascular malformation is difficult to diagnose due to its rarity, but because in otologic surgical procedures there is a danger it could cause hemorrhaging or other complications or, if obstructed, result in insufficient venous blood drainage from the brain, one should be mindful of this anomaly especially when treating hearing impaired children with syndromes.

References

1 Hall BD: Choanal atresia and associated multiple anomalies. J Pediatr 1979;95:395–398.
2 Verloes A: Updated diagnostic criteria for CHARGE syndrome: a proposal. Am J Med Genet A 2005;133:306–308.
3 Millan Ruiz D, Gailloud P, Yilmaz H, et al: The petrosquamosal sinus in humans. J Anat 2006;209:711–720.
4 Wysocki J: Morphology of the temporal canal and postglenoid foramen with reference to the size of the jugular foramen in man and selected species of animals. Folia Morphol 2002;61:199–208.
5 Marsot-Dupuch K, Gayet-Delacroix M, Elmaleh-Berges M, et al: The petrosquamosal sinus: CT and MR findings of a rare emissary vein. Am J Neuroradiol 2001;22:1186–1193.
6 Song JJ, Kwon SK, Cho CG, Park SW: Skull base vascular anomaly in CHARGE syndrome: A case report and review. Int J Otorhinolaryngol 2008;72:535–539.

Points

❶ When skull base malformation is involved, it sometimes is accompanied by vascular malformations such as sigmoid sinus anomalies or persistence or enlargement of the PSS.

❷ PSS and PGF can be the cause of complications in otologic surgical procedures, so it is important to use imaging to make a full prior evaluation.

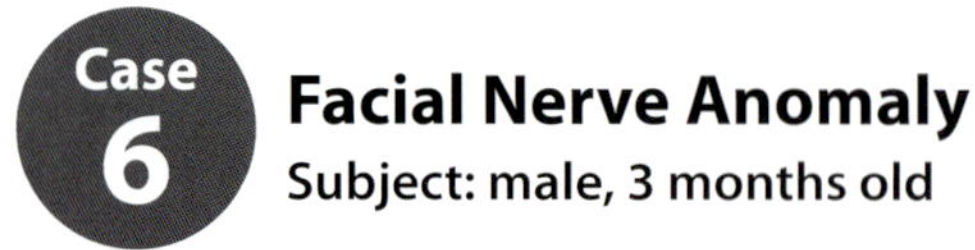

Case 6

Facial Nerve Anomaly

Subject: male, 3 months old

■ History and Clinical Findings

There were no particular problems at birth, but the mother noticed that the child had trouble closing his right eye and that when he smiled the right corner of his mouth did not rise, so she had him examined by a local doctor who referred him to our department. Because the subject was an infant and could not yet intentionally make facial expressions, a detailed evaluation was difficult, but based on his expressions made while laughing or crying, he was diagnosed as grade 5 on the House-Brackmann scale.

■ Patient CT and MRI Findings

Mastoid air cell development is judged to be normal for this age on both sides. Observing the right facial nerve along its path from the internal auditory canal, the labyrinthine segment (fig. 20:4) displays no abnormalities, but from the geniculate ganglion (fig. 20:4) and tympanic segment to the second genu (fig. 20:3) and in the proximal portion of the mastoid segment (fig. 20:2), an enlargement of the neural canal is apparent compared to the normal control. The diameter of the facial nerve changes slightly in each segment, but the normal value for the diameter of the facial nerve distal to the tympanic segment is reported as 1.42 mm in neonates and an average of 1.87 mm in infants [1]. In this case, the diameter of the same segment of the facial nerve as measured on the image is 3.1 mm—roughly twice normal. On the other hand, no anomalies were found in the ossicles, including the incudostapedial joint and the superstructure of the stapes. Also, in the distal portion of the mastoid segment, the bony tube is bifurcated (fig. 20:1).

For this case, an MRI was also taken under general anesthesia using an intravenous anesthetic. In a contrast-enhanced MRI, the swollen facial nerve with contrast enhancement can be observed from the geniculate ganglion and tympanic segment to the mastoid segment (fig. 21:1). At the same time, a clear contrast enhancement can be seen in the middle ear cavity (fig. 21:1), showing strong otitis media.

Because symptoms of otitis media did not improve even with treatment using antibiotics and intravenous administration of steroids, a mastoidectomy was performed to directly observe and decompress the facial nerve.

■ Surgical Findings and Postoperative Course

A mastoidectomy and posterior tympanotomy were performed, at which point no ossicular abnormalities were discernible. When the incus was temporarily extracted to observe the tympanic segment of the facial nerve, it was discovered that the bony tube was absent from the geniculate ganglion to the second genu, exposing the tympanic segment of the facial nerve in the tympanic cavity. A decompression was performed from the mastoid segment to the stylomastoid foramen to expose the facial nerve, whereupon it was confirmed that the nerve was divided in two in the distal portion of the mastoid segment. Response of the facial muscles to intraoperative electrical stimulation was clear on stimulation of both branches of the nerve, in both the tympanic and the mastoid segments. When the nerve's epineurium and perineurium were incised from the tympanic segment to the mastoid segment (the area of pronounced neuronal swelling) to further decompress the nerve, swelling in the edematous nerve became more pronounced, but no tumor was visible. When electrical stimulation was applied directly to the nerve, it produced stronger facial muscle contraction than when applied through the perineurium. The incus was returned to its original position and a steroid-soaked gelatin sponge interned over the nerve to complete the operation.

■ Postoperative MRI and Clinical Course

Six months after facial nerve decompression surgery another contrast-enhanced MRI exam was performed. The otitis media observed preoperatively had healed and the contrast enhancement for the tympanic and mastoid segments of the facial nerve had abated (fig. 21:2).

Postoperatively, facial nerve function gradually improved to a grade 2 on the House-Brackman scale, as of two years after surgery.

■ Congenital Facial Nerve Anomalies

As mentioned in the section on EAC atresia and stenosis in this chapter, abnormal location of the facial nerve path often accompany external auditory canal anomalies. There are also reports of facial nerve bifurcation in cases of severe systemic deformity such as multiple anomalies [2, 3] and chromosomal abnormality [4]. A case such as this, however, in which there is a morphological defect to the facial nerve with no other defects beyond the ear, is extremely rare [5]. The facial nerve differentiates from the neural crest and otic vesicle in the fourth week of embryonic development and is complete after eight weeks, but the nerve's bony tube originates from the second branchial arch, with formation starting around the end of the fifth month. The distal portion of the mastoid segment in particular continues to extend peripherally after birth along with temporal bone development. The tip of the long process of the incus and the stapes also originate from the second branchial arch, and combined malformations of these structures and the facial nerve have been reported [6]. However, the present case is unique in that there were no anomalies of the ossicles. Initially, I concluded that the bifurcation of the distal region of the facial nerve's mastoid segment was a deformity. Certainly one does not see this kind of bifurcation of the facial nerve between the mastoid segment and the stylomastoid foramen in adults. But on examination of CT images in multiple cases of other young infants around one year old without facial paralysis or middle or external ear anomalies, it became clear that images showing bifurcation were not uncommon (fig. 20:n1), so perhaps this finding may be considered as within the normal range of the developmental process for the mastoid segment of the temporal bone.

Patient CT Findings

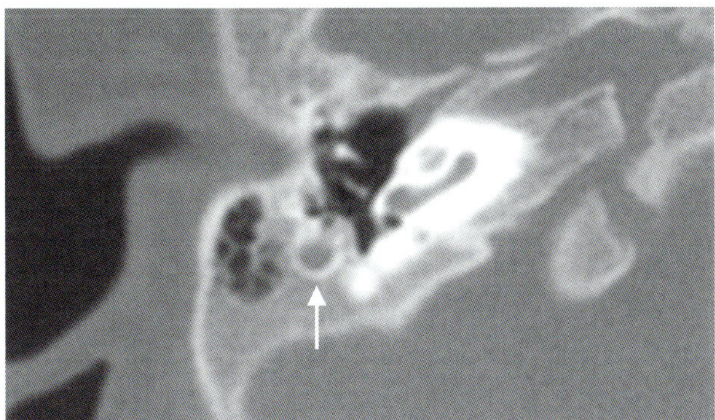

1. axial image

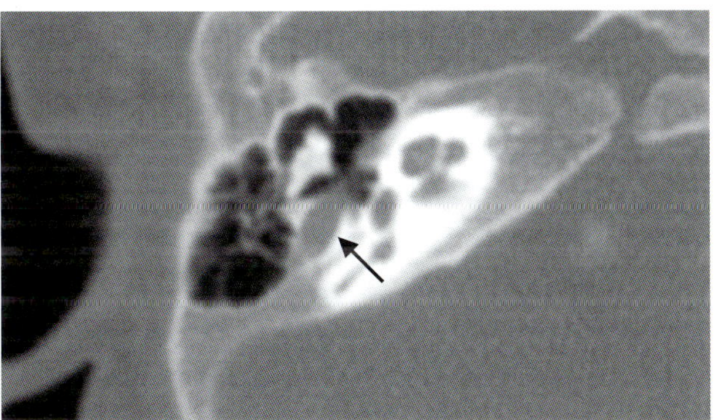

2. axial image

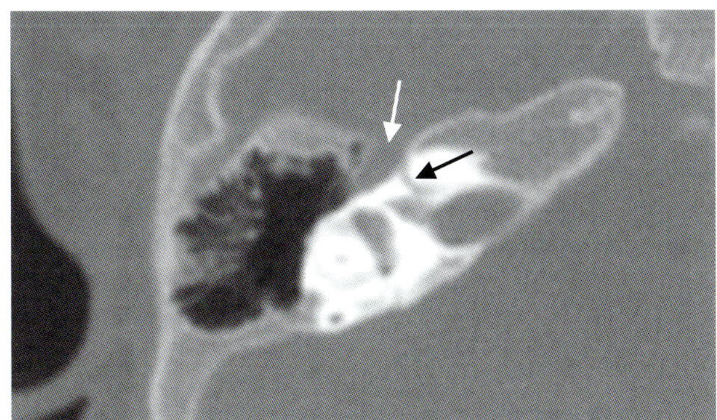

3. axial image

4. axial image

Normal Control CT Findings

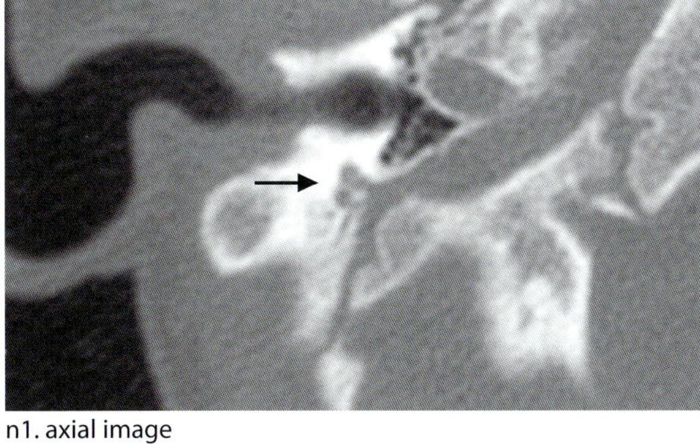

n1. axial image

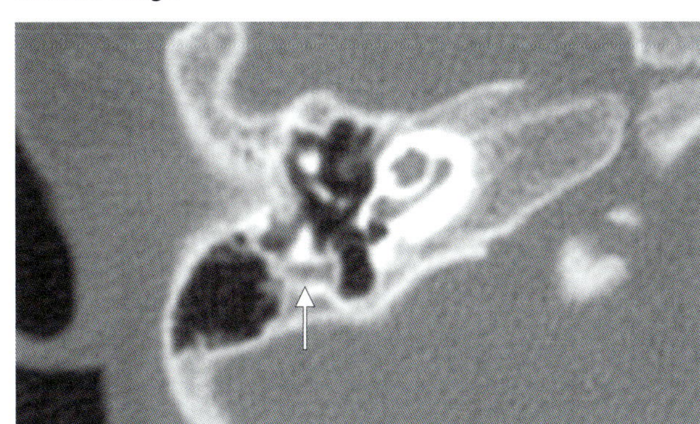

n2. axial image

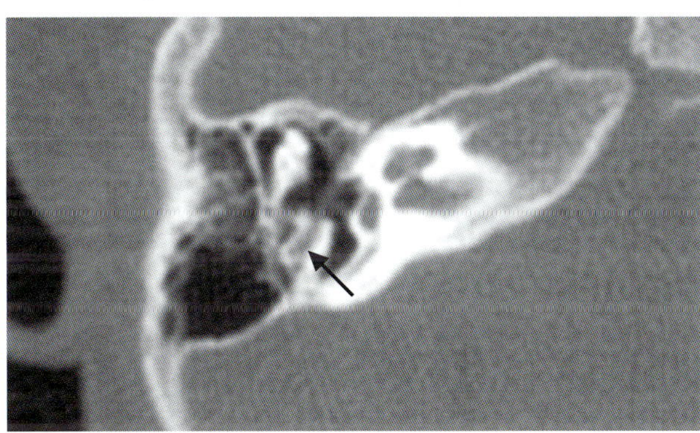

n3. axial image

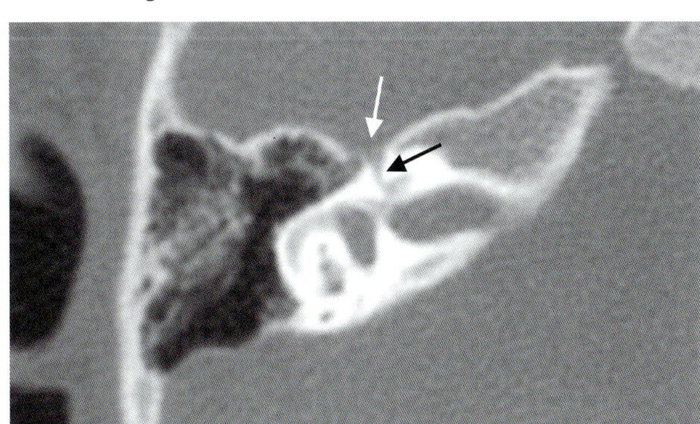

n4. axial image

Fig. 20. (Case 6) Right ear CT: preoperative

[Patient CT Findings]

The labyrinthine segment of the facial nerve (4: ↙) displays no abnormalities, but from the geniculate ganglion (4: ⇓) and tympanic segment to the second genu (3: ↖) and in the proximal portion of the mastoid segment (2: ⇑) an enlargement of the neural canal is apparent. In the distal portion of the mastoid segment the bony tube bifurcates (1: →).

《Normal Control CT Findings》

n1: → The distal part of the facial nerve's mastoid segment is sometimes bifurcated in young infants, even in normal control samples. n2: ⇑ proximal portion of mastoid segment. n3: ↖ second genu. n4: ⇓ geniculate ganglion, ↙ labyrinthine segment.

Patient MRI Findings

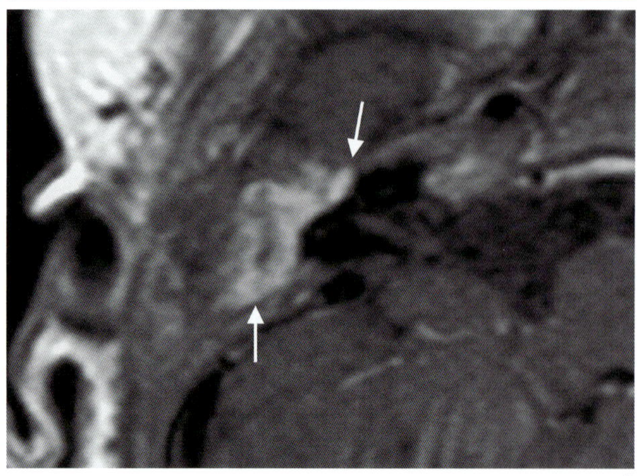 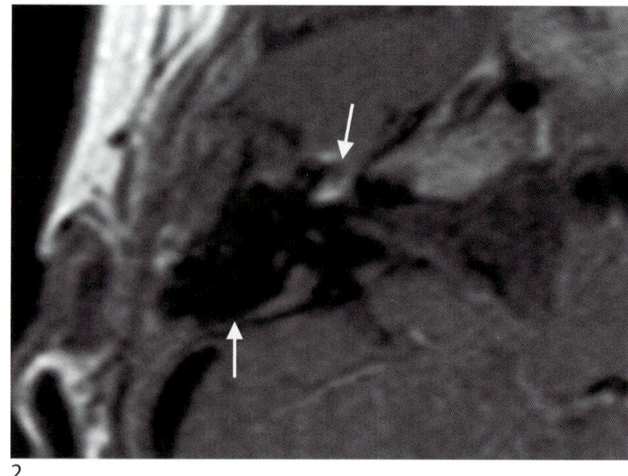

Fig. 21. (Case 6) Right ear contrast-enhanced MRI: 1 = preoperative, 2 = six months after facial nerve decompression surgery

[Patient MRI Findings]

In a contrast-enhanced MRI, the swollen facial nerve with contrast enhancement can be observed from the geniculate ganglion and tympanic segment to the vicinity of the mastoid segment (1: ⇓). At the same time, a clear contrast enhancement can be seen in the middle ear cavity (1: ⇑), indicating otitis media. In another contrast-enhanced MRI exam performed six months after facial nerve decompression surgery, the otitis media observed preoperatively had healed (2: ⇑) and the contrast enhancement for the tympanic and mastoid segments of the facial nerve had abated (2: ⇓).

Facial paralysis accompanies facial nerve anomalies involving aplasia or extreme hypoplasia [3], but in cases reported by Takahashi et al [6], the only symptom was hearing loss due to attendant ossicular deformities, with no accompanying facial paralysis despite the existence of facial nerve path anomaly and bifurcation. In a report by Glastombury et al [5], all three cases were accompanied by congenital hearing loss, with two cases displaying facial paralysis since birth. However, whether or not the paralysis in these cases was congenital cannot be confirmed, as their histories included such factors as forceps delivery and physical trauma. In the present case, snapshots taken of the infant since birth showed no asymmetry, indicating that the paralysis was probably acquired. The fact that complications due to otitis media were present at the time the MRI was taken, the facial nerve's bony tube was absent in the tympanic segment and the nerve exposed in the middle ear, and the contrast enhancement reduced and nerve function recovered after decompression, it is possible that this case of facial paralysis was caused by neuritis that had spread to the nerve from otitis media, though because the previous CT image indicated no finding of otitis media we cannot be certain. In cases such as this, in which not just morphology but also the possibility of inflammation or tumor is being considered, both simple and contrast-enhanced MRI are required.

References

1 Nakashima S, Sando I, Takahashi H, Fujita S: Computer-aided 3-D reconstruction and measurement of the facial canal and facial nerve. I. Cross-sectional area and diameter: preliminary report. Laryngoscope 1993;103:1150–1156.

2 Sando I, English GM, Hemenway WG: Congenital anomalies of the facial nerve and stapes: a human temporal bone report. Laryngoscope 1968;78:316–323.

3 Takahara T, Momota T, Okuno H: Sentensei ganmenshinkei mahi shorei no sokutokotsu ganmenshinkei byohen. (Histopathology of temporal bone and facial nerve in a case of congenital facial nerve paralysis.) Facial N Res Jpn 1987;7:67–70. (in Japanese.)

4 Koyama S, Iino Y, Kaga K, et al: Sentensei ijoji ni okeru ganmenshinkei no ijo —sokutokotsu byori hyohon ni yoru kento. (Facial nerve anomalies of children with congenital anomalies.) Nippon Jibiinkoka Gakkai Kaiho (Tokyo) 1998;101:192–197. (in Japanese.)

5 Glastonbury CM, Fischbein NJ, Harnsberger HR, et al: Congenital bifurcation of the intratemporal facial nerve. Am J Neuroradiol 2003; 24:1334–1337.

6 Takahashi H, Kawanishi M, Maetani T: Abnormal branching of facial nerve with ossicular anomalies: report of two cases. Am J Otol 1998; 19:850–853.

Points

❶ In infant facial paralysis there is a possibility of facial nerve anomalies.

❷ In this case the facial nerve anomaly was isolated, but care must be taken to determine if there are combined malformations of the tip of the long process of the incus or the superstructure of the stapes, which originate from the second branchial arch.

❸ A contrast-enhanced MRI is useful in diagnosing neuritis, but requires general anesthesia in young infants.

③ Inner Ear

Congenital Malformation of the Inner Ear

Congenital malformations of the inner ear can cause a variety of deficits in hearing and vestibular function. Recently congenital malformations are often discovered in newborn hearing screening tests, but in cases of mild hearing loss where the tests were not performed, deficiency symptoms may be unclear and remain unnoticed until the child is older. Also, one must be cautious as hearing loss that progresses after birth may not be picked up in neonatal screening. In cases of severe hearing loss, a doctor will eventually be consulted when the parents notice unresponsiveness to sound or delayed language development, or if abnormalities are identified during a regular physical exam. On the other hand, with congenital peripheral vestibular dysfunction, it is often difficult to determine whether symptoms such as delayed walking deviate from the normal range of individual developmental variations, making it more difficult to arrive at a definitive diagnosis than with hearing loss.

Malformations of the inner ear account for around 20% of congenital hearing loss [1], making it a major cause of disease. As with other causes, in cases of hearing loss due to inner ear malformation early diagnosis and intervention is important. Particularly in cases of severe to profound hearing loss with a high probability that a cochlear implant will be required, an accurate evaluation of the malformation is required not only for diagnosis and classification but also for surgical planning. Points to keep in mind when performing cochlear implantation in cases of inner ear malformation will be covered in detail in each of the cases in this chapter.

Genesis of the Inner Ear

Genesis of a normal inner ear begins around the third week of gestation with the formation of the otic placode, which forms a depression that becomes the otic pit, which in turn becomes the otic vesicle and separates around the fourth week. The otic vesicle divides into the masses that will form the basis for each component of the inner ear, which then enlarge and differentiate to form discrete shapes until the precise structure is complete. The bony labyrinth is basically formed first, with the formation of the membranous labyrinth following later.

Looking first at the cochlea, at around the fifth week of embryonic development the cochlear duct begins to extend from the saccule, reaching completion between the ninth and tenth weeks with approx. 2.5 turns. In the membranous labyrinth, the sensory cells arise in the organ of Corti starting at seven weeks and are complete at around 24 weeks, at which point the fetus is capable of hearing sounds. With the vestibular system, as the endolymphatic duct extends from the dorsal surface of the otic vesicle around the end of the fourth week, the eminences which will form the basis for the semicircular canals appear. In the seventh week, the vestibule specializes into the utricle and the saccule, and around the end of the eighth week the mesenchymal tissue of first the anterior and posterior semicircular canals, then the lateral semicircular canal, is absorbed and they become tubular [2].

After nine weeks, the mesenchymal tissue around the otic vesicle becomes cartilage and after ten weeks the cartilage around the membranous labyrinth is absorbed and replaced with fluid and the perilymphatic space is formed. From around 15 weeks the cartilage around the labyrinth begins to ossify, and this process is completed in the 23rd week, with overall completion of the inner ear at around 26 weeks.

Histopathological Classification of Inner Ear Malformation

Histopathologically, inner ear malformation may be classified [3] as 1) Michel aplasia: the inner ears is completely failure of development of the inner ear; 2) Mondini dysplasia: the cochlea is flat, the cochlear duct is short, the modiolus is hypoplastic, the auditory and vestibular sense organs and nerves are immature, the vestibule is large, the semicircular canals are wide, small, or missing, and the endolymphatic sac is bulbous; 3) Bing-Siebenmann dysplasia: normal bony labyrinth with underdeveloped membranous labyrinth; 4) Scheibe dysplasia: disorder of the membranous labyrinth of the saccule and cochlea, with normal development of the utricle and semicircular canals and 5) Alexander dysplasia: aplasia of the cochlear membranous labyrinth, especially when accompanied by high-frequency hearing loss due to abnormalities in the basal turn [4]. This classification system is based on findings of microscopic observations on histopathological temporal bone sections, however diagnosis of inner ear malformation in everyday clinical settings is performed using temporal bone CT and MRI examination so it is not possible to use the above classification as is. Current CT and MRI spatial resolution and contrast resolution permits observation of the modiolus and the septum between the cochlear turns, but because the membranous labyrinth and sensory cells are not depicted, in clinical imaging examination it is not possible to distinguish between 3) to 5) above, namely Bing-Siebenmann, Scheibe, and Alexander dysplasia. This classification system also makes no reference to inner ear malformations in which the cochlea and vestibule are fused in an undifferentiated cyst (explained later as common cavity deformity). Moreover, 1) Michel aplasia is rare, so as a result the majority of inner ear malformations encountered everyday are 2) Mondini dysplasia, rendering this classification system meaningless. Given this state of affairs it is apparent that, in addition to histopathological classification, a classification system of inner ear malformations based on clinical imaging findings is also required.

Classification Based on Clinical Imaging

The Jackler-Luxford-House classification system (table 3) [1] indicates the basic thinking behind classification of inner ear malformations based on clinical imaging findings, and up to now has served as the standard in this field. Category II, relating to the bony labyrinth and membranous labyrinth, is epoch-making in that it systematically classifies inner ear malformations based on findings for the cochlea, vestibule, vestibular aqueduct, and cochlear canaliculus that can be observed by imaging, allowing the inner ear malformation classification system previously centered on histopathological classification to be applied clinically. Furthermore, based on the Jackler classification system, Sennaroglu and Saatci have introduced changes to create a more practical system overall (table 4) [5], particularly by clearly distinguishing between Mondini dysplasia (incomplete partition type II) and a similar but embryologically more immature malformation (incomplete partition type I). Henceforth we will follow the Sennaroglu and Saatci classification when describing inner ear malformations from a clinical imaging perspective.

Classification of inner ear malformation, particularly the severity of cochlea malformation, using temporal bone CT imaging is shown in table 4-(1). The earlier the arrested development that causes the malformation occurs, the more advanced the malformation.

The most serious malformation is Michel aplasia, in which the inner ear is unformed, but this is due to an anomaly around the third week of embryonic development and as previously mentioned is rare. The next most serious malformation is cochlear aplasia, which is thought to result from problems occurring slightly after the third week.

Next, due to an anomaly occurring around the fourth week of embryonic development, the primodium of both the cochlea and vestibule is formed, but thereafter does not differentiate so the inner ear becomes a single, cystic structure. This is referred to as common cavity deformity. With common cavity deformity, there is a wide variation in the overall size of the cavity and the relative sizes of the areas corresponding to the cochlea and the vestibule.

In the next category, incomplete partition type I (IP-I), the vestibule, semicircular canals, and cochlea are clearly separated and formed to some extent but, even though the contours of the basal and upper turns of the cochlea are present, the septa separating cochlear turns and the modiolus are not discernible on the CT image. IP-I is thought to occur due to an anomaly in the fifth week of embryonic development. If inner ear development is impeded in the sixth week, the inner ear is divided into cochlea and vestibule, but their development is arrested before reaching maturity and the turns of the cochlea are slightly undersized and the vestibule and semicircular canals are either aplastic or hypoplastic, resulting in what is referred to as cochleovestibular hypoplasia.

Table 3. Jackler-Luxford-House classification of congenital malformations of the inner ear

I. Malformations limited to the membranous labyrinth

A. Complete membranous labyrinthine dysplasia
B. Limited membranous labyrinthine dysplasia
   i. Cochleosaccular dysplasia (Scheibe)
   ii. Cochlear basal turn dysplasia (Alexander)

II. Malformations of the osseous and membranous labyrinths

A. Complete labyrinthine aplasia (Michel)
B. Cochlear anomalies
   i. Cochlear aplasia
   ii. Cochlear hypoplasia
   iii. Incomplete partition (Mondini)
   iv. Common cavity
C. Labyrinthine anomalies
   i. Semicircular canal dysplasia
   ii. Semicircular canal aplasia
D. Aqueductal anomalies
   i. Enlargement of the vestibular aqueduct
   ii. Enlargement of the cochlear aqueduct
E. Abnormalities of the internal auditory canal
   i. Narrow internal auditory canal
   ii. Wide internal auditory canal

From Jackler, Luxford and House [1]

Table 4. Sennaroglu-Saatci classification of congenital malformation of the inner ear

Cochlear malformations
Cochlear malformations include the following: 1) Michel deformity. There is complete absence of all cochlear and vestibular structures. 2) Cochlear aplasia. The cochlea is completely absent. 3) Common cavity deformity. There is a cystic cavity representing the cochlea and vestibule, but without showing any differentiation into cochlea and vestibule. 4) Cochlear hypoplasia. Malformation is further differentiated so that the cochlea and vestibule are separate from each other but their dimensions are smaller than normal. Hypoplastic cochlea resembles a small bud off the internal auditory canal (IAC). 5) Incomplete partition type I (IP-I). The cochlea is lacking the entire modiolus and cribriform area, resulting in a cystic appearance. This is accompanied by a large cystic vestibule. 6) Incomplete partition type II (IP-II) (Mondini deformity). The cochlea consists of 1.5 turns, in which the middle and apical turns coalesce to form a cystic apex, accompanied by a dilated vestibule and enlarged VA.
Vestibular malformations
Vestibular malformations include Michel deformity, common cavity, absent vestibule, hypoplastic vestibule, and dilated vestibule.
Semicircular canal malformations
Semicircular canal malformations are described as absent, hypoplastic, or enlarged.
Internal auditory canal malformations
Internal auditory canal malformations are described as absent, narrow, or enlarged.
Vestibular and cochlear aqueduct findings
Vestibular and cochlear aqueduct abnormalities are described as enlarged or normal.

From Sennaroglu and Saatci [5]

Finally, incomplete partition type II (IP-II), which arises in the seventh week of embryonic development, is the mildest type of malformation in this classification system. In this malformation, 1.5 or more turns of the cochlea are formed and the septum between the basal and upper turns is clearly visible, but the part above the basal turn is cystic. The modiolus can be ascertained at the basal turn. On the other hand, in the vestibular system, malformation of the semicircular canals is insignificant and there is only slight enlargement of the vestibule, but it is accompanied by enlargement of the vestibular aqueduct. These findings are in accordance with findings from cases of inner ear malformation reported by Carlo Mondini in 1791 [6]. Mondini dysplasia is the most well-known inner ear malformation, but because this term has not necessarily been used according to its strict definition, here it tends to be understood as a blanket term for various different deformities. In Sennaroglu's research [5], he clearly defines the mildest category of malformation and accurately applies this definition to reported cases of Mondini dysplasia. In this sense as well, the Sennaroglu classification system is highly significant.

A note of caution, however: when viewing inner ear malformations in their entirety, there are many cases that are difficult to explain solely through the mechanism of arrested development during a specific period in the embryonic process. For example, there are cases in which the vestibule and semicircular canals are completely unformed, even though the cochlea has formed 1.5 turns, or in which only the vestibular aqueduct is enlarged, even though CT imaging indicates no anomalies whatsoever in the other components of the labyrinth. These exceptions imply the existence of some other internal factor involving, for example, a genetic mutation that selectively affects a specific part of the inner ear. In other words, there exist malformations in which multiple components of the inner ear are simultaneously damaged during the embryonic process (Sennaroglu calls these multi-branch abnormalities), those in which abnormalities occur independently in specific components (single-branch abnormalities), and also those in which the two coincide. Consequently, strictly speaking, one cannot obtain a complete evaluation of inner ear malformation unless one divides the inner ear into its various components and describes in further detail the degree of malformation in each, as is done in the Jackler classification system (table 3-II). However, such a strict approach is excessive for the majority of inner ear malformations. Since most cases conform to one of the categories shown in table 4-(1), the most practical approach in clinical terms is first to determine roughly which of the stages between Michel aplasia and IP-II applies, then if this is insufficient, append more detailed findings and, in cases that do not fall within the framework of systematic anomalies, individually record the anomalies for each part of the inner ear.

Complete formation of the inner ear follows a process of development, growth, and ossification. In malformations of the inner ear it is important first to determine whether or not development has taken place, then the extent of growth, as increase in size also affects final inner ear morphology. In the inner ear of a normal adult, the outer diameter of the basal turn of the cochlea is approx. 7 mm, the diameter of a cross-section of the basal turn just under 2 mm, and the height of the modiolus approx. 5 mm. The size of a normal vestibule is 4–5 mm anteroposteriorly and approximately 6 mm mediolaterally, and the outer diameter of the semicircular canals is 6–7 mm [7]. The diameter of the internal auditory canal is approx. 5 mm anteroposteriorly and approx. 4.5 mm vertically, with a length of approx. 11 mm [8]. In most cases involving malformations of the inner ear, categorization is determined by irregularities to the shape itself, but in determining, for example, the size of the cavity in common cavity deformity, the existence of vestibule enlargement or lateral semicircular canal hypoplasty for IP-II malformation, or the presence of stenosis for internal auditory canal anomalies, measurement values for each component are useful for attaining a more detailed understanding of characteristics with each category.

Role of CT and MRI in Diagnosis of Inner Ear Anomalies

Structurally the inner ear is composed of a membranous labyrinth inside a bony labyrinth, but the structures that actually sense sound and acceleration are the hair cells of the membranous labyrinth. Consequently the membranous labyrinth is important in functional terms, and it would be ideal if it were depicted in medical images. However, as stated previously, there is a limit to spacial resolution with current MRI performance, so it is impossible to differentiate the content of the bony labyrinth so long as there is no fibrosis. Also, in actual clinical practice, imaging of the temporal bone is often carried out to diagnose hearing loss, and occasionally also to check for malformations of the middle ear, and this requires CT imaging. For depicting the overall morphology of the inner ear both CT and MRI are roughly equal, but whereas bony tissues are not shown in MR images, CT also permits observation of malformations of the auditory ossicles, making CT the superior diagnostic tool. CT is the appropriate first choice in imaging for hearing impaired patients in which congenital malformation is suspected.

However recent years have seen a dramatic increase in cochlear implantations, making it important in cases of inner ear malformation not only simply to record the morphological classification, but also to evaluate from a functional perspective regarding the propriety and estimated prognosis of a cochlear implantation. For this reason, an MRI is necessary to evaluate the condition of structures other than the bones of the inner ear, including cranial nerve VIII, the cochlear nerve, and if possible, inside the modiolus. In this section we present cases of varying degrees of inner ear malformation and examine them using temporal bone CT images in combination with soft tissue findings obtained from MR images, to convey the procedure and focal points of comprehensive imaging diagnosis.

References

1 Jackler RK, Luxford WM, House WF: Congenital malformation of the inner ear. Laryngoscope 1987; 97 (suppl 40):2–14.

2 Swartz JD, Mukherji SK: Chapter 5 The inner ear and otodystrophy. 4th edition. Imaging of the temporal bone. Thieme, New York, 2009.

3 Schuknecht HF: Pathology of the ear. Second edition. Lea and Febiger, Philadelphia, 1993.

4 Ormerod FC: The pathology of congenital deafness. J Lryngol Otol 1960;74:919–950.

5 Sennaroglu L, Saatci I: A new classification for cochleovestibular malformations. Laryngoscope 2002;112:2230–2241.

6 Mondini C: Anatomical surdi nedi sectio. De Bononiensi Scientiarum et Artium Instituto Arque Acadamia Commentarii, Borogna 1791; 7:419 (quoted from reference 4).

7 Lang J: Anatomy of the brainstem and the lower cranial nerves, vessels, and surrounding structures. Am J Otol Supplement 1985;1–19.

8 McClay JE, Tandy RT, Grundfast K, et al: Major and minor temporal bone abnormalities in children with and without congenital sensorineural hearing loss. Arch Otolaryngol Head Neck Surg 2002; 128:664–671.

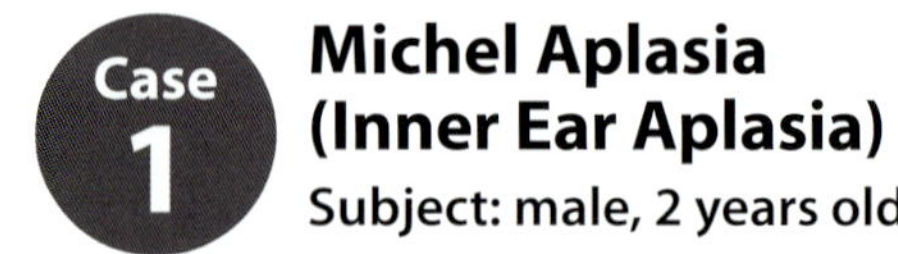

Michel Aplasia (Inner Ear Aplasia)

Subject: male, 2 years old

■ History and Clinical Findings

The subject was born at 40 weeks gestation. No particular abnormalities were detected in the perinatal period. A pediatric exam one month after birth identified deficient reaction to sound and an ABR was carried out at three months, at which time it was confirmed that there was no response to 105 dB NHL stimulation in either ear. Pediatrically, aside from mild motor retardation, there were no other obvious problems. A hearing aid was fitted at a rehabilitation center, but with no effect, so the subject was referred to our department to determine whether a cochlear implant would be appropriate. There were no abnormalities of the auricle, external auditory canal, or tympanic membrane. There was nothing of note in the family history.

■ Patient CT Findings

The cochlea and vestibule are completely unobservable (fig. 22:1–4, fig. 24:1–3). The high-density bone mass of the labyrinth visible in the normal control images (fig. 22:n2–n4, fig. 24:n1–n3) are barely visible in this case in the vicinity of the internal auditory canal (fig. 22:2–4) and the superior part of the anterior semicircular canal (fig. 23, fig. 24:4). Normally, the structures of the inner ear and internal auditory canal are located between the middle ear and the intracranial space, but in this case as one moves medially in from the middle ear, one passes through a single bony wall before directly entering the intracranial space (fig. 24:3).

The internal auditory canal is located more inferiorly than normal (fig. 22:2&3, fig. 24:2) and, following its contents, one finds that it turns into the geniculate ganglion (fig. 22:2, fig. 24:1), then, after running slightly posteriorly (fig. 22:1), turns inferiorly and becomes the stylomastoid foramen (fig. 22:1, fig. 24:3). Also, it can be confirmed on the MR image that the space inside the internal auditory canal contains only the facial nerve (fig. 25:1, indicated by the numeral 7). The overall path of the facial nerve and position of the stylomastoid foramen is significantly anterior to normal (fig. 22:n1). The tympanic segment (fig. 24:2) is also more inferior than normal (fig. 24:n2). Cranial nerve VIII (cochlear and vestibular nerves) is completely unobservable.

Observing the structures of the middle ear, among the ossicles the malleus and incus show no defects, however the stapes is almost nonexistent, with merely a portion of the head of the stapes present.

A small portion of the arch of the upper extremity of the anterior semicircular canal is present (fig. 23:2&3, fig. 24:4), so it does not represent complete aplasia. Therefore, this case could be described as "cochlear aplasia, vestibular aplasia, lateral and posterior semicircular canal aplasia, anterior semicircular canal hypoplasia." However, aside from the vestigial presence of a portion of the anterior semicircular canal, the majority of the inner ear is aplastic and displays many of the characteristic image findings of inner ear aplasia, so it has been presented here

| **Patient CT Findings** | **Normal Control CT Findings** |

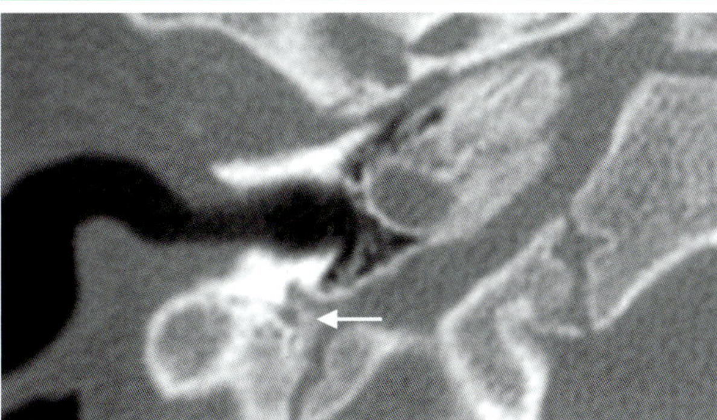

1. axial image   n1. axial image

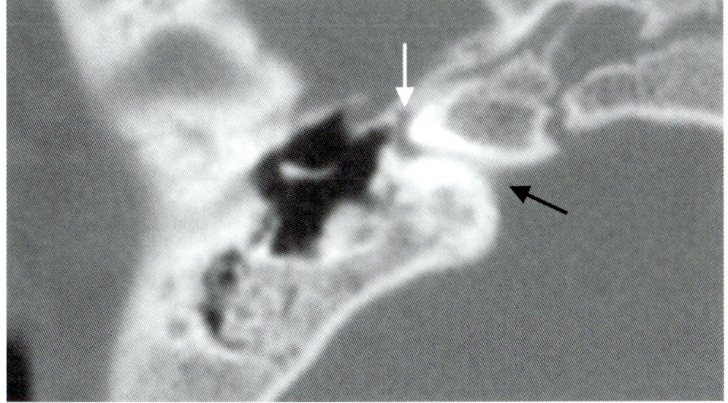
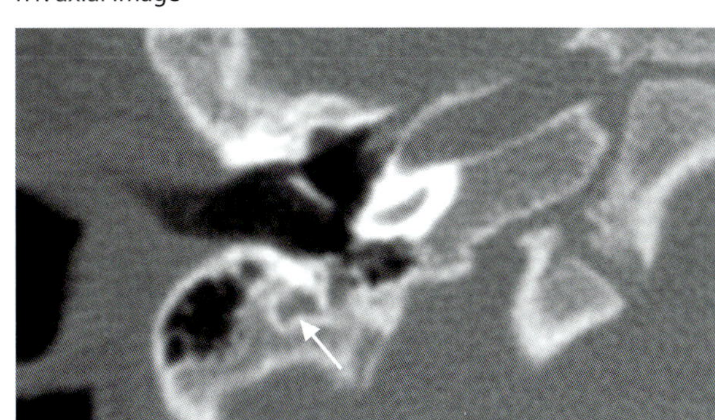

2. axial image   n2. axial image

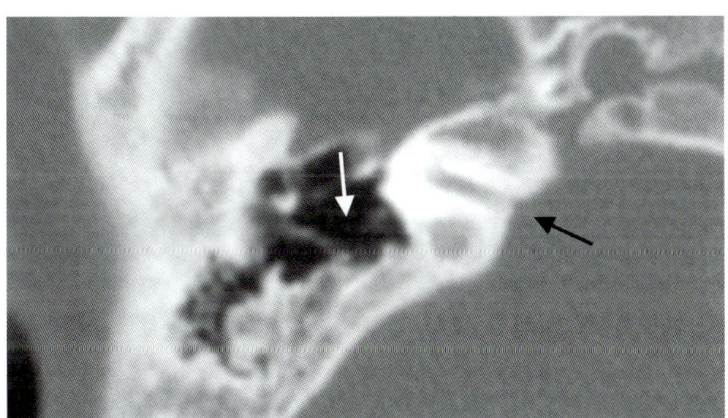
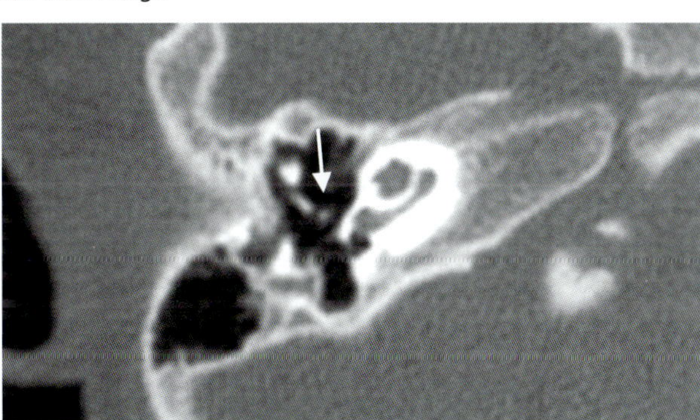

3. axial image   n3. axial image

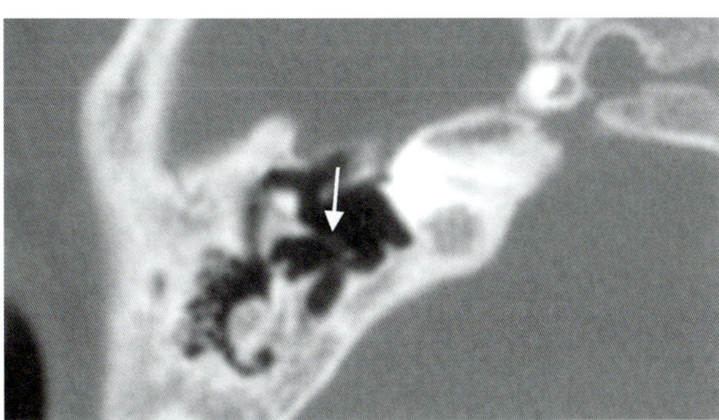
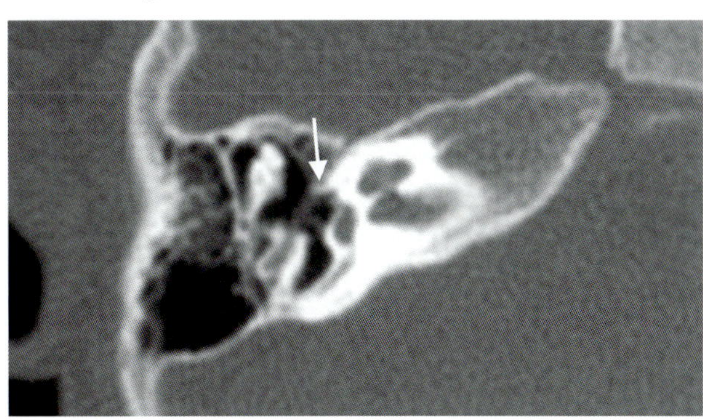

4. axial image   n4. axial image

Fig. 22. (Case 1) CT

〖Patient CT Findings〗

The cochlea and vestibule are completely unobservable (1–4). The high-density bone mass of the labyrinth visible in the normal control images (n2–n4) is barely visible in this case in the vicinity of the internal auditory canal (2–4) and the superior part of the anterior semicircular canal (Fig. 23). The internal auditory canal is located more inferiorly than normal (2, 3: ↖) and, following its contents, one finds that it turns into the geniculate ganglion (2: ↧), then, after running slightly posteriorly (1: ↘), turns inferiorly and becomes the stylomastoid foramen (1: ←). The overall path of the facial nerve and position of the stylomastoid foramen are significantly anterior to normal (n1: ←). Observing the structures of the middle ear, among the ossicles the malleus and incus show no defects, however the stapes is almost nonexistent (4: ↧), with merely a portion of the head of the stapes present (3: ↧)

《Normal Control CT Findings》

n1: ← stylomastoid foramen. n2: ↘ mastoid segment of facial nerve. n3, n4: ↧ tympanic segment of the facial nerve and stapes.

Patient CT Findings

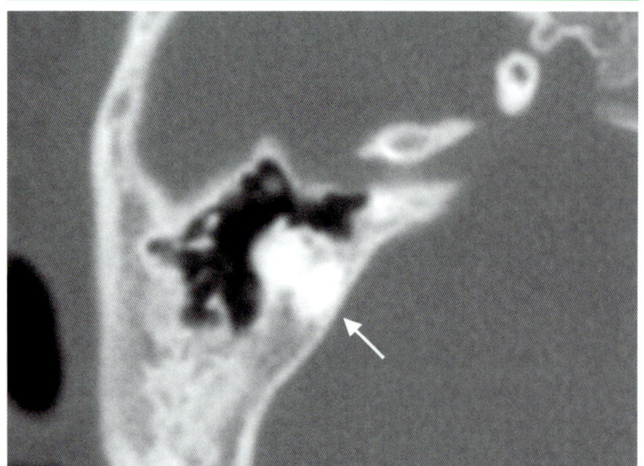

1. axial image

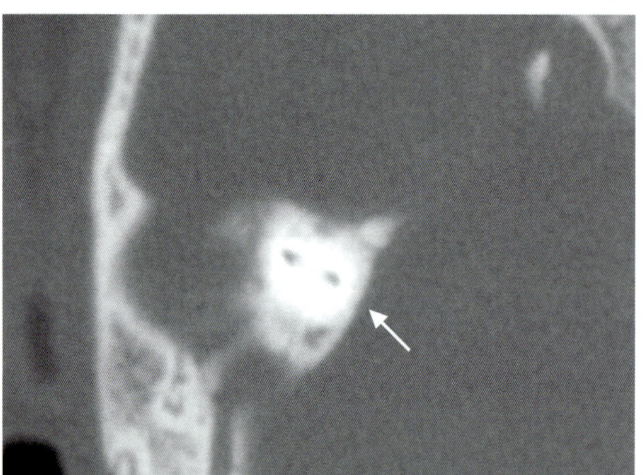

2. axial image

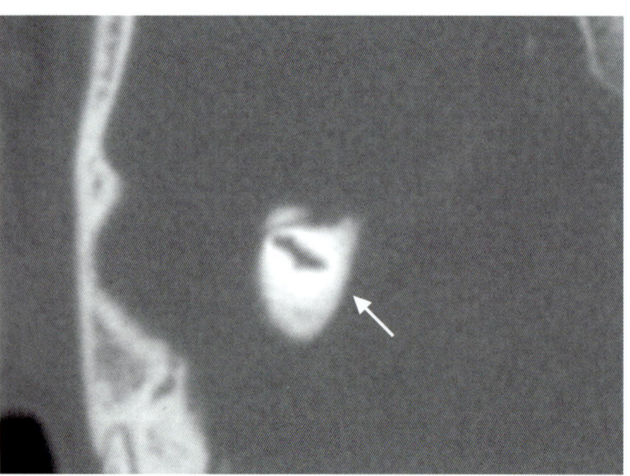

3. axial image

Normal Control CT Findings

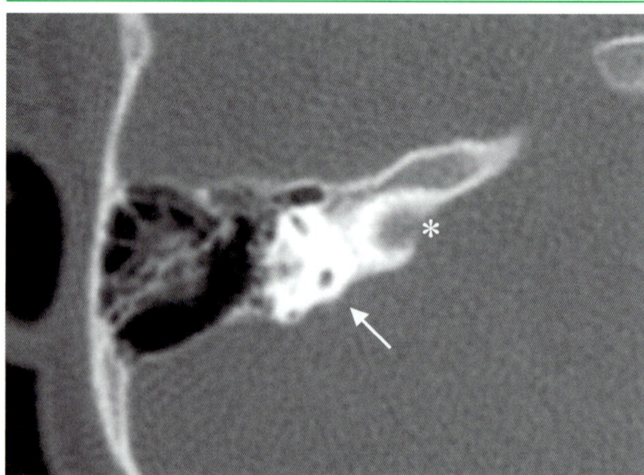

n1. axial image

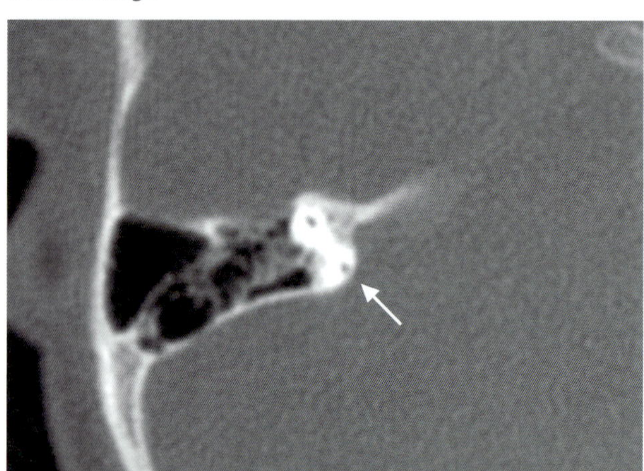

n2. axial image

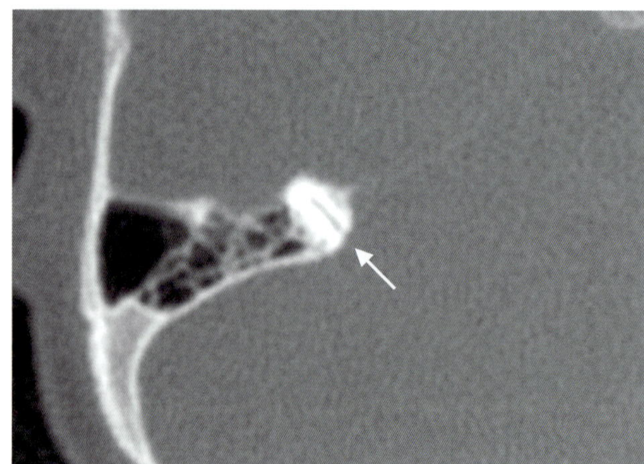

n3. axial image

Fig. 23. (Case 1) CT

[Patient CT Findings]

In this case, the area below the anterior semicircular canal's base is not formed (1: ✎), but a small portion of the arch of its upper extremity is present (2, 3: ✎).

《Normal Control CT Findings》

n1–n3: ✎ anterior semicircular canal; ✿ internal auditory canal.

Patient CT Findings | Normal Control CT Findings

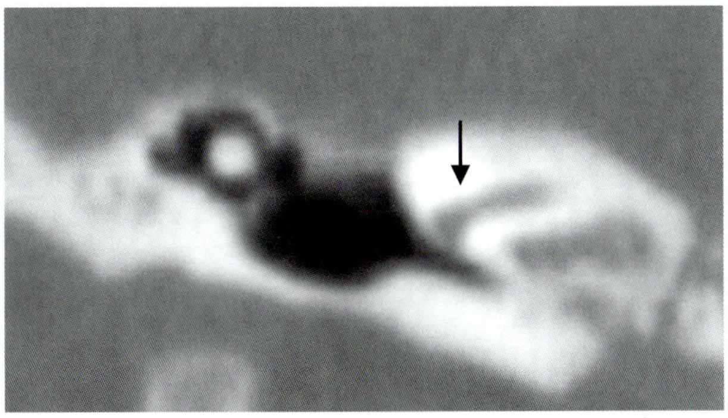

1. coronal image

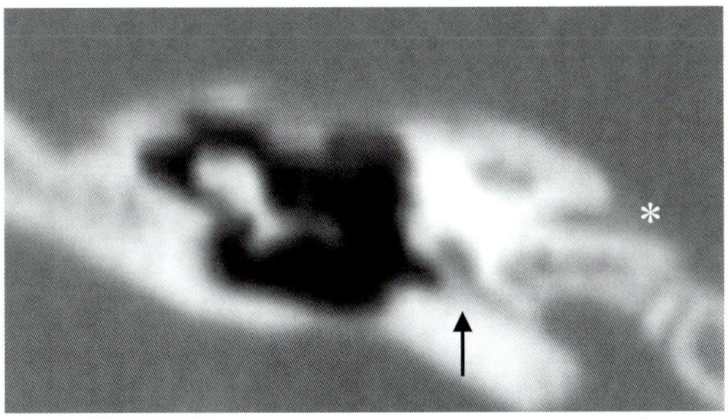

n1. coronal image

2. coronal image

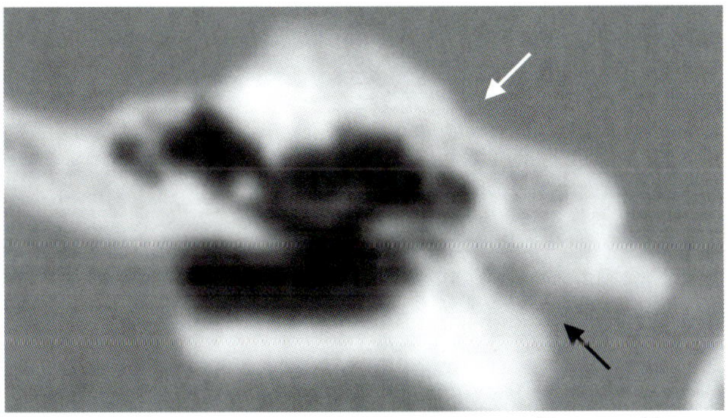

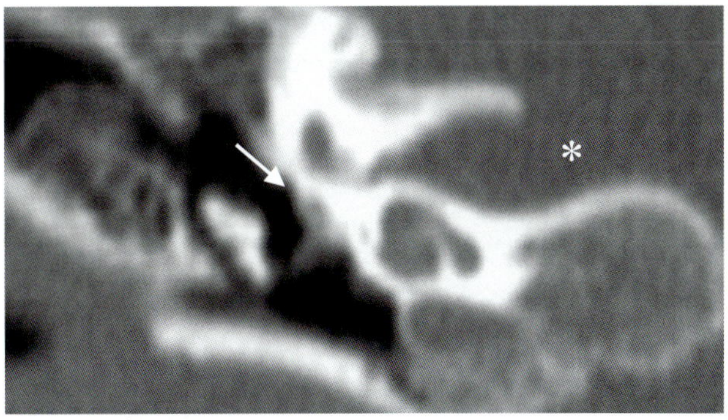

n2. coronal image

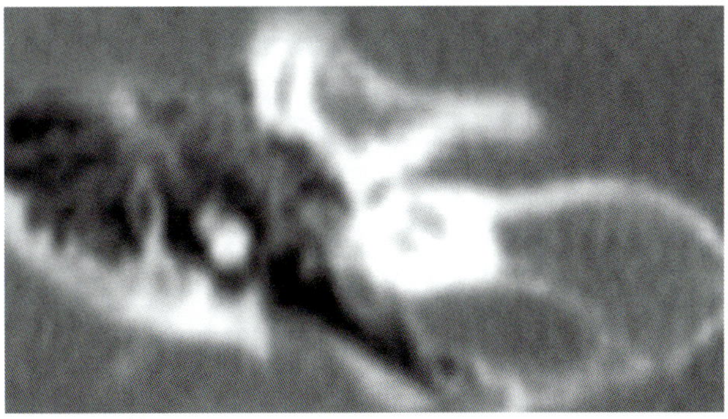

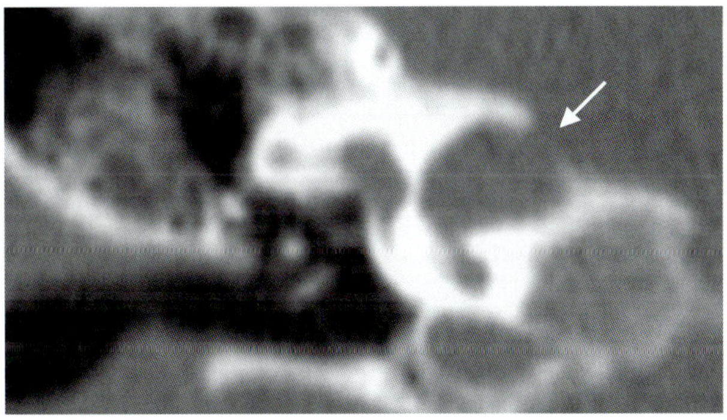

3. coronal image

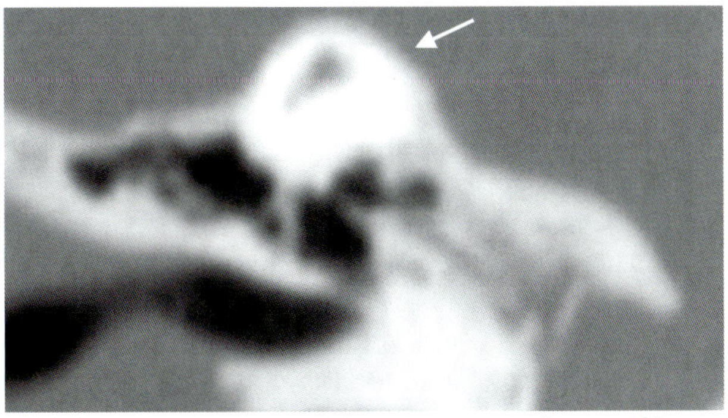

n3. coronal image

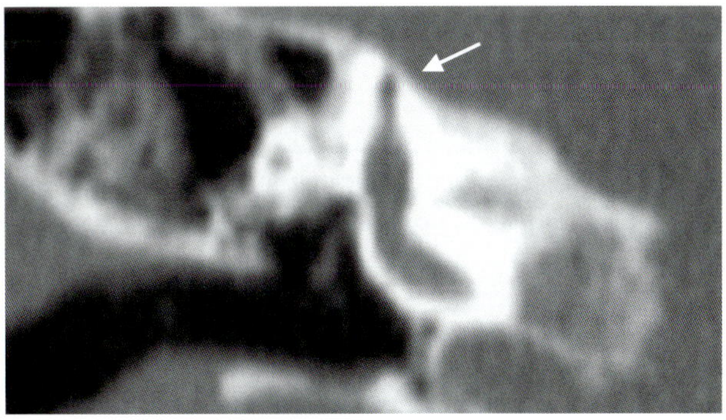

4. coronal image

n4. coronal image

Fig. 24. (Case 1) CT

[Patient CT Findings]

The bone mass of the labyrinth is barely visible in the vicinity of the internal auditory canal and the superior part of the anterior semicircular canal (4: ✐). Normally, the structures of the inner ear and internal auditory canal are located between the middle ear and the intracranial space, but in this case as one moves medially in from the middle ear, one passes through a single bony wall before directly entering the intracranial space (3: ✐). The internal auditory canal is located more inferiorly than normal (2: ✿) and turns into the geniculate ganglion (1: ↓) then, after running slightly posteriorly, turns inferiorly and becomes the stylomastoid foramen (3: ↘). The tympanic segment (2: ↑) is also more inferior than normal (n2: ↘). In this case, a small portion of the arch of the upper extremity of the anterior semicircular canal is present (4: ✐), so it does not represent complete aplasia.

《Normal Control CT Findings》

n1: foremost part of the bony capsule of the inner ear. n2: ↘ geniculate ganglion; ✿ internal auditory canal. n3: ✐ internal auditory canal. n4: ✐ anterior semicircular canal.

Patient MRI Findings

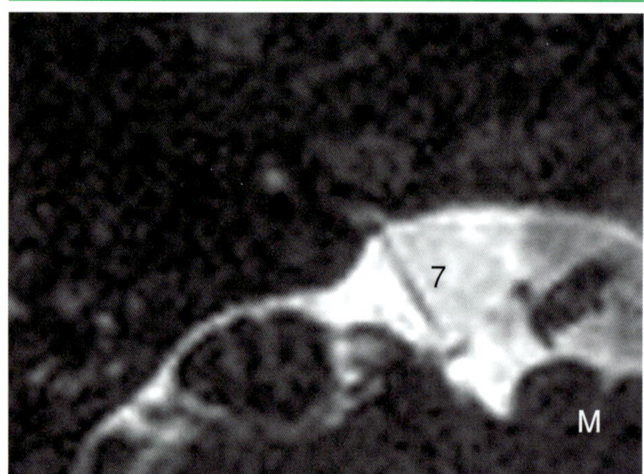

1. axial image

Normal Control MRI Findings

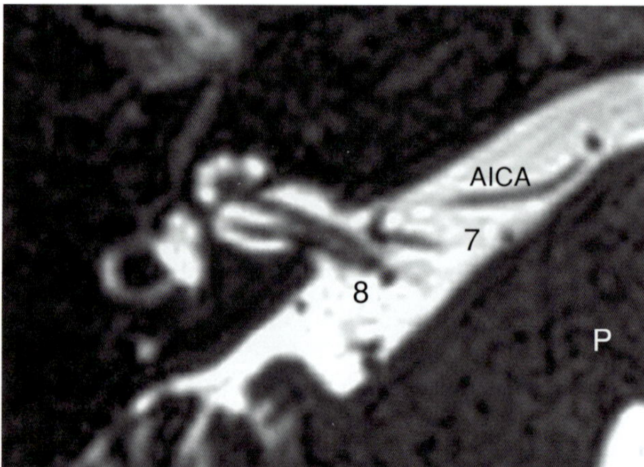

n1. axial image

Fig. 25. (Case 1) MRI

[Patient MRI Findings]
The space inside the internal auditory canal contains only the facial nerve (1: numeral **7**). 1: **M** indicates the medulla oblongata.

《Normal Control MRI Findings》
In n1, the numeral **7** indicates the facial nerve, **8** indicates cranial nerve VIII, **AICA** indicates the anterior inferior cerebellar artery, and P indicates the pons.

as Michel aplasia. Because there is no area corresponding to the ampulla of the anterior semicircular canal it lacks the function of a semicircular canal, and so, as inner ear function can be considered to be completely absent, in functional terms this case belongs in the category of inner ear aplasia.

■ Michel Aplasia

Reported by Michel in 1863, Michel aplasia is the most severe inner ear malformation [1], caused by arrested inner ear development around the third week of embryonic development. In a normal temporal bone, arrangement of the parts of the ear is, from lateral to medial, the external auditory canal, the middle ear, the inner ear, and the internal auditory canal, but in Michel aplasia the inner ear is absent, with corresponding lateral thinning of the temporal bone. Cases have been reported both in which the inner ear is completely absent and in which, as in this case, it is hypoplastic containing only the facial nerve [2]. As a rule there are no abnormalities of the middle ear, but among the ossicles there is always abnormality of the stapes, including absence or deformation. The path of the facial nerve also deviates inferiorly and anteriorly to normal [3].

When diagnosing Michel aplasia, caution must be exercised to differentiate it from cases in which the inner ear was formed, but has ossified as a result of labyrinthitis due to meningitis or other causes, preventing confirmation of the inner ear in a CT image. As can be seen in this case, in Michel aplasia the bony capsule of the inner ear is essentially absent, with the internal auditory canal either hypoplastic or aplastic. Malformation of the stapes is also frequently observed [1]. Consequently, in cases where a bone mass corresponding to the inner ear is present, the internal auditory canal is normal, and there is no abnormality of the stapes, most likely it is not inner ear aplasia but postnatal inner ear ossification.

References

1 Michel P: Mémoire sur les anomalies congénitales de l'oreille interne. Gazette Méd de Strasbourg 1863;23:55–58.
2 Ozgen B, Oguz KK, Atas A, Sennaroglu L: Complete labyrinthine aplasia: clinical and radiologic findings with review of the literature. AJNR Am J Neuroradiol 2009;30:774–780.
3 Romo LV, Curtin HD: Anomalous facial nerve canal with cochlear malformations. Am J Neuroradiol 2001;223:838–844.

Points

❶ Michel aplasia is accompanied by hypoplasia or aplasia of the bony capsule of the inner ear.

❷ The internal auditory canal is either hypoplastic or aplastic, and cranial nerve VIII is also absent.

❸ The path of the facial nerve is abnormal, and malformation of the stapes is frequent.

❹ Caution is required to differentiate Michel aplasia from acquired inner ear ossification.

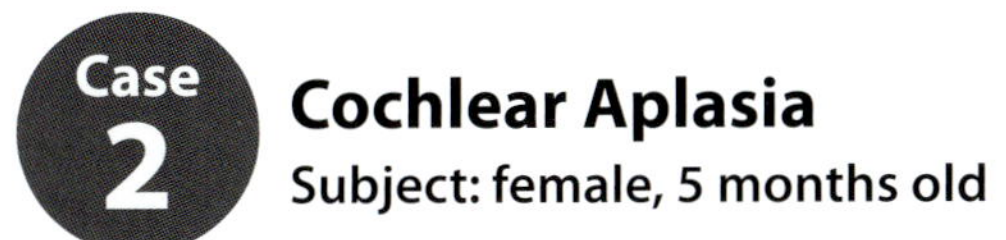

Cochlear Aplasia

Subject: female, 5 months old

■ History and Clinical Findings

Newborn hearing screening indicated a need for detailed bilateral examination and the subject received ABR testing at two and three months after birth, but all tests showed no response in either ear (105 dB NHL stimulation). Pediatric examination revealed microcephaly, developmental retardation, and corpus callosum hypoplasia. The subject was referred to our department to determine whether she was compatible for a cochlear implant and for general detailed examination relating to hearing loss. ASSR showed bilateral unresponsiveness for 110 dB at all frequencies, nor was there a response for Behavioral Observation Audiometry (BOA). No abnormalities were observed in the auricle or external auditory canal, but otitis media with effusion was present in both ears.

■ Patient CT Findings

The cochlea is completely absent, and in the location where it would normally be observed there is only the margin of the bony capsule of the vestibule (fig. 26:1, 2). On the other hand, the vestibule is present, but the lateral and anterior semicircular canals are fused and cystic, with the loops unformed. The structure corresponding to the posterior semicircular canal is not visible (fig. 26:3, 4). Particularly when viewing the coronal images (fig. 27), one can grasp that, even though the so-called pars superior of the inner ear is formed to some extent (fig. 27:3, 4), the pars inferior is almost completely absent (fig. 27:1). The internal auditory canal (fig. 26:3, 4; fig. 27:1–3) is located more anteriorly and inferiorly than normal and is short and narrow.

On examination of the middle ear, the ossicles in this case are almost normal and the malleus, incus, and stapes can all be observed (fig. 26:2–4; fig. 27: 1–4), but except for the epitympanum and mastoid antrum the pneumatic cavities are undeveloped and filled with soft tissue density, including the tympanic cavity. Clinically, because this subject has recurrent acute otitis media, the soft tissue density is assumed to be effusion. The labyrinthine segment of the facial nerve cannot be ascertained, and the tympanic segment cannot be identified due to effusion in the tympanic cavity. For the mastoid segment, a structure that one may assume to be the facial canal is visible lateroposterior to the tympanic cavity (fig. 26:1).

■ Cochlear Aplasia

Cochlear aplasia is the next most severe inner ear malformation after inner ear aplasia, with abnormality thought to arise around the fourth week of embryonic development. In both Michel aplasia and the cochlear aplasia shown here it is difficult to acquire hearing sensation, and because neither the space to implant an electrode nor the cochlear nerve are present, a cochlear implant is not compatible. However, in recent years, Auditory Brainstem Implant (ABI) surgery has been attempted in cases like this, and it has been reported that a definite hearing sensation can be obtained [1]. ABI was first used on cases of neurofibromatosis type 2 (NF2), but recently is increasingly being applied in cases other than NF2, including severe inner ear malformations such as those shown here. However, compared to acquired ossification of the cochlea, the results for ABI on severe inner ear malformation are relatively poor [2]. The reason for this is not clear but, in addition to the fact that severe inner ear malformation is often accompanied by multiple disabilities, it is possible that congenital deficit of the primary auditory nerve for the cochlea has some sort of negative effect on the development or function of the cochlear nucleus.

References

1 Sennaroglu L, Ziyal I, Atas A, et al: Preliminary results of auditory brainstem implantation in prelingually deaf children with inner ear malformations including severe stenosis of the cochlear aperture and aplasia of the cochlear nerve. Otol Neurotol 2009;30:708–715.
2 Colletti V, Shannon R, Carner M, et al: Outcomes in nontumor adults fitted with the auditory brainstem implant: 10 Years' Experience. Otology & Neurotology 2009;30:614–618.

Patient CT Findings

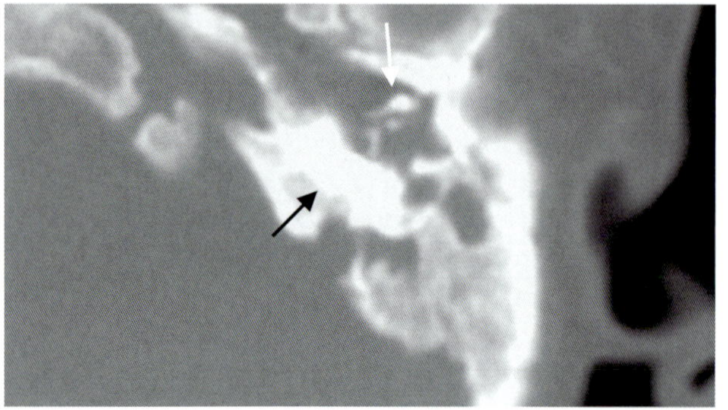

1. axial image

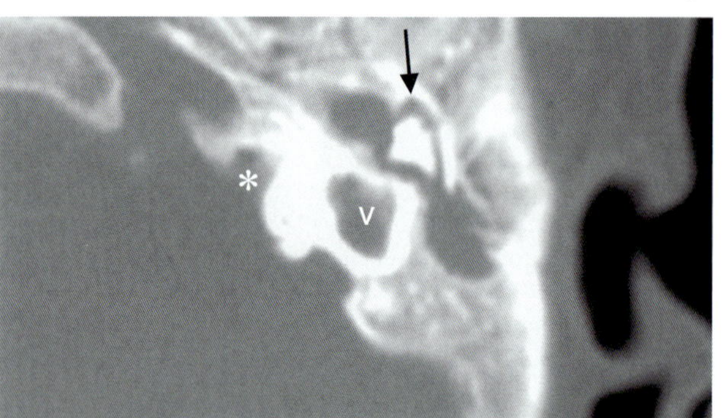

2. axial image

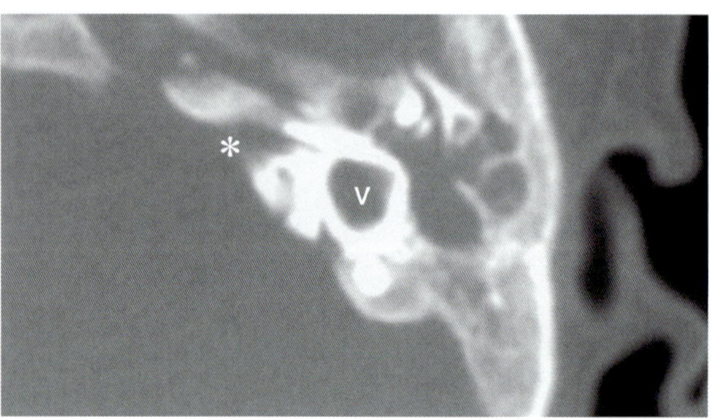

3. axial image

4. axial image

Normal Control CT Findings

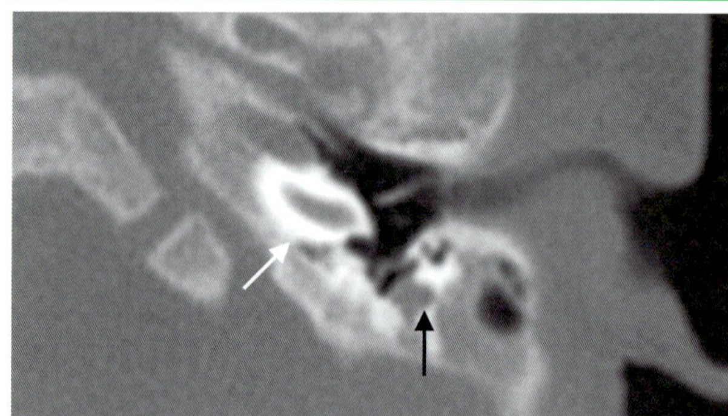

n1. axial image

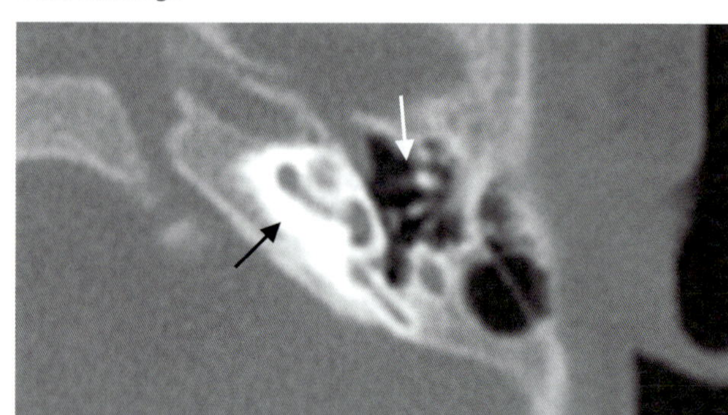

n2. axial image

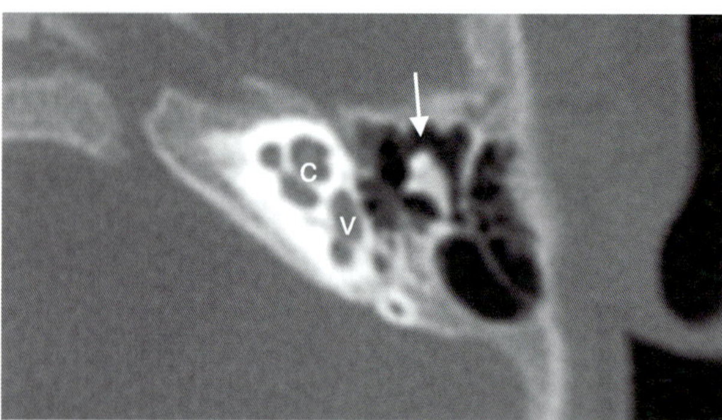

n3. axial image

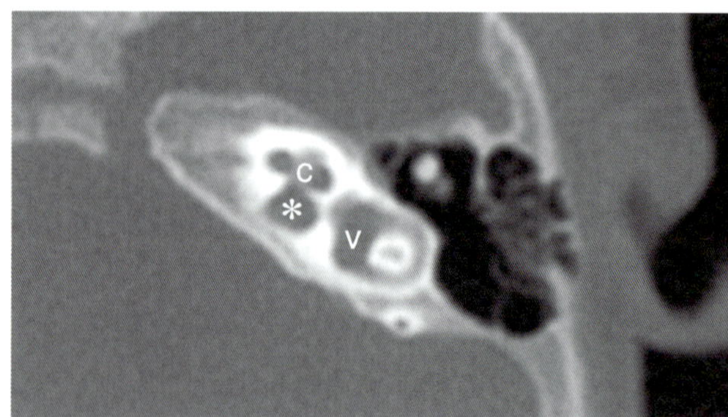

n4. axial image

Fig. 26. (Case 2) CT

[Patient CT Findings]

The cochlea is completely absent, presenting only the margin of the bony capsule of the vestibule (1, 2: ↗). The vestibule is present, but the semicircular canals are undifferentiated (3, 4: **V**). The internal auditory canal (3, 4: ✿) is located more anteriorly and inferiorly than normal and is short and narrow. The ossicles in this case are almost normal and the malleus, incus, and stapes can all be observed (2: ⇓ ; 3: ↓), but except for the epitympanum and mastoid antrum the pneumatic cavities are undeveloped and filled with soft tissue density, including the tympanic cavity. In the mastoid segment, a structure that one may assume to be the facial canal is visible lateroposterior to the tympanic cavity (1: ↑).

《Normal Control CT Findings》

n1: ↗ cochlea; ↑ mastoid segment of facial nerve. n2: ↗ cochlea; ⇓ ossicles. n3: ⇓ malleus, incus; **C** cochlea; **V** vestibule. n4: **C** cochlea; **V** vestibule; ✿ internal auditory canal.

Patient CT Findings

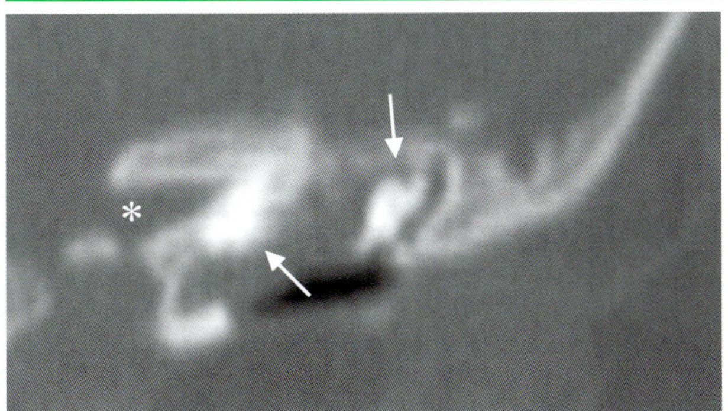

1. coronal image

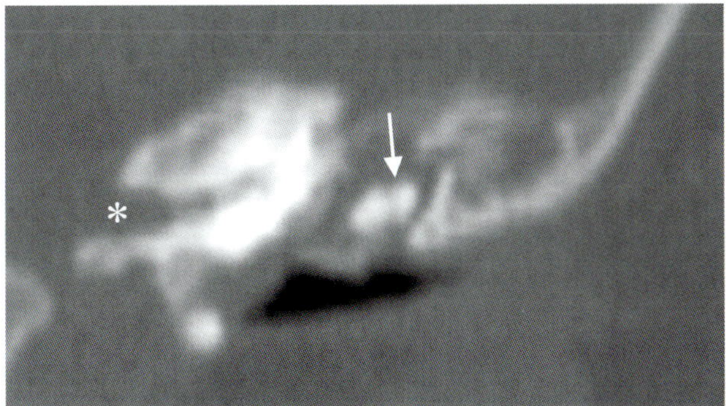

2. coronal image

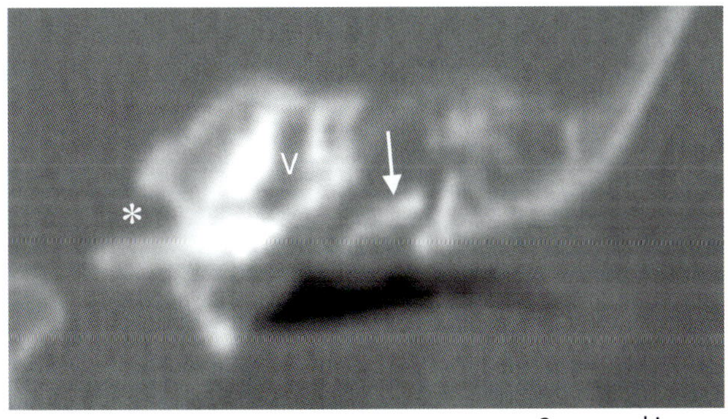

3. coronal image

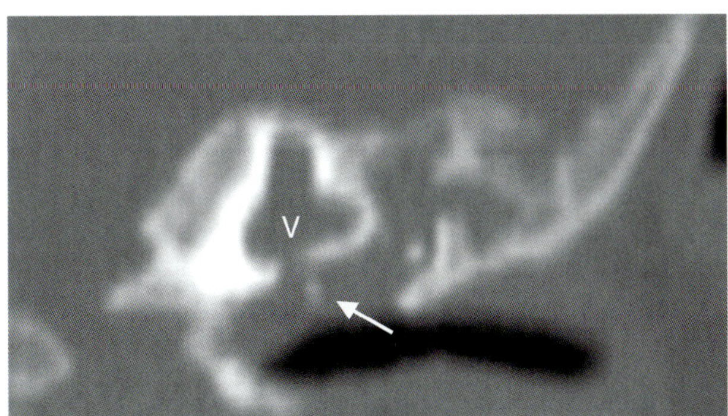

4. coronal image

Normal Control CT Findings

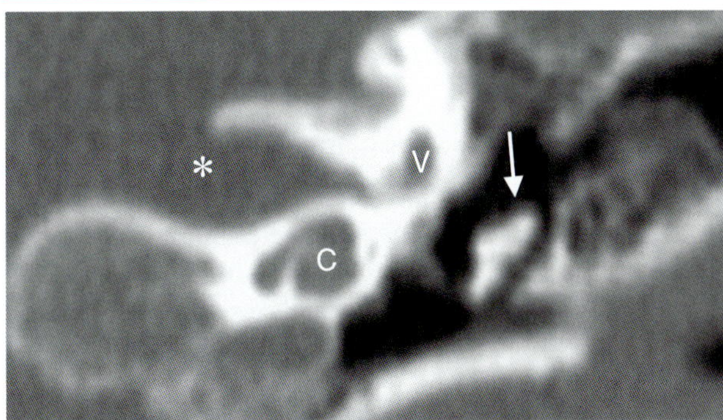

n1. coronal image

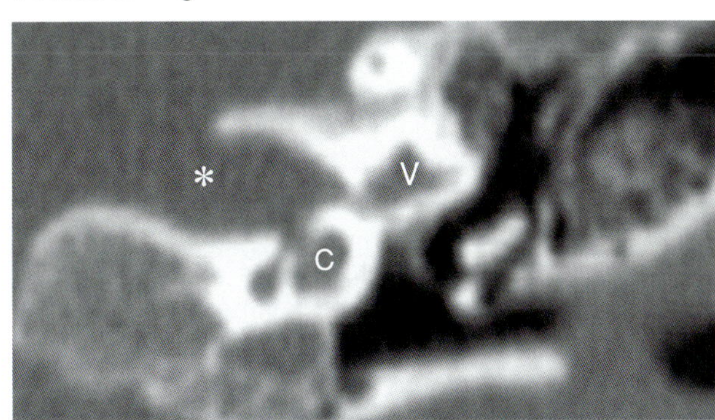

n2. coronal image

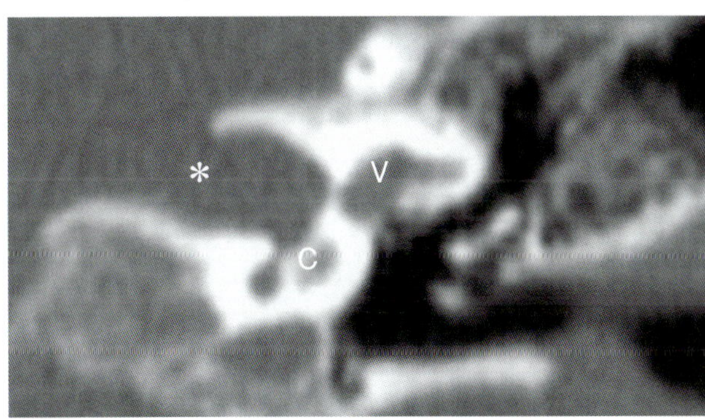

n3. coronal image

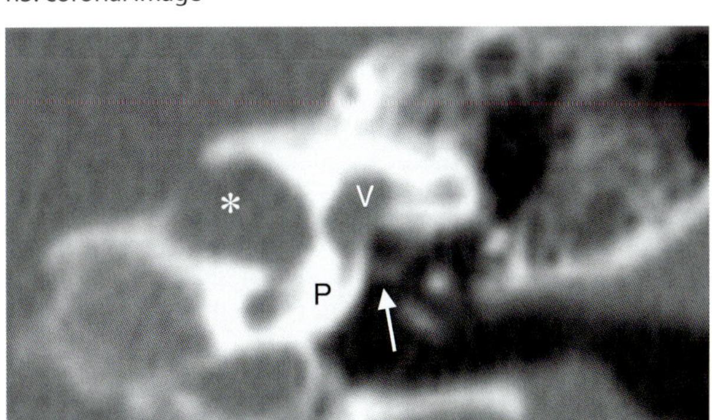

n4. coronal image

Fig. 27. (Case 2) CT

[Patient CT Findings]

In the inner ear, even though the so-called pars superior is formed to some extent (3, 4: **V**), the pars inferior is almost completely absent (1: ✎). The lateral and anterior semicircular canals are fused and sacculated, with the loops unformed (4: **V**). The internal auditory canal (1–3: ✿) is located more anteriorly and inferiorly than normal and is short and narrow. On examination of the middle ear, the ossicles in this case are almost normal and the malleus, incus, and stapes can all be observed (1–3: ↓ ; 4: ✎), but except for the epitympanum and mastoid antrum the pneumatic cavities are undeveloped and filled with soft tissue density, including the tympanic cavity.

《Normal Control CT Findings》

n1: **V** vestibule; **C** cochlea; ↓ ossicles; ✿ internal auditory canal. Repeated in n2, n3, and n4. n4: **P** promontory; ↑ stapes.

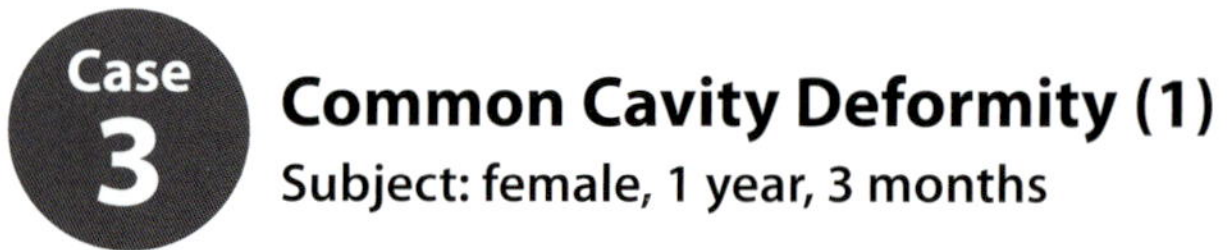

Case 3 — Common Cavity Deformity (1)

Subject: female, 1 year, 3 months

■ History and Clinical Findings

There were no particular perinatal abnormalities. The subject did not undergo newborn hearing screening. At around one year the subject was examined by a local otolaryngologist to address worries about delayed language development, then subject to auditory testing in the otolaryngology department of a general hospital. The subject was unresponsive to both ABR and ASSR, and was fitted with a hearing aid as an initial step. However, the hearing aid was ineffective, so the subject was brought to our department to determine candidacy for a cochlear implant. There were no abnormalities of the auricle or external auditory canal. The tympanic membrane itself displayed no abnormalities, but there was otitis media with effusion in the right ear along with a history of recurring otitis media. There were no developmental abnormalities except for delays in language and social interaction due to hearing loss.

■ Patient CT Findings

Findings are for the right ear. First, examining the axial images, the area corresponding to the cochlea is smaller than the normal control (fig. 28:1) and forms a common cavity with no separation from the vestibule. The vestibule and lateral semicircular canal form a single cavity (fig. 28:2–4), but the anterior and posterior semicircular canals are looped (fig. 28:2, 3, 4). Between this common cavity and the internal auditory canal, a thin bony partition can be found (fig. 28:2). The labyrinthine segment of the facial nerve is separated more than usual anteriorly from the internal auditory canal (fig. 28:1), while the tympanic segment is located immediately lateral to the common cavity and runs posterior to the inferior side of the prominence of the lateral semicircular canal. Overall air cell development of the middle ear is inhibited, but the ossicles display no clear abnormalities.

Next, examining the coronal images, it is readily apparent that the space corresponding to the cochlea is slightly protruding inferiorly from the cavity. Also, one can clearly see that, while the lateral semicircular canal is cystic, the anterior semicircular canal forms a separate loop (fig. 28:4).

■ Patient MRI Findings

Axial MR images for the left and right ears are shown in fig. 29:1R and 1L. Both sides form a common cavity with uniform T2 hyperintense signal inside the cavity and the modiolus, membranous labyrinth, and other structures indiscernible. The partition between the inner ear cavity and the internal auditory canal is clear on the right (fig. 29:1R), but unclear on the left (fig. 29:1L), with the possibility that the internal auditory canal and the common cavity are connected. In considering fenestration of the inner ear during cochlear implant surgery, because the left ear displays a high apparent risk for cerebrospinal fluid leakage (a "gusher") or meningitis due to retrograde infection from the middle ear, we settled on the right ear

as more appropriate for surgery.

Examining the 3-dimensional reconstructed MR image (fig. 29:2R, 2L), the overall morphology and points of abnormality are easily discerned. The area corresponding to the cystic lateral semicircular canal displays almost no left-right difference, but the pars inferior, which corresponds to the cochlea, is more solidly formed on the right. Also, on examination of the semicircular canals, while in the right ear the posterior and anterior semicircular canals are separated and have a common crus (fig. 29:2R), in the left ear the two form a single, undifferentiated loop (fig. 29:2L). These minor disparities between the left and right ears are difficult to spot through observation of axial images alone.

■ Surgical Findings

Cochlear implantation was performed on the right ear, as it was determined from image findings that the probability of a gusher was lower on this side, overall differentiation of the inner ear was slightly more advanced than the left side, and the area corresponding to the cochlea was slightly larger. A mastoidectomy and posterior tympanotomy were performed, the incudostapedial joint severed and the incus extracted, and an approx. 2.5 mm diameter fenestration performed on the common cavity in the anterior end of the lateral semicircular canal prominence. No gusher occurred, and a straight electrode bent in the shape of a U was inserted through the fenestrated portion. During surgery we tried to find a way to implant the electrode as deeply as possible, but due to such factors as the electrode's tendency to spring straight we concluded the operation with it positioned slightly more shallowly than our original objective (fig. 30:1a, 1b, 1c). In postoperative mapping, the electrodes induced nystagmus in response to auditory stimulation, and it was established through verification of the CT images that the problem occurred on the portion contacting the area immediately lateral to the floor of the internal auditory canal. The effectiveness of the cochlear implant was examined with these electrodes disabled. The result was that, while response to sound was apparent, it was insufficient, and revision surgery was performed one year after initial surgery.

In revision surgery, we widely opened the area in the common cavity corresponding to the lateral semicircular canal and directly viewed the cavity's interior (fig. 30:2b). A thin bony partition was ascertained on the floor of the internal auditory canal (through which cerebrospinal fluid was faintly visible), and the electrode bent in the shape of a U was laid anteroinfeior to it. The wide fenestration allowed us to deliberately install the electrode on the anteroinferior segment of the cavity and stabilize it (fig. 30:2c). In the postoperative CT image as well, it was confirmed that the electrode was installed in the position assumed to correspond to the cochlea on the anteroinferior segment of the common cavity (fig. 30:2a, 2b). Postoperatively, a remarkable improvement in sound response compared to the results of the initial operation was obtained using the 12 electrodes in the central region of the array. However, leakage of stimulation current from the electrodes in the tip and base of the array near the fenestrated part of the cavity stimulated the facial nerve, so the device is being used with these electrodes disabled.

Patient CT Findings	**Normal Control CT Findings**

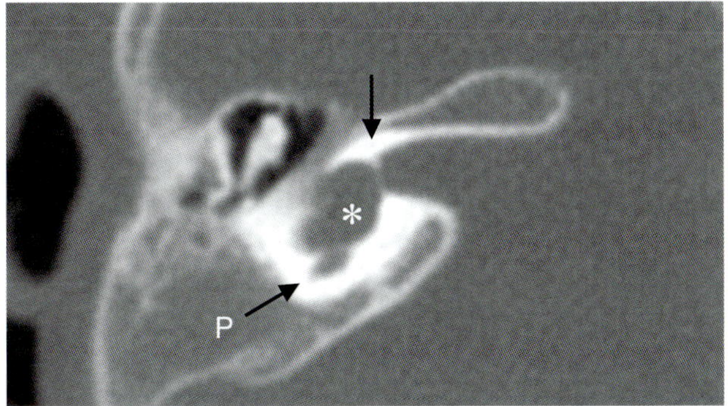

1. axial image

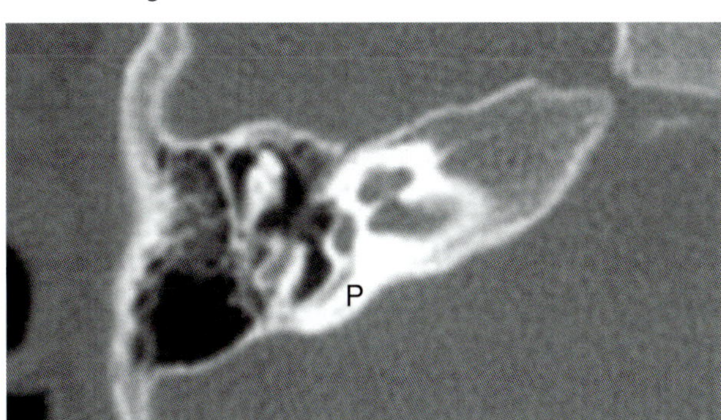

n1. axial image

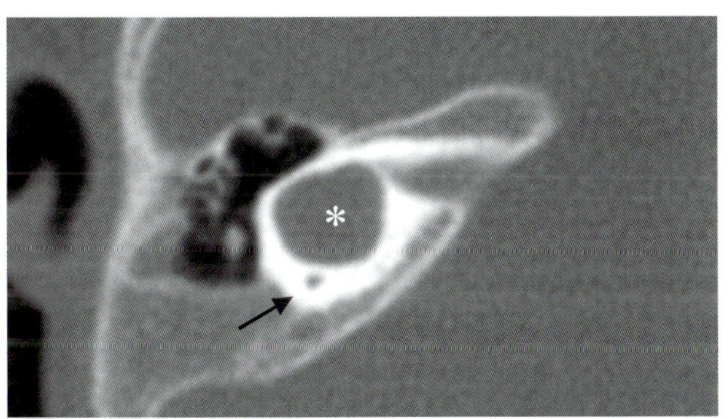

2. axial image

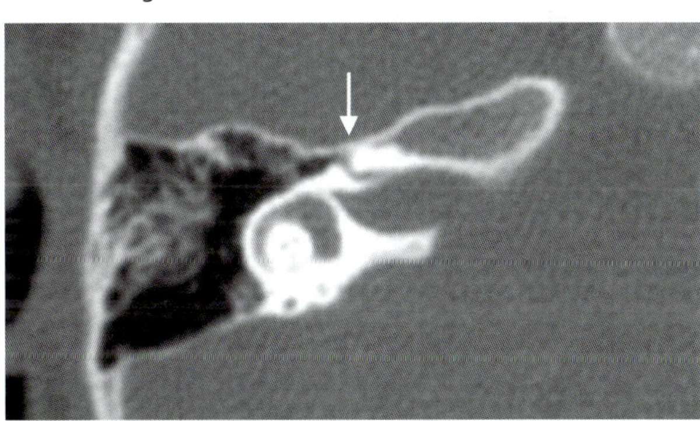

n2. axial image

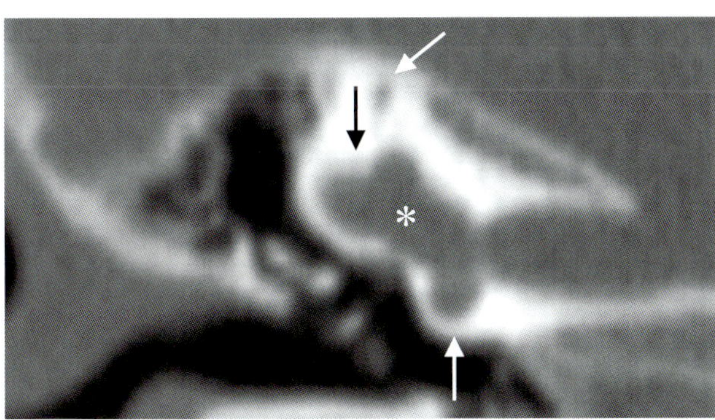

3. axial image

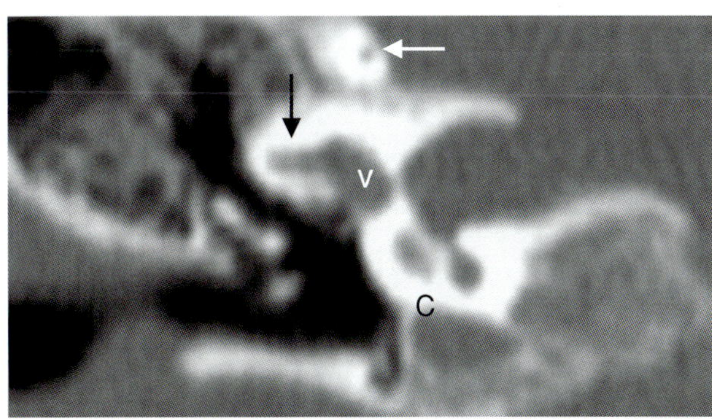

n3. axial image

4. coronal image   n4. coronal image

Fig. 28. (Case 3) CT

[Patient CT Findings]

The area corresponding to the cochlea is smaller than the normal control (1: ↖) and forms a common cavity with no separation from the vestibule. The vestibule and lateral semicircular canal form a single cavity (2–4: ✳), but the anterior and posterior semicircular canals are looped (2: **P** ↗, 3: ↗, 4· ✐) Between this common cavity and the internal auditory canal, a thin bony partition can be found (2: ↓). The labyrinthine segment of the facial nerve is separated more than usual anteriorly from the internal auditory canal (1: ↧). Overall air cell development of the middle ear is inhibited, but the ossicles display no clear abnormalities. It is readily apparent that the space corresponding to the cochlea (4: ↑) is slightly protruding inferiorly from the cavity. One can clearly see that, while the lateral semicircular canal is cystic (4: ↓), the anterior semicircular canal forms a separate loop (4: ✐).

《Normal Control CT Findings》

n1: ↖ cochlea. n2: **P** posterior semicircular canal. n3: ↧ labyrinthine segment of facial nerve. n4: ↓ lateral semicircular canal; ↩ anterior semicircular canal; **V** vestibule; **C** cochlea.

Patient MRI and 3-Dimensional Reconstructed MRI Findings

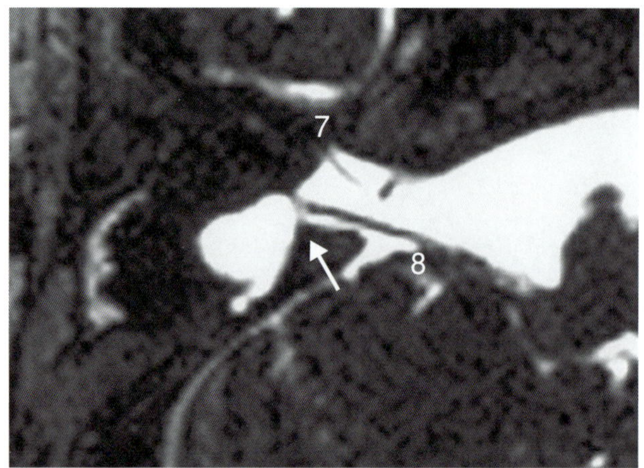

1R. axial image

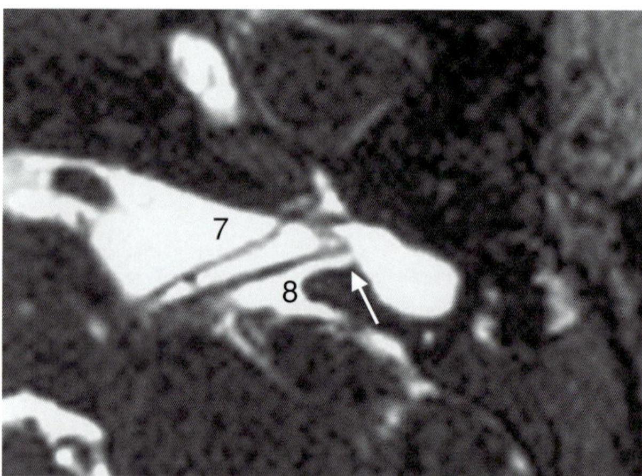

1L. axial image

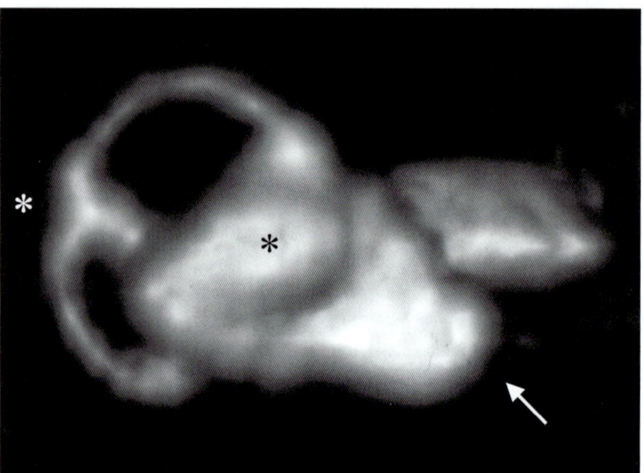

2R. 3-dimensional reconstructed MRI

2L. 3-dimensional reconstructed MRI

Fig. 29. (Case 3) MRI, 3-dimensional reconstructed MRI

[Patient MRI and 3-Dimensional Reconstructed MRI Findings]

Both sides form a common cavity with uniform T2 hyperintense signal inside the cavity and the modiolus, membranous labyrinth, and other structures indiscernible. The partition between the inner ear cavity and the internal auditory canal is clear on the right (1R: ⬉), but unclear on the left (1L: ⬉), with the possibility that the internal auditory canal and the common cavity are connected. In considering fenestration of the inner ear during cochlear implant surgery, the left ear displays a high apparent risk of cerebrospinal fluid leakage (a "gusher") or meningitis due to retrograde infection from the middle ear. The area corresponding to the cystic lateral semicircular canal (2R, 2L: ✱) displays almost no left-right difference, but the pars inferior (2R: ⬉, 2L: ⬈), which corresponds to the cochlea, is more solidly formed on the right. On examination of the semicircular canals, while in the right ear the posterior and anterior semicircular canals are separated and have a common crus (2R: ✿), in the left ear the two form a single, undifferentiated loop (2L: ✿).

Patient CT and X-Ray Findings

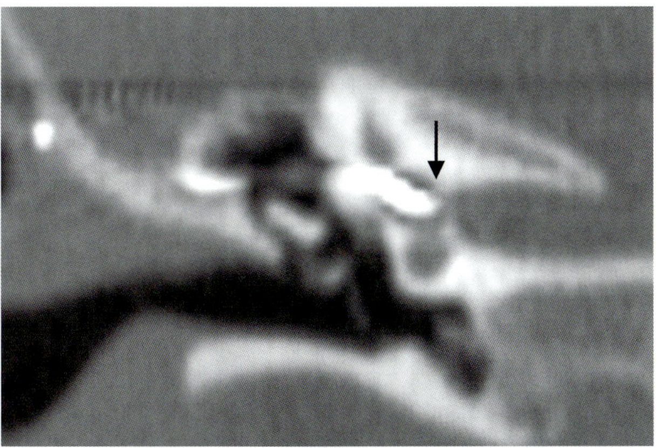

1a.   CT: Initial surgery

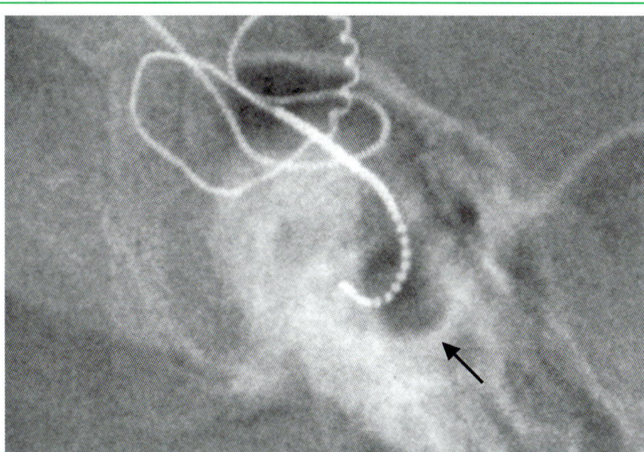

1c.   X-ray: Initial surgery

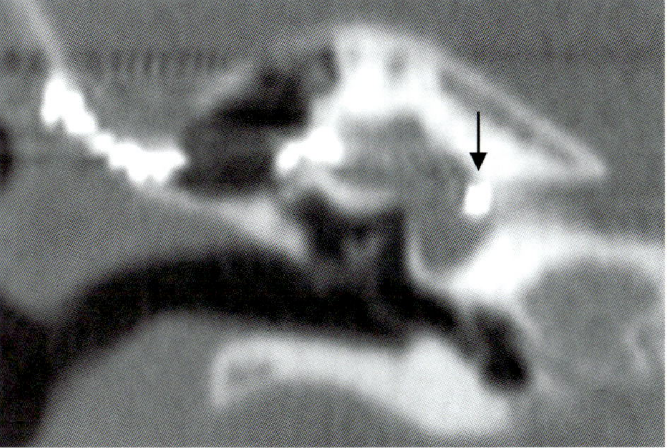

1b.   CT: Initial surgery

[Patient CT and X-Ray Findings—1]

Initial Surgery: An approx. 2.5 mm diameter fenestration was performed on the common cavity in the anterior end of the lateral semicircular canal prominence. A straight electrode bent in the shape of a U was inserted through the fenestrated portion. During surgery we tried to find a way to implant the electrode as deeply as possible, but due to such factors as the electrode's tendency to spring straight we concluded the operation with it positioned slightly more shallowly than our original objective (1a:↓, 1b:↓, 1c:↖).

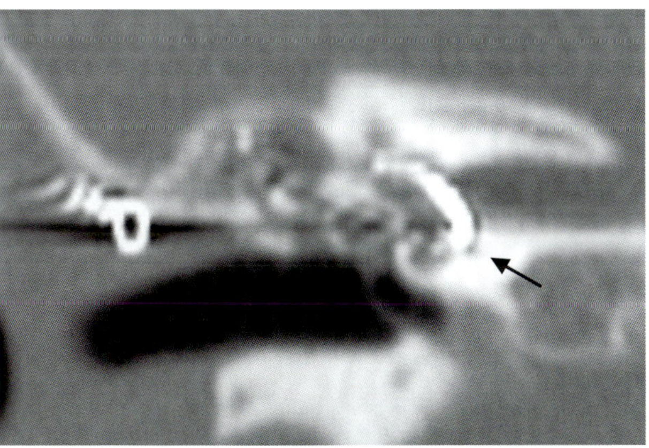

2a.   CT: Revision surgery

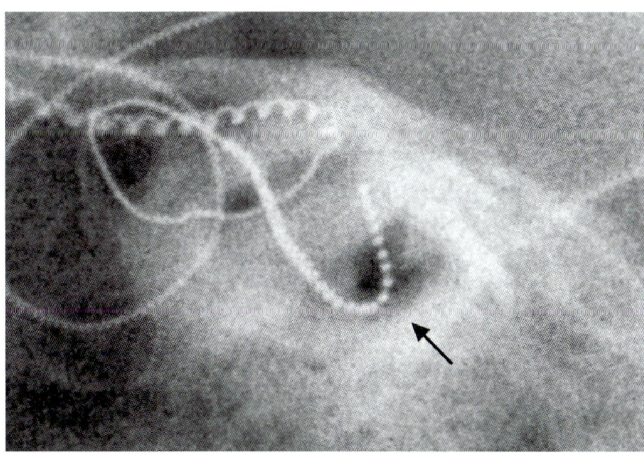

2c.   X-ray: Revision surgery

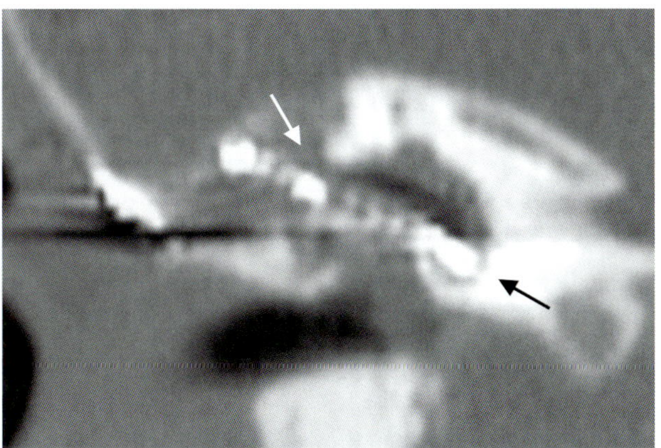

2b.   CT: Revision surgery

[Patient CT and X-Ray Findings—2]

Revision Surgery: In revision surgery, we widely opened the area in the common cavity corresponding to the lateral semicircular canal and directly viewed the cavity's interior (2b: ↘). A thin bony partition was ascertained on the floor of the internal auditory canal, and the electrode bent in the shape of a U was laid anteroinferior to it. The wide fenestration allowed us to deliberately install the electrode on the anteroinferior segment of the cavity and stabilize it (2c: ↖). In the postoperative CT image as well, it was confirmed that the electrode is installed in the position assumed to correspond to the cochlea on the anteroinferior segment of the common cavity (2a: ↖, 2b: ↖).

Fig. 30. (Case 3) CT, X-ray

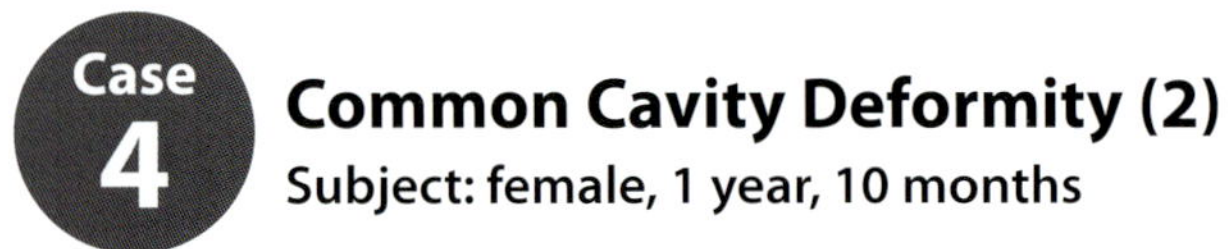

Case 4 — **Common Cavity Deformity (2)**
Subject: female, 1 year, 10 months

■ History and Clinical Findings

At around one year five months, the subject's parents noticed that her language development was delayed. At the 18-month physical exam, hearing loss was identified and the subject underwent testing at a pediatric hospital, where she was diagnosed with severe hearing loss due to bilateral inner ear malformation. The infant patient was fitted with a hearing aid, but disliked it and resisted wearing it regularly. The subject was referred to our department at one year ten months to determine the indication for cochlear implant surgery. Both ears were unresponsive to ABR and ASSR, and even with COR no auditory response was observed at maximum sound stimulus level.

■ Patient CT Findings

The cochlea and vestibule are undifferentiated, forming a common cavity (fig. 31:2–4). The center area of the common cavity is slightly indented, and generally, the anteroinferior portion may be thought to correspond to the cochlea and the posterosuperior portion to the vestibule. The vestibular part is cystic overall, with only the posterior semicircular canal (fig. 31:2, 3) partially formed. As in Case 3, the path of the labyrinthine segment of the facial nerve is abnormal, running anteriorly starting from slightly anterior and medial position of the internal auditory canal (fig. 31:3). A bony partition can be observed between the common cavity and the internal auditory canal (fig. 31:3). In the coronal image, normally both the position and the shape of the vestibule and cochlea can be clearly determined (fig. 31:n4), but in this case, it is impossible to morphologically differentiate between the pars inferior of the cochlea and the pars superior of the vestibule (fig. 31:4).

Turning our attention to the middle ear, we find that mastoid air cell development is favorable and there are no anomalies of the malleus and incus. However, although normally the footplate of the stapes can be observed in the oval window (fig. 31:n2), in this case it cannot be ascertained. Also, a small soft tissue density mass is present lateral to the area corresponding to the oval window, continuous with the common cavity (fig. 31:1, 2, 4). This mass, which is further examined in the MRI findings, could be either a congenital cholesteatoma or a herniation of the inner ear structure.

■ Patient MRI Findings

The common cavity shows high T2 signal intensity due to labyrinthine fluid, but some low T2 signal structures are observed, which may be some sort of membranous labyrinth. The mass lateral to the oval window mentioned in the section on CT findings is T2 hyperintense and continuous with the common cavity (fig. 32:1), leading us to suspect herniation of inner ear structure. The structure marked P in figure 32:2 and 3 is a single vertical semicircular canal continuous to the posterior or anterior semicircular canal.

Cranial nerves VII and VIII can be observed inside the internal auditory canal (fig. 32:2, 3: 7 and 8), but division of cranial nerve VIII into the cochlear nerve and vestibular nerve cannot be confirmed. As suggested in the CT findings, the facial nerve runs slightly anteriorly starting from slightly central to the fundus (fig. 32:2: 7). The common cavity is independent of the internal auditory canal, separated by a thick septum (fig. 32:2).

■ Surgical Findings

At two years one month, cochlear implant surgery was performed on the right ear using a straight electrode. A mastoidectomy with posterior tympanotomy was carried out and the incudostapedial joint severed. The long process of the incus was deformed and curved, and the footplate of the stapes between the anterior and posterior limbs was absent. A thin, sacculated structure was herniated and protruding laterally; when incised, it exuded clear labyrinthine fluid. The incus was removed to secure a broad field of view of the posterior half of the epitympanum and an approx. 2.5 mm diameter fenestration performed in the vicinity of the anterior end of the lateral semicircular canal prominence to examine the cavity's interior (fig. 33:1).

A spiderweb-like membrane of soft tissue was present inside the common cavity. This was appropriately transected so as not to interfere with electrode insertion. The size of the common cavity had previously been measured on the images and the electrode bent into a loop to enable it to cover a broad area of the anterior portion of the cavity, then inserted through the fenestration (fig. 33:1). It was confirmed through the fenestration that the electrode was in contact along the cavity wall (fig. 33:2) and the cavity was filled with muscle pieces and fascia. The oval window in particular was filled with soft tissue from inside the cavity so as to occlude the defective area on the footplate of the stapes. Intraoperative X-ray images confirmed that the electrode had been positioned as planned and the bend was smooth (fig. 33:3). Neural Response Telemetry (NRT) testing confirmed a clear response from the cochlear nerve with electrical stimulation of all electrodes (fig. 33:4).

Patient CT Findings

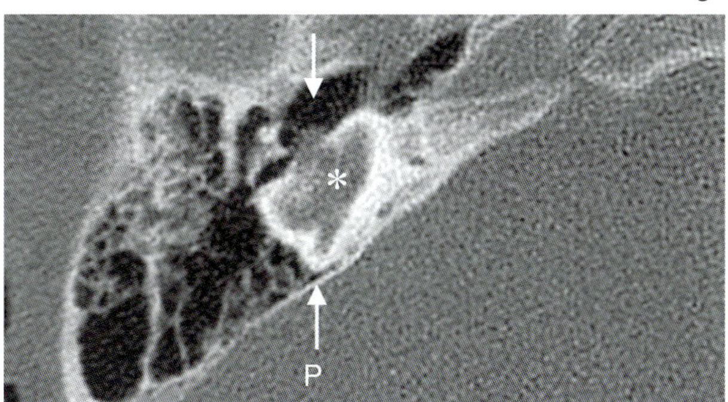

1. axial image

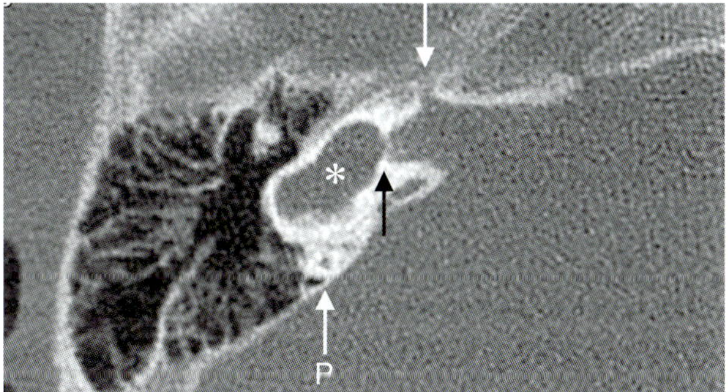

2. axial image

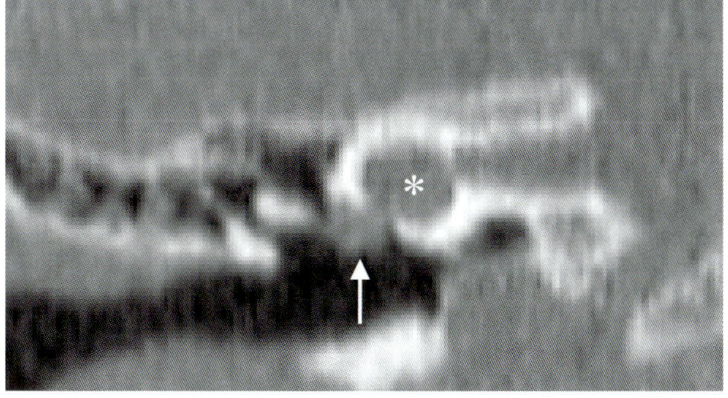

3. axial image

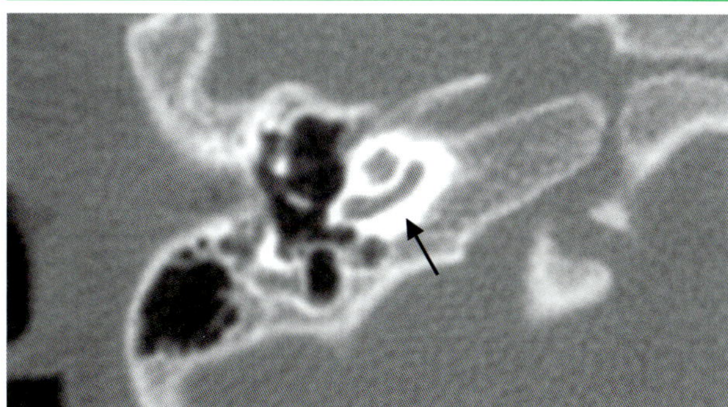

4. coronal image

Normal Control CT Findings

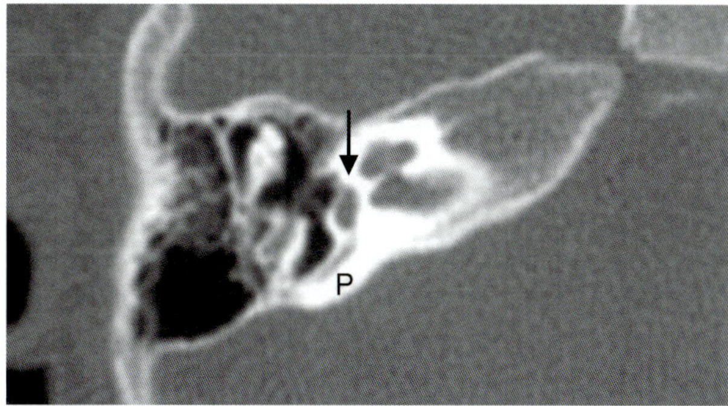

n1. axial image

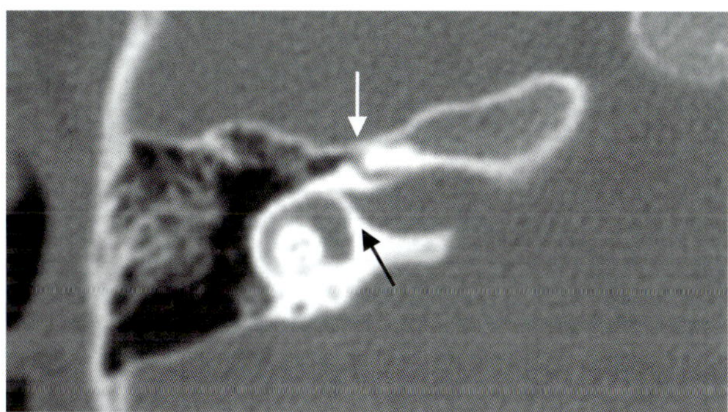

n2. axial image

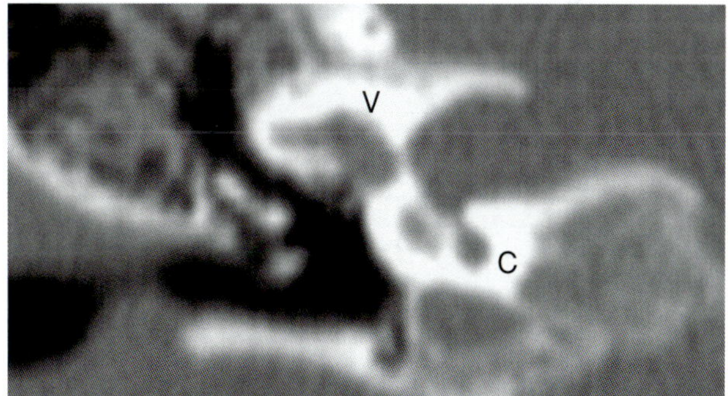

n3. axial image

n4. coronal image

Fig. 31. (Case 4) CT

[Patient CT Findings]

The cochlea and vestibule are undifferentiated, forming a common cavity (2–4: ✿). The center area of the common cavity is slightly indented, and generally, the anteroinferior portion may be thought to correspond to the cochlea and the posterosuperior portion to the vestibule. The vestibular part is cystic overall, with only the posterior semicircular canal (2, 3: **P** ⇑) partially formed. The path of the labyrinthine segment of the facial nerve is abnormal, running anteriorly starting from slightly anterior and medial position of the internal auditory canal (3: ⇓). A bony partition can be observed between the common cavity and the internal auditory canal (3: ⇑). In the coronal image, it is impossible to morphologically differentiate between the pars inferior of the cochlea and the pars

superior of the vestibule (4: ✿). Mastoid air cell development is favorable and there are no anomalies of the malleus and incus, however the footplate of the stapes cannot be ascertained. Also, a small soft tissue density mass is present lateral to the area corresponding to the oval window, continuous with the common cavity (1, 2: ⇓; 4: ⇑).

《Normal Control CT Findings》

n1: ↘ cochlea. n2: ↓ oval window, footplate of stapes; **P** posterior semicircular canal. n3: ⇓ labyrinthine segment of facial nerve; ↘ bony wall of internal auditory canal floor. n4: **V** vestibule; **C** cochlea.

Patient MRI Findings

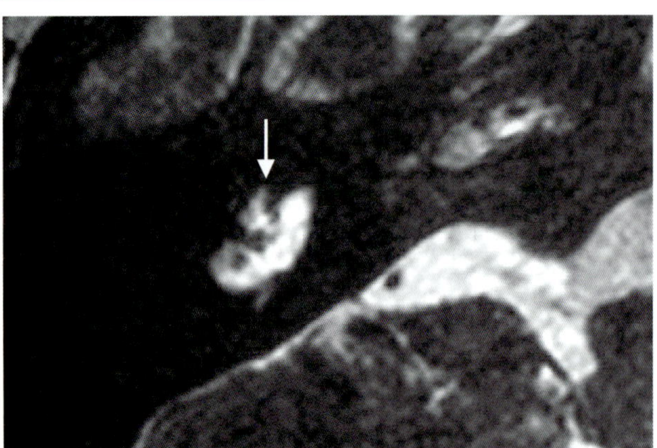

1. axial image

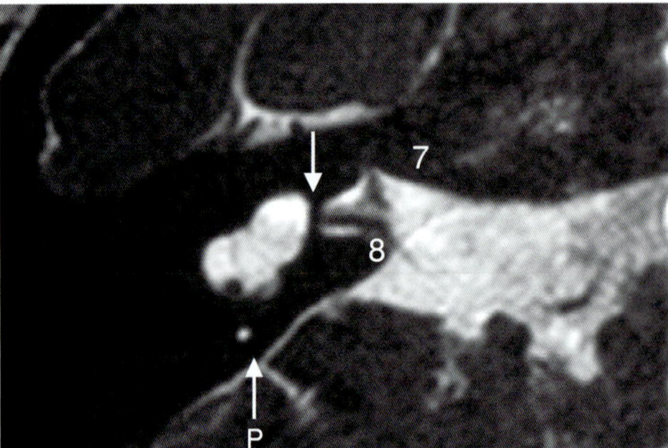

2. axial image

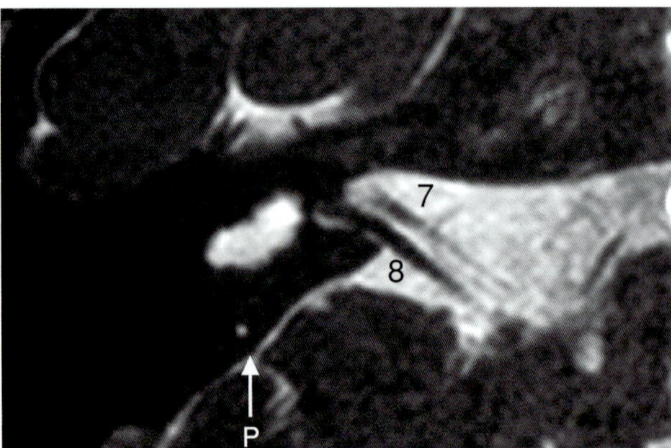

3. axial image

Fig. 32. (Case 4) MRI

〖Patient MRI Findings〗

The common cavity shows high T2 singal intensity due to labyrinthine fluid, but some low T2 signal structures are observed, which may be some sort of membranous labyrinth formation. The mass lateral to the oval window is T2 hyperintense and continuous with the common cavity (1: ⇓), and herniation of inner ear structure is suspected. The structure marked **P** in 2 and 3 is a single vertical semicircular canal continuous to the posterior or anterior semicircular canal. Cranial nerves VII and VIII can be observed inside the internal auditory canal (2, 3: **7** and **8**), but division of cranial nerve VIII into the cochlear nerve and vestibular nerve cannot be confirmed. The facial nerve runs slightly anteriorly starting from slightly central to the fundus (2: **7**). The common cavity is independent of the internal auditory canal, separated by a thick septum (2: ⇓).

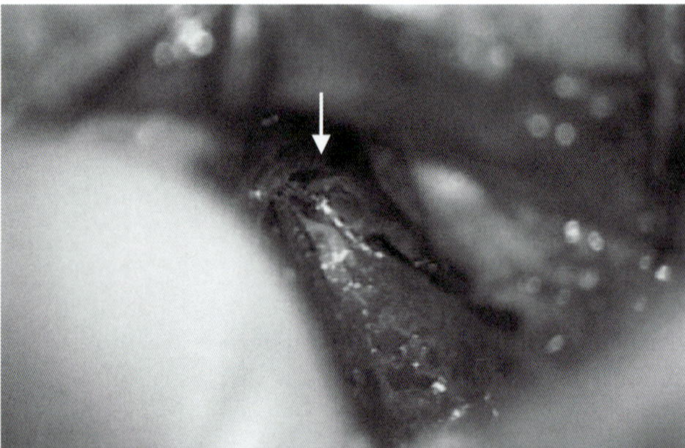

1. Intraoperative findings: The common cavity is fenestrated on the anterior end of the area corresponding to the vestibule and the electrode (↓) inserted.

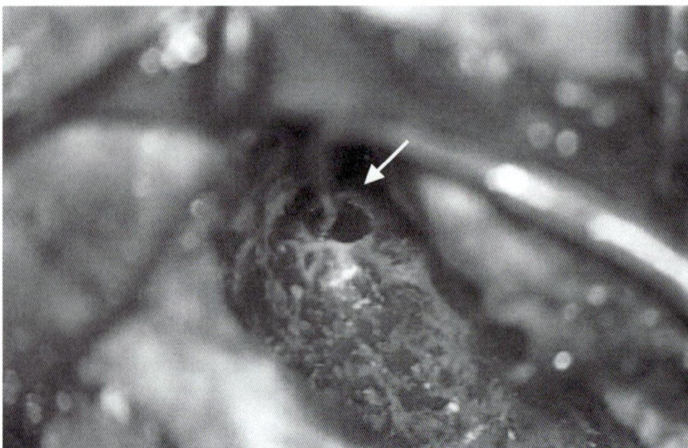

2. Intraoperative findings: Insertion of the cochlear implant electrode (↙) has just been completed.

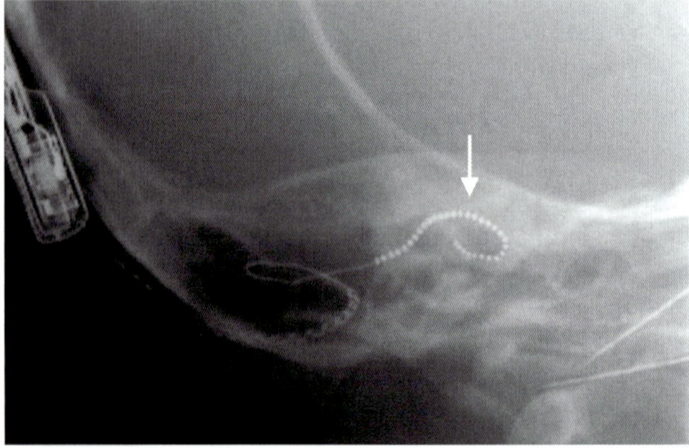

3. Intraoperative X-ray image: ↓ indicates the electrode array in the common cavity.

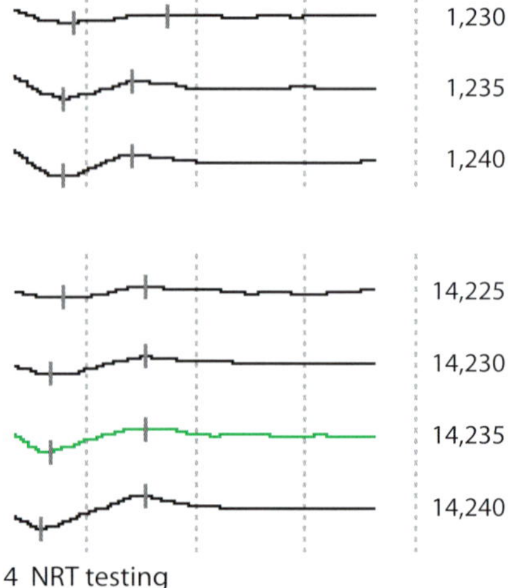

4 NRT testing

Fig. 33. (Case 4) Right ear cochlear implant surgery findings

Aplasia of Cochlear Upper Turns and Semicircular Canals with Cochlear Nerve Canal Stenosis

Case 5

Subject: female, 3 years old

■ History and Clinical Findings

This child did not undergo newborn hearing screening. Since just after one year old the parents had been worried by the child's unclear response to sound, and when even at two years she had not begun speaking they took her to an otolaryngology department of a general hospital. There she was diagnosed with severe hearing loss after ABR testing showed no response on either side with a stimulation of 105 dB NHL, whereupon the hospital referred the subject to our department for further testing. In COR testing no significant response was observed at 110 dB and, taking other findings into consideration, we recommended cochlear implantation. Since the family were concerned about the risks of surgical treatment, the subject was fitted with a hearing aid. It was confirmed that language development could not be obtained with a hearing aid, and the subject underwent cochlear implantation at the age of three.

■ Patient CT Findings

The temporal bone CT images taken during the initial medical examination by our department presented approximately the same findings for both ears. The results for the left ear are presented here. The cochlea's basal turn is thicker than normal (fig. 34:1**C**) and the upper turns can hardly be identified. The vestibule is present (fig. 34:2), but the semicircular canals are not identified (fig 34:3) except for a vestige of the posterior semicircular canal (fig 34:1).

Also, the structure of the area between the fundus of the internal auditory canal and the cochlea demands special attention in this case. Normally the cochlear base portion of the internal auditory canal, referred to as the cochlear area, is seen as a broad opening on CT images (fig. 34:n2) where the cochlear nerve fibers pass through a cribriform plate, but in this case only a narrow tube connects the fundus of the internal auditory canal with the modiolus (fig. 34:2). This type of tubular structure does not have a proper anatomical name as it does not exist in normal anatomy, but it is sometimes referred to as the cochlear nerve canal. When it is constricted, the cochlear implant efficacy is reduced, so it is important to check its condition when evaluating clinical images. This matter is discussed in further detail in the section titled "Anomalies of the internal auditory canal."

■ Patient MRI and 3-Dimensional Reconstructed MRI Findings

The modiolus can be ascertained (fig. 35:1). The individual nerves within the internal auditory canal cannot be identified as clearly as usual, but it is impossible to determine whether this is due to the nerves not being properly captured in the imaging slice or to a morphological abnormality in the nerves themselves. At the cerebellopontine angle, normally cranial nerve (CN) VIII is depicted thicker than CN VII, but here it is the reverse and CN VII is thicker, indicating the possibility that CN VIII (fig. 35:1) is atrophied or hypoplastic.

Observing the 3-dimensional reconstructed MR image of the inner ear, the overall abnormal condition is readily apparent. The cochlea in this case (fig. 35:2) ends after around 1.5 turns overall (①, ②). Compared to the normal control image, which has a second turn (fig. 35:n2, ②) and an apical turn (✳), it is clear that the upper turn is deficient. As seen in the CT images, hypoplasia of the vestibular system is conspicuous (fig. 35:2), with only a slight distention in the area assumed to be the base of the ampullae of the posterior and anterior semicircular canals.

■ Surgical Findings

Cochlear implantation was performed on the left ear. Normally in cases of inner ear malformation, use of a straight electrode array is recommended. This is because the design of a pre-curved electrode is based on the shape of a normal cochlea, so in cases of malformation it is uncertain whether or not the electrode can be properly inserted in accordance with the condition of the structure of the cochlea for each individual case. However, in this case, the modiolus was clearly present and the structure of the first turn, while slightly thicker than usual, appeared to be normal, so a pre-curved electrode was used. As a result, the electrode could be inserted smoothly without complication, and intraoperative X-ray confirmed that it had been suitably inserted in place.

Postoperative response to sound was fair, and the threshold level with cochlear implant stabilized at 45 dB.

<table>
<tr><td align="center">Patient CT Findings</td><td align="center">Normal Control CT Findings</td></tr>
<tr><td>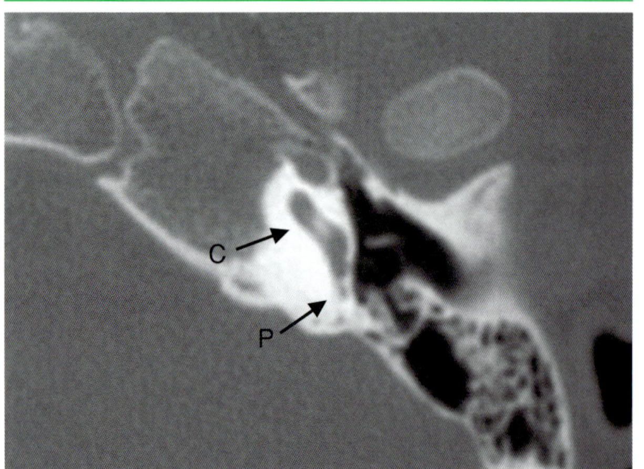</td><td>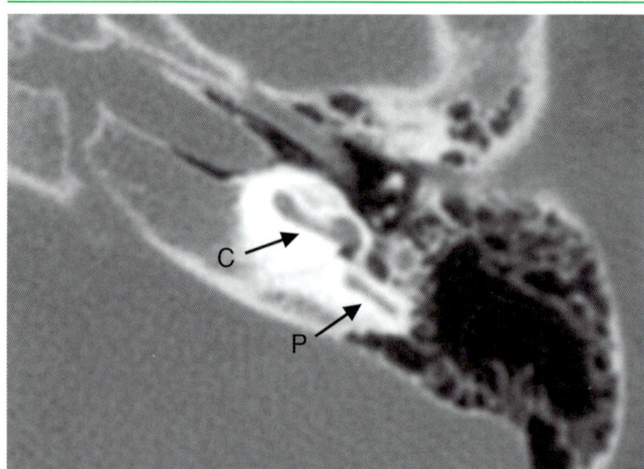</td></tr>
<tr><td>1. axial image</td><td>n1. axial image</td></tr>
<tr><td>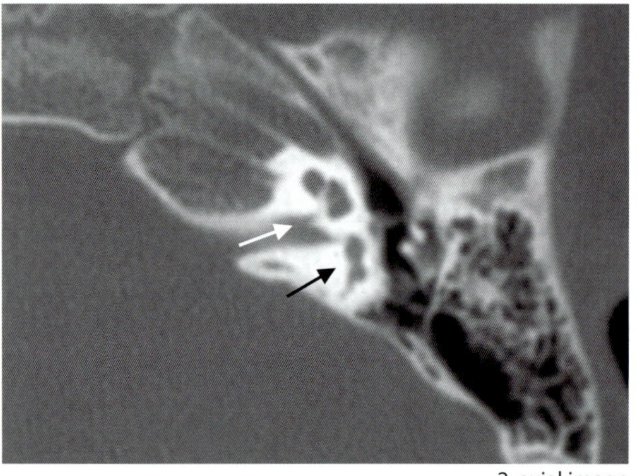</td><td>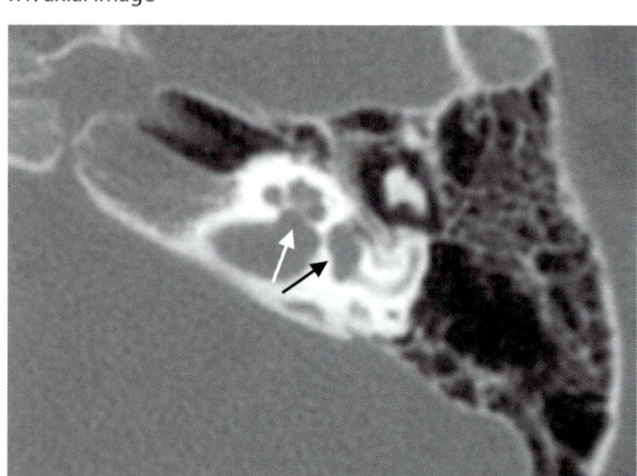</td></tr>
<tr><td>2. axial image</td><td>n2. axial image</td></tr>
<tr><td>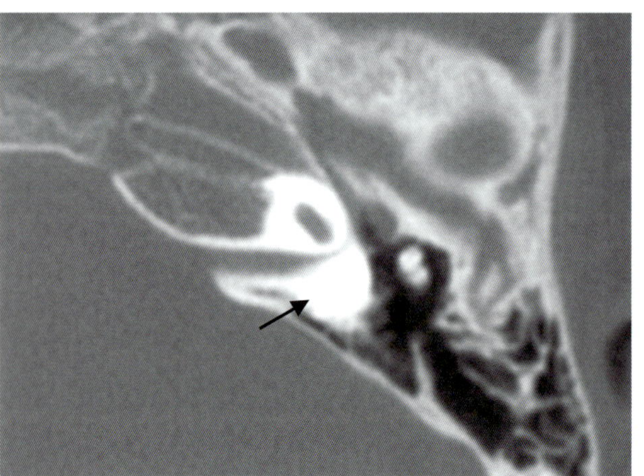</td><td>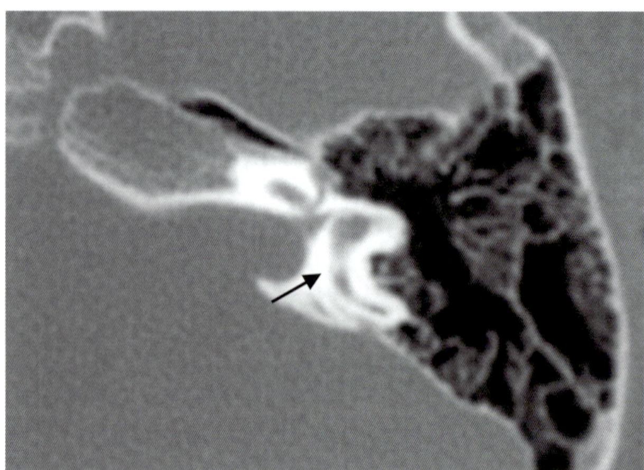</td></tr>
<tr><td>3. axial image</td><td>n3. axial image</td></tr>
</table>

Fig. 34. (Case 5) CT

[Patient CT Findings]

The cochlea's basal turn is thicker than normal (1: **C** ↗) and the upper turns can hardly be identified. Of the semicircular canals, only a vestige of the posterior semicircular canal can be seen (1: **P** ↗). The vestibule is present (2: ↗), but the semicircular canals are not identified (3: ↗). Normally the cochlear base portion of the internal auditory canal, referred to as the cochlear area, is seen as a broad opening on CT images (n2: ⇡) where the cochlear nerve fibers pass through a cribriform plate, but in this case only a narrow tube connects the fundus of the internal auditory canal with the modiolus (2: ⇗).

《Normal Control CT Findings》

n1: **C** ↗ cochlea; **P** ↗ posterior semicircular canal. n2: ⇗ cochlear area on fundus of internal auditory canal; ↗ vestibule. n3: ↗ vestibule, semicircular canals.

Patient MRI and 3-Dimensional Reconstructed MRI Findings

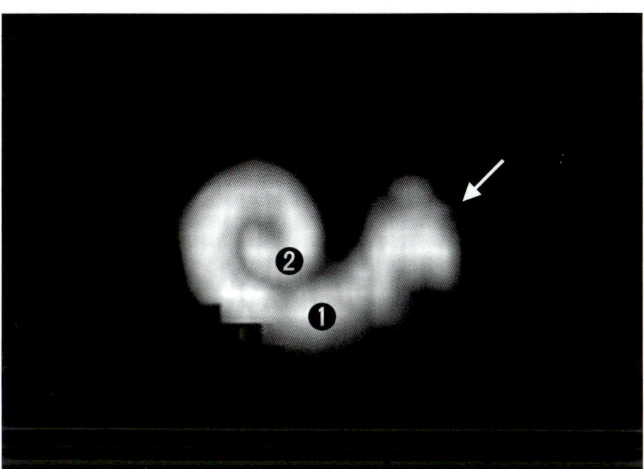

1. axial image

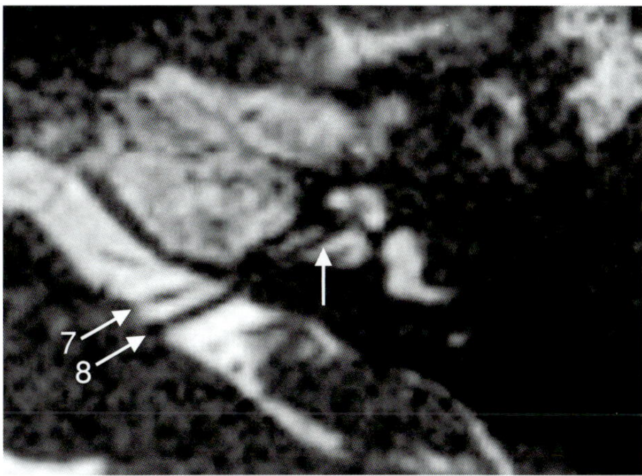

2. 3 dimensional reconstructed MRI

Normal Control MRI and 3-Dimensional Reconstructed MRI Findings

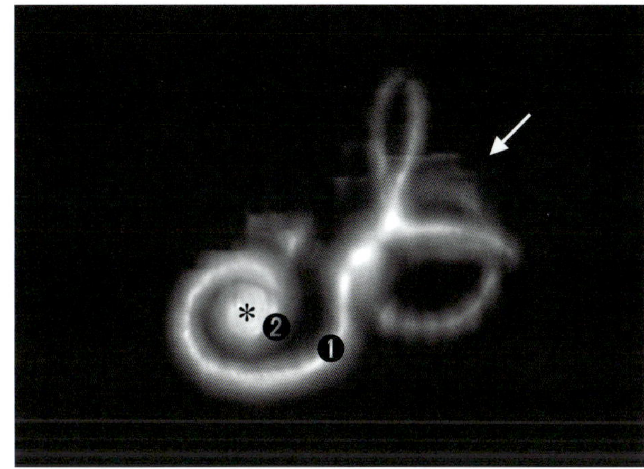

n1. axial image

n2. 3-dimensional reconstructed MRI

Fig. 35. (Case 5) MRI, 3-dimensional reconstructed MRI

[Patient MRI and 3-Dimensional Reconstructed MRI Findings]

The modiolus can be ascertained (1: ✐). The individual nerves within the internal auditory canal cannot be identified as clearly as usual. At the cerebellopontine angle, normally cranial nerve (CN) VIII is depicted thicker than CN VII, but here it is the reverse and CN VII is thicker (1: **7** ✐), indicating the possibility that CN VIII (1: **8** ✐) is atrophied or hypoplastic. The cochlea (2) ends after around 1.5 turns overall (①, ②). Compared to the normal control image, which has a second turn (n2: ②) and an apical turn (✳), it is clear that the upper turn is deficient. Hypoplasia of the vestibular system is conspicuous (2: ✐), with only a slight distention in the area assumed to be the base of the ampullae of the posterior and anterior semicircular canals.

《Normal Control MRI and 3-Dimensional Reconstructed MRI Findings》

n1: **7** ✐ facial nerve; **8** ✐ cranial nerve VIII; ↑ cochlear nerve.
n2: ① start of turn at base of cochlea; ② start of second turn; ✳ apical turn.

Case 6

Incomplete Partition Type I (IP-I): Case of Cochlear Implantation Revision
Subject: male, 3 years old

■ History and Clinical Findings

Newborn hearing screening revealed the need for further testing and the subject received a detailed examination in the otolaryngology department of a local general hospital. He was then fitted with and began wearing a hearing aid. At the time, the threshold value while wearing a hearing aid was 40–50 dB and at first language development was observed, but gradually hearing deteriorated and the effects of the hearing aid diminished, so at three years old the subject was referred to our department. In our initial exam, hearing level was 120–130 dB in the right ear and 110–120 dB in the left ear. Aided thresholds were 50 dB at 500 Hz, 65 dB at 1,000 Hz, and off the scale at 2,000 Hz and above. The developmental quotients on the Kyoto Scale of Psychological Development were as follows: Posture-Movement: 100; Cognitive-Adaptive: 94; Language-Social: 64, with developmental delay shown only in language and socialization. It was a typical profile for a hearing-impaired child without accompanying general developmental retardation. It was decided that a cochlear implant would be indicated and surgery should be performed.

■ Patient CT and MRI Findings

In CT images of the temporal bones, inner ear malformations are observed on both sides. On the right side, the basal turn and upper turn of the cochlea are unseparated and cystic (fig. 36:1R). The lateral semicircular canal is also cystic (fig. 36:2R), with the vertical semicircular canal existing separately from this cystic vestibule. The reason we refer to this structure as the "vertical semicircular canal" here is because in this case there is no common crus and the posterior and anterior semicircular canals are unified as a single semicircular canal vertical to the horizontal plane. The right inner ear is an incomplete partition type I according to the Sennaroglu-Saatci classification. On the MRI of the right side, a partition is faintly visible between the inner ear and the internal auditory canal (fig. 36:3R). Meanwhile, on the left side, the basal turn of the cochlea is thicker than normal (fig. 36:1L), and the second turn and beyond is cystic. The vestibule and lateral semicircular canal form a single cyst (fig. 36:2L), but the vertical semicircular canal is separate from it. The left ear is also diagnosed as an incomplete partition type I. On the left side, no partition is visible between the internal auditory canal and the cochlea (fig. 36:3L), so it is possible that cerebrospinal fluid is freely exchanged with the inner ear and a cerebrospinal fluid gusher is anticipated if fenestration of the cochlea is performed during cochlear implantation.

In the MR images of the cochlea, a hypointense area corresponding to the modiolus is faintly visible (fig. 36:3L). Normally, this area is hypointense due to both the bony structure of the modiolus and the cochlear nerve and spiral ganglion cells inside. However, here we have already determined from the CT images that there is no bony modiolus, so the hypointense signal in the central part of the cochlea observable on the MRI is probably the cochlear nerve and spiral ganglion cells.

Observing the 3-dimensional reconstructed MR images for this case (fig. 37:R, L), the vestibular part is formed nearly the same on both sides. For the cochlea, however, whereas on the right side (R) the cochlea has approx. 1.5 turns overall and is cystic in the upper part, on the left side (L) the basal turn is almost completely formed and the second turn and beyond is cystic, leading us to believe that the left side is slightly more differentiated than the right.

■ Surgical Findings and Postoperative Course

Cochlear implantation was performed on the left ear. A mastoidectomy was performed and the opening of the posterior tympanotomy made wider than usual in anticipation of the need for steps to be taken later in the event of a gusher. Cerebrospinal fluid erupted on fenestration of the basal turn of the cochlea, but the eruption weakened after a short time and the cochlear implant electrode (straight type) was inserted. The area between the fenestration and the electrode was then filled with pieces of temporalis fascia and sealed and fixed using fibrin glue. After waiting to confirm that there was no eruption of cerebrospinal fluid, surgery was concluded. The postoperative course went well, favorable hearing was obtained, and language acquisition was promoted.

However, two years after the operation, facial spasms started to occur with sound stimulation, and speech perception scores began to deteriorate. On viewing simple X-ray images of the electrode, in the intraoperative image taken during the initial surgery full insertion could be confirmed (fig. 38:a), but in the image taken after the occurrence of facial spasms it was apparent that the electrode had slipped out slightly (fig. 38:b). The cochlear implant installed in the initial surgery was extracted, and this time a cochlear implant with a curved electrode was implanted (fig. 38:c). This approach was followed because, in this case, the left cochlea had a modiolus, so it was surmised that a curved electrode would provide more efficient nerve stimulation than a straight one. We also hypothesized that latent cerebrospinal pressure might have pushed the electrode array out of the cochlea, and hoped that a curved electrode around the modiolus would help maintain the electrode in a stable position. The postoperative course went well, with no stimulation of the facial nerve, and the electrode array remained stable.

Patient CT and MRI Findings

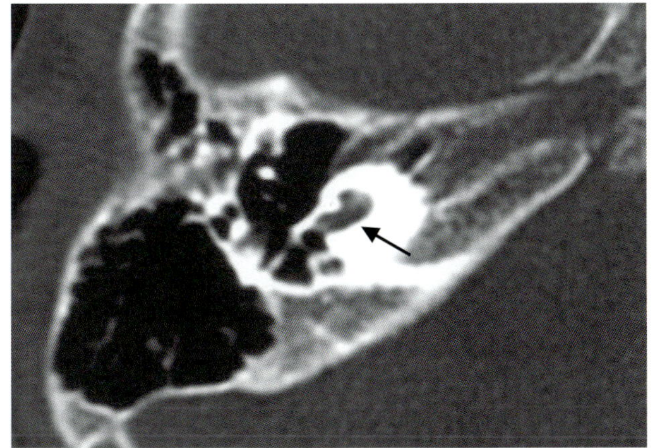

1R. CT: axial image

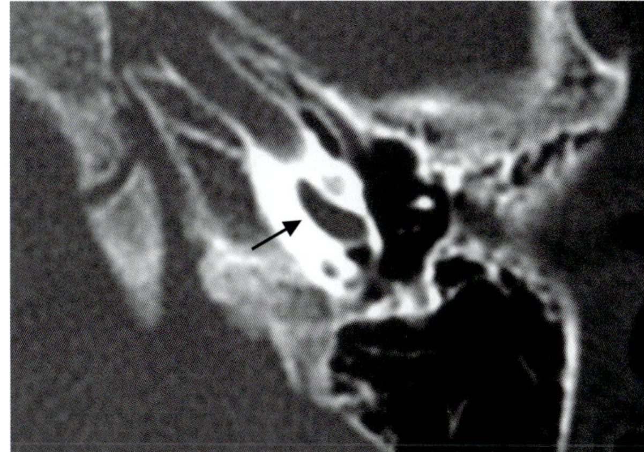

1L. CT: axial image

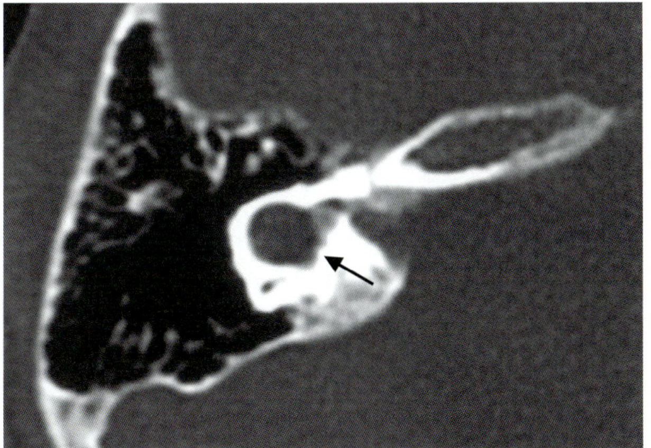

2R. CT: axial image

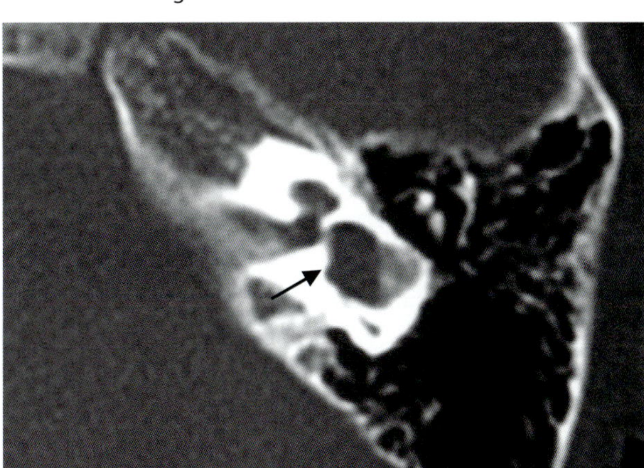

2L. CT: axial image

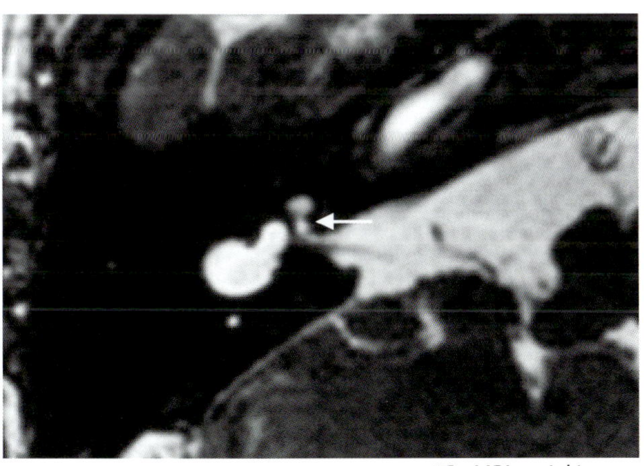

3R. MRI: axial image

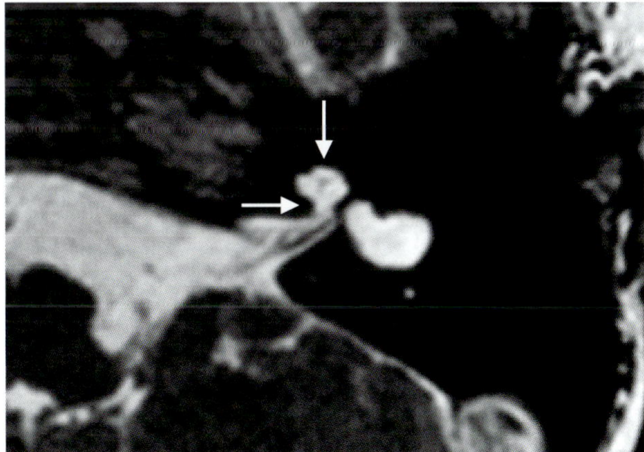

3L. MRI: axial image

Fig. 36. (Case 6) CT and MRI

〔Patient CT and MRI Findings〕

On the right side, the basal turn and upper turn of the cochlea are unseparated and cystic (1R: ↖). The lateral semicircular canal is also cystic (2R: ↖), with the vertical semicircular canal existing separately from this cystic vestibule. The right inner ear is an incomplete partition type I according to the Sennaroglu-Saatci classification. On the MRI a partition is faintly visible between the inner ear and the internal auditory canal (3R: ⇐).

Meanwhile, on the left side, the basal turn of the cochlea is thicker than normal, and the second turn and beyond is cystic. The vestibule and lateral semicircular canal form a single cyst (2L: ↗), but the vertical semicircular canal is separate

from it. The left ear is also diagnosed as an incomplete partition type I. On the left side, no partition is visible between the internal auditory canal and the cochlea (3L: ⇨). In the MR images of the cochlea, a hypointense area corresponding to the modiolus is faintly visible (3L: ⇓). Normally, this area is hypointense due to both the bony structure of the modiolus and the cochlear nerve and spiral ganglion cells inside. However, here we have already determined from the CT images that there is no bony modiolus, so the hypointense signal in the central part of the cochlea that can be observed on the MRI is probably the cochlear nerve and spiral ganglion cells.

Patient 3-Dimensional Reconstructed MRI Findings

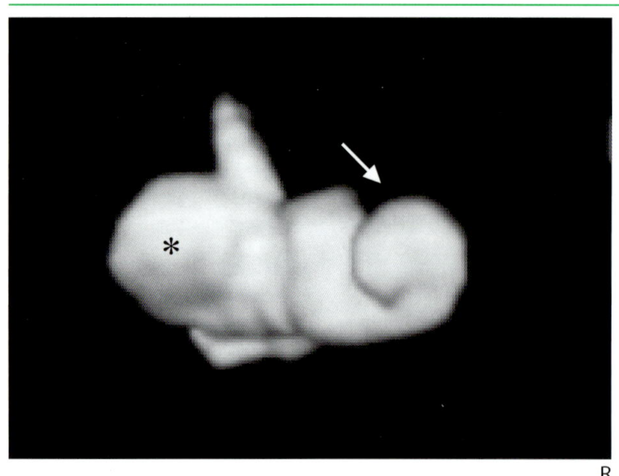
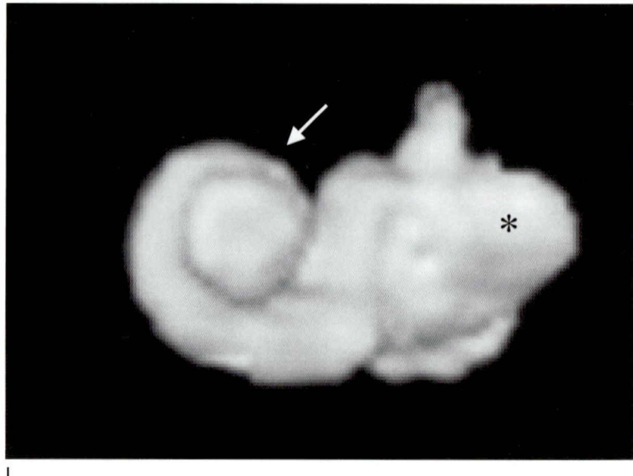

Fig. 37. (Case 6) 3-dimensional reconstructed MRI

[Patient 3-Dimensional Reconstructed MRI Findings]

Observing the 3-dimensional reconstructed MR images (R, L), the vestibular part (∗) is formed nearly the same on both sides. For the cochlea, however, whereas on the right side (R: ↘) the cochlea has approx. 1.5 turns overall and is cystic in the upper part, on the left side (L: ↗) the basal turn is almost completely formed and the second turn and beyond is cystic, leading us to believe that the left side is slightly more differentiated than the right.

Patient X-Ray Image Findings

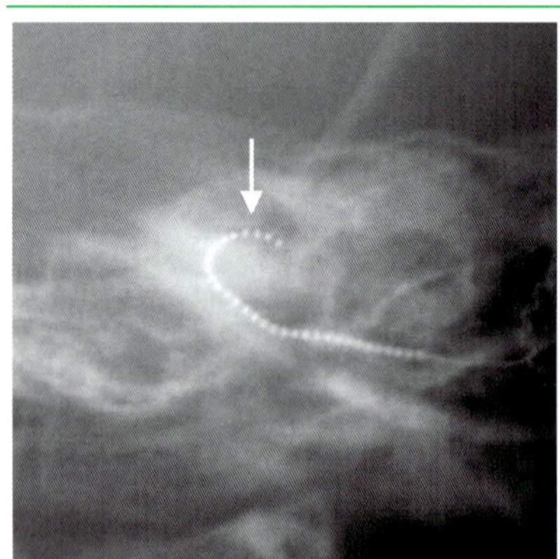
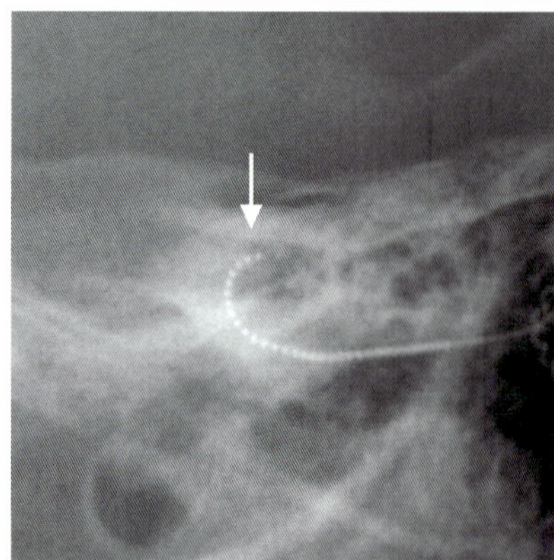
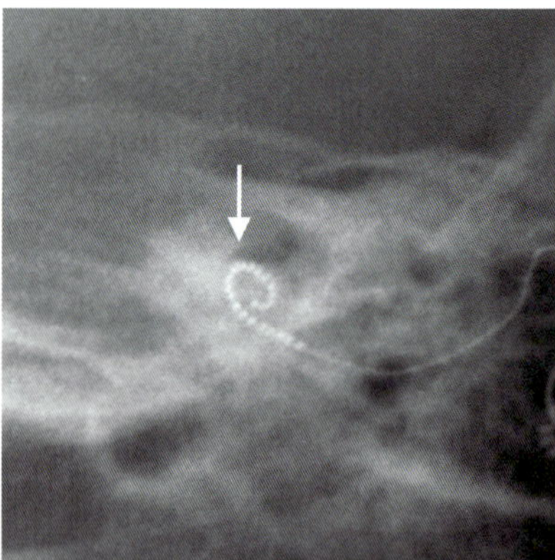

a. Initial implant (straight electrode)

b. Initial implant (same electrode as image left): facial spasms occurring

c. current implant (curved electrode)

Fig. 38. (Case 6) Postoperative X-ray images

[Patient X-Ray Image Findings]

In the intraoperative image taken during the initial surgery, full insertion could be confirmed (a: ↓), but in the image taken after the occurrence of facial spasms it was apparent that the electrode had slipped out slightly (b: ↓). The cochlear implant installed in the initial surgery was extracted, and this time a cochlear implant with a curved electrode was implanted (c: ↓).

Case 7

Incomplete Partition Type II (IP-II): Mondini Dysplasia (Enlarged Vestibular Aqueduct)

Subject: female, 7 years old

■ History and Clinical Findings

Newborn hearing screening revealed the need for further testing in both ears. The subject underwent hearing test and imaging and was diagnosed with moderate hearing loss accompanied by bilateral inner ear malformation. She was first examined by our department at three years ten months for detailed testing and evaluation of indication for a cochlear implant in the future. There were no findings of abnormality in the tympanic membranes in either ear, pure tone averages were 78.3 dB right and 93.3 dB left (fig. 39a), and spoken language had been favorably acquired through use of hearing aids in both ears, with no speech distortion. However, the subject's hearing level in both ears later showed a gradual decline, with repeated cycles of deterioration and improvement (fig. 39b), until at seven years for no particular reason hearing in both ears deteriorated, making it impossible for the subject to hear lessons at school or communicate with her peers, so she once again came to our department with her parents for consultation. At this time she exhibited bilateral deafness and completely lacked speech perception. After steroid therapy and follow-up study, cochlear implant surgery was performed on the left ear.

■ Patient CT Findings

There were no abnormalities of the external ear, middle ear, or ossicles in either ear. The findings presented are for the left ear, as findings for both ears were essentially the same. In the inner ear, whereas normally in the cochlea the structure of one or more turns can be identified after the second turn over the basal turn (fig. 40:n1, n2), in this case the basal turn is slightly thicker than normal and the upper turns form a single cavity with no partition visible between them and the modiolus (fig. 40:1). Examining the coronal image, it is readily apparent that the upper turns of the cochlea in this case are a single cystic mass (fig. 41:1). In the normal control image, observe that the structure is further divided in the second turn and beyond (fig. 41:n1). Overall 3-dimensional morphology of the inner ear will be covered in the MRI section.

The horizontal semicircular canal is slightly hypoplastic and the vestibule (fig. 40:2) is larger than normal (fig. 40:n2), but the most remarkable finding is the abnormally enlarged vestibular aqueduct. Normally the vestibular aqueduct is depicted as a line posterior to the posterior semicircular canal (fig. 40:n1, n2) and the endolymphatic sac cannot be directly observed, though it is positioned in a depression on the surface of the petrous bone (fig. 40:1). On the other hand, in this case the structure corresponding to the endolymphatic sac is clearly observable as a crevice on the posterior surface of the petrous part (fig. 40:1–3), and both the vestibular aqueduct itself and the opening to the posterior cranial fossa are extremely wide. Also, normally the origin of the vestibular aqueduct is exceedingly thin in the vestibule and invariably only partially depicted on a CT image, not becoming clearly visible until it has travelled several millimeters posteriorly (fig. 40:n3). In this case, though, one can plainly see the aqueduct leading directly medioposteriorly from the base of the common crus (fig. 40:3). However, the endolymphatic sac itself and its contents cannot be observed in the CT images because there is not enough density difference between them and the dura or the cerebrospinal fluid of the posterior cranial fossa posterior to them. The axial section diameter of the vestibular aqueduct in this case is 2.3 mm (fig. 40:4).

■ Patient MRI and 3-Dimensional Reconstructed MRI Findings

The clinically relevant points to focus attention on in the MR images for this case are the 3-dimensional morphology of the inner ear, the cochlear nerve, the vestibular aqueduct, and the endolymphatic sac.

First, examining the overall morphology of the inner ear, the insufficient turns of the cochlea could be diagnosed in the CT images, but can be more directly evaluated in the 3-dimensional reconstructed MRI. The basal turn of the cochlea in this case (fig. 41:2 ①) is little different from the normal control (fig. 41:n2 ①), but although in the normal control there is further structure (fig. 41:n2 *) superior to the second turn (fig. 41:n2 ②), in this case the area superior to the second turn is a single, cystic mass (fig. 41:2 ②).

The cochlear nerve is of normal thickness and clearly

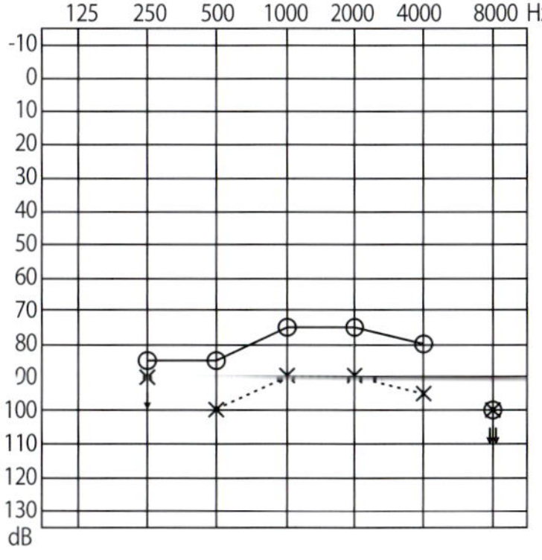

a. 3 years, 10 months

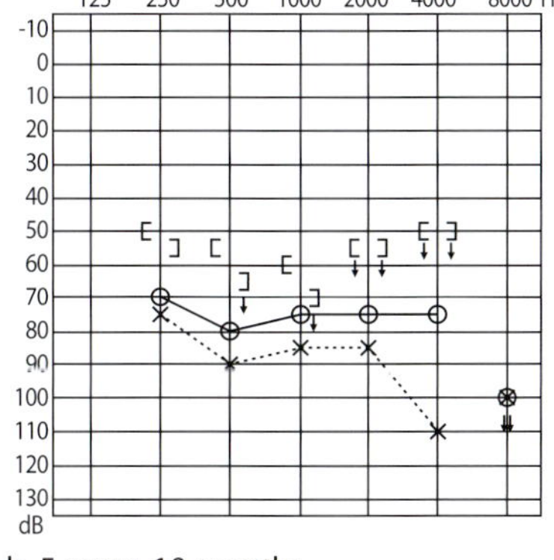

b. 5 years, 10 months

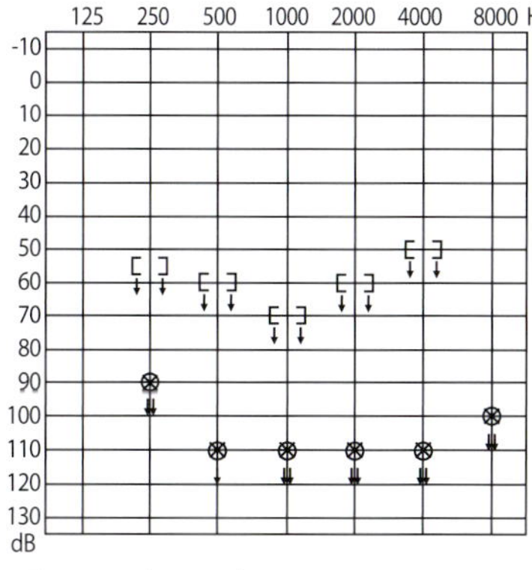

c. 7 years, 4 months

Fig. 39. (Case 7) Audiogram

Patient CT Findings

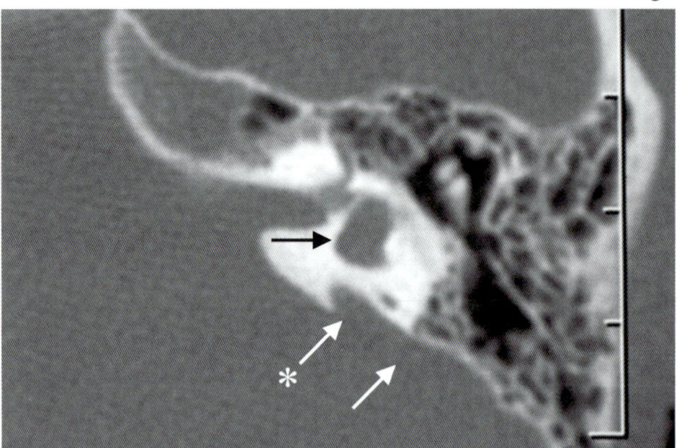

1. axial image

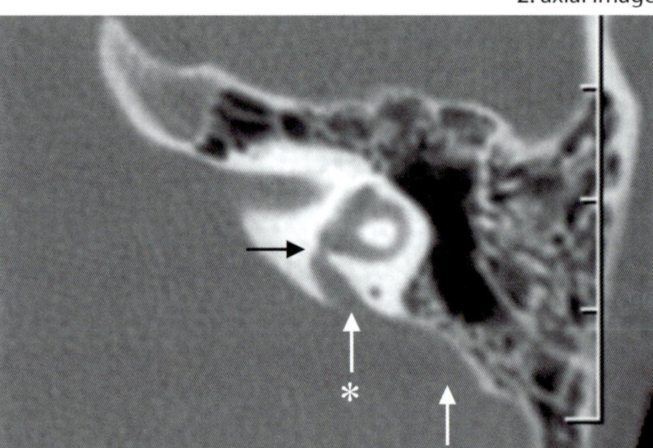

2. axial image

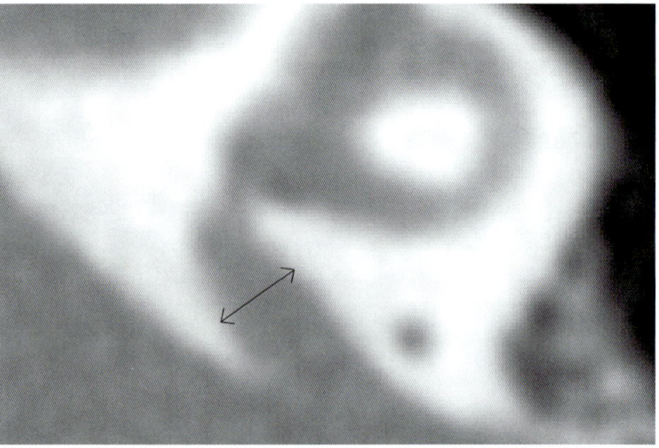

3. axial image

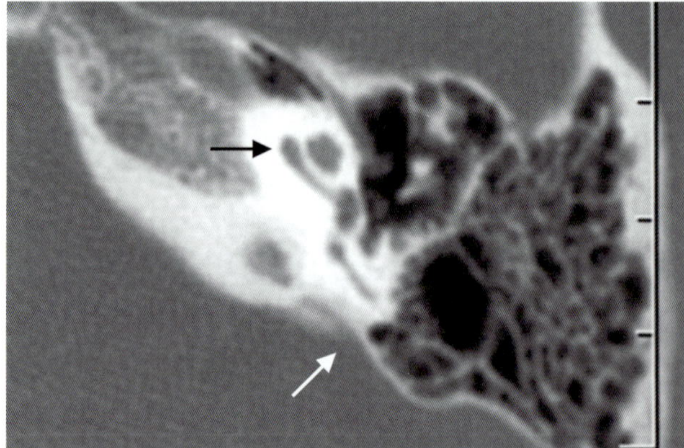

4. axial section diameter of
the vestibular aqueduct

Fig. 40. (Case 7) CT

[Patient CT Findings]

In this case the basal turn of the cochlea is slightly thicker than normal and the upper turns form a single cavity with no

Normal Control CT Findings

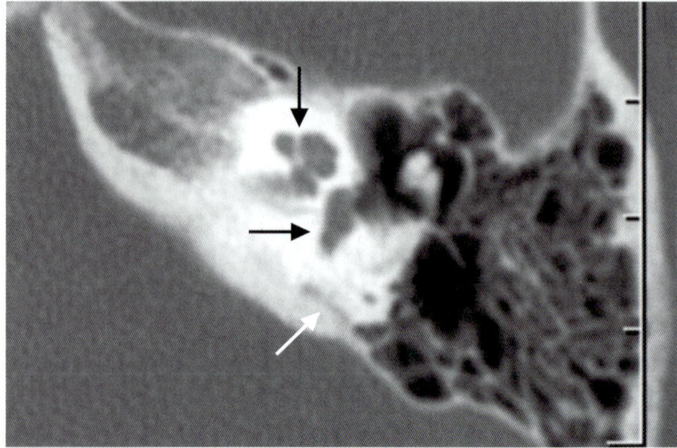

n1. axial image

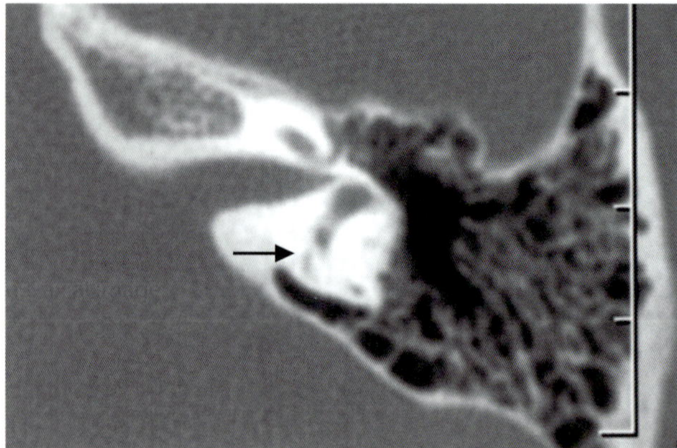

n2. axial image

n3. axial image

partition visible between them and the modiolus (1: →). The horizontal semicircular canal is slightly hypoplastic and the vestibule (2: →) is larger than normal (n2: →), but the most remarkable finding is the abnormally enlarged vestibular aqueduct. In this case the structure corresponding to the endolymphatic sac is clearly visible as a crevice on the posterior surface of the petrous part (1–3: ↗↑), and both the vestibular aqueduct itself and the opening to the posterior cranial fossa are extremely wide (2, 3: ↗↑ with ❀). Also, one can plainly see the aqueduct leading directly medioposteriorly from the base of the common crus (3: →). The axial section diameter of the vestibular aqueduct in this case is 2.3 mm (4: ↗).

《Normal Control CT Findings》

The structure of one or more turns can be identified over the basal turn (n1: →, n2: ↓). n2: → vestibule; ↗ vestibular aqueduct. Normally the origin of the vestibular aqueduct is exceedingly thin in the vestibule and invariably only partially depicted on a CT image, not becoming clearly visible until it has travelled several millimeters posteriorly (n3: →).

Patient CT and 3-Dimensional Reconstructed MRI Findings

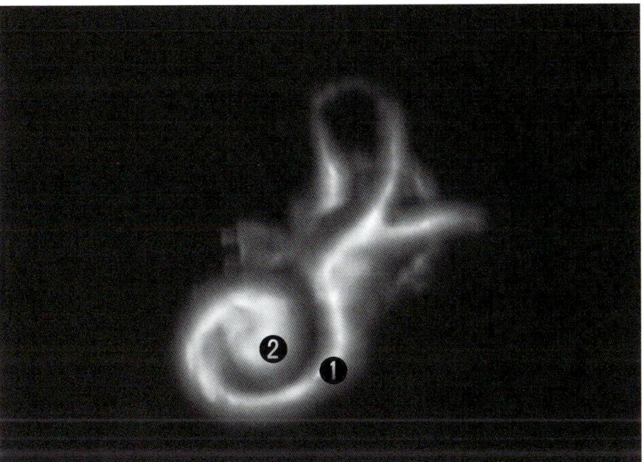

1. coronal image

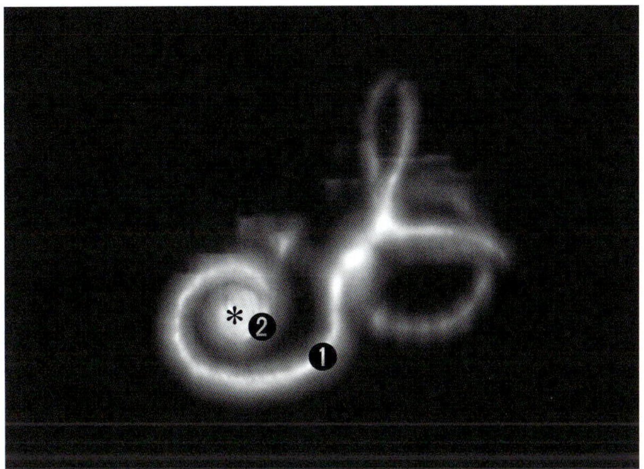

2. 3 dimensional reconstructed MRI

Normal Control CT and 3-Dimensional Reconstructed MRI Findings

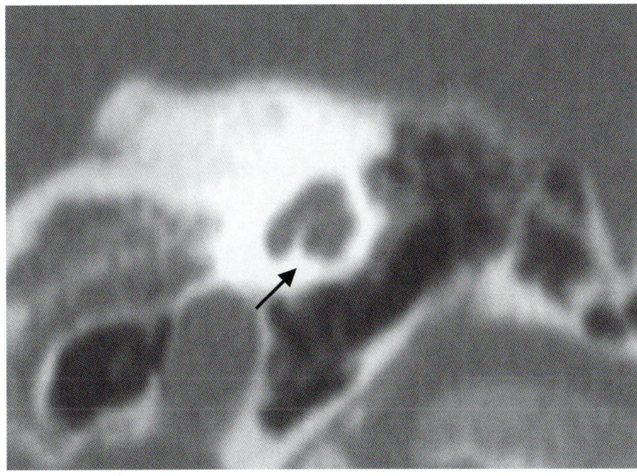

n1. coronal image

n2. 3-dimensional reconstructed MRI

Fig. 41. (Case 7) CT and 3-dimensional reconstructed MRI

[Patient CT and 3-Dimensional Reconstructed MRI Findings]

It is clear that the upper turns of the cochlea form a single cavity (1: ↑).The basal turn of the cochlea in this case (2 ①) is little different from the normal control (n2 ①), but although in the normal control there is further structure superior to the second turn (n2 ②), in this case the area superior to the second turn is a single, cystic mass (2 ②).

《Normal Control CT and 3-Dimensional Reconstructed MRI Findings》

In the normal cochlea, observe that the structure is further divided in the second turn and beyond (n1: ↗). n2: ① origin of basal turn; ② origin of second turn; * apical turn.

---

depicted (fig. 42:1). No atrophy or other abnormality can be ascertained, at least in the images, and the modiolus is also clearly visible (fig. 42:1). The fact that cochlear nerve morphology is normal suggests that we can expect electrical stimulation via a cochlear implant to be fully effective.

Furthermore, because the soft tissue contrast is much higher in the MRI than the CT images, it is possible to observe not only the vestibular aqueduct, but the endolymphatic sac itself. The endolymphatic sac in this case is T2 hyperintense and T1 hypointense in the proximal part, with similar intensity to cerebrospinal fluid, but in the distal part it is T1 isointense and T2 iso- to hypointense (fig. 42:1–3), indicating a possible accumulation of viscous fluid rich in protein, etc. In other words, we find that the characteristics of the fluid content vary depending on the part within the abnormally enlarged endolymphatic sac. Reports of this sort of accumulation of T1 hyperintense fluid in the endolymphatic sac in a case of

enlarged vestibular aqueduct have already been seen elsewhere [1].

■ Surgical Findings

Cochlear implant surgery was performed on the left ear. There were no findings out of the ordinary during the mastoidectomy and posterior tympanotomy. Upon fenestration of the basal turn of the cochlea there was a pulsating discharge of lymph fluid, but the discharge ceased soon afterward. The cochlear implant, which employed a curved electrode that curls around the modiolus, was inserted as usual with no complications. Response of the cochlear nerve to cochlear implant stimulation during surgery was favorable.

The postoperative course was favorable, a broad dynamic range was obtained in cochlear implant mapping, and a final maximum discrimination score of 100% (monosyllabic speech perception test) was achieved.

Patient MRI Findings

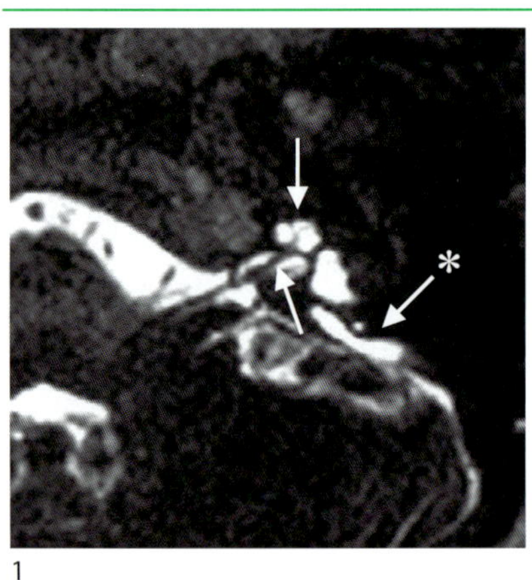
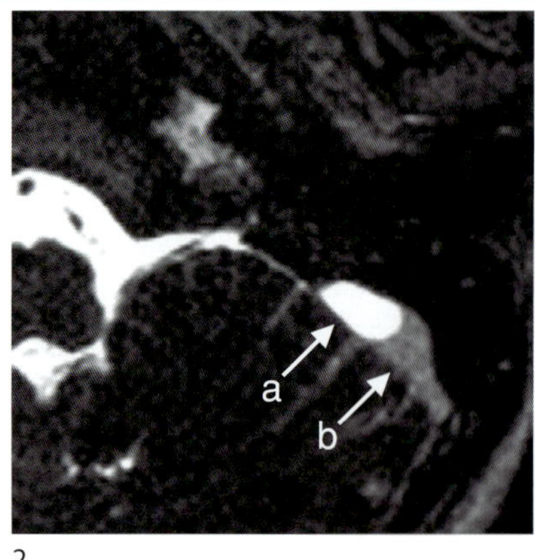
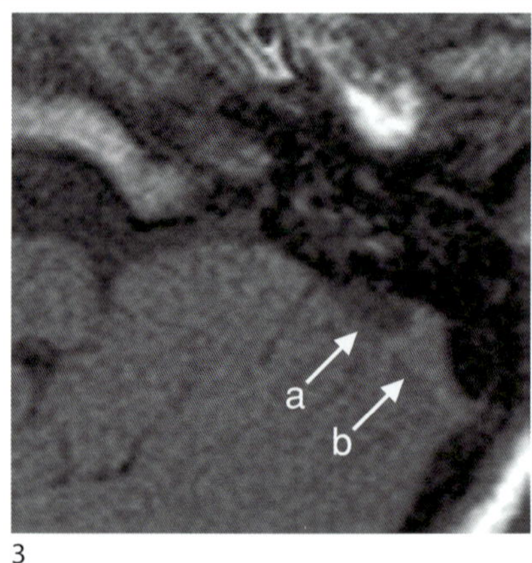

Fig. 42. (Case 7) MRI

[Patient MRI Findings]
The cochlear nerve is of normal thickness and clearly depicted (1: ⌇). No atrophy or other abnormality can be ascertained, at least in the images, and the modiolus is also clearly visible (1: ⬇). The endolymphatic sac is T2 hyperintense and T1 hypointense in the proximal part, with similar characteristics to cerebrospinal fluid (1: ✿ ✐; 2&3: **a** ↗), but in the distal part it is T1 isointense and T2 iso- to hypointense (2&3: **b** ↗), indicating a possible accumulation of viscous fluid rich in protein, etc.

■ Enlarged Vestibular Aqueduct Syndrome and the Anatomy of the Vestibular Aqueduct and Endolymphatic Sac

The vestibular aqueduct branches from the utricular and saccular ducts and exits from the medioposterior part of the vestibule, diverting medially around the common crus then running posterior to the posterior semicircular canal from medial to posterior before transitioning into the endolymphatic sac. The part of the vestibular aqueduct immediately after its origin in the medioposterior part of the vestibule is called the isthmus, or narrowest part. Ogura et al have reported [2] the measurement values for the vestibular aqueduct as follows: average overall length: 8.7 mm; average width at opening to posterior cranial fossa: 6.2 mm; average diameter at isthmus: 0.3 mm. The average spatial resolution for temporal bone CT images currently in general clinical use is around 0.3 mm on the XY plane and 0.6 mm in the Z direction, which are the settings of nearly all the CT images appearing in this book. Under these imaging conditions, it is difficult to clearly depict the isthmus of the vestibular aqueduct in the normal control sample due to the partial volume effect of the surrounding bony tissue. However, pathological enlargement of the vestibular aqueduct and endolymphatic sac can be clearly observed in CT images. The problem here is determining what degree of enlargement is abnormal. Valvassori and Clemis were the first to propose the disease concept of "large vestibular aqueduct syndrome" after examining the vestibular aqueduct in temporal bone tomograms and showing that, when the point midway between the common crus and the opening to the posterior surface of the petrous part had a diameter of 1.5 mm or greater, this constituted abnormal enlargement and such cases were almost always accompanied by hearing loss [3]. On the other hand, in a recent report by Madden et al, the condition of the vestibular aqueduct was measured in temporal bone CT axial images of cases with no sensorineural hearing loss due to injury, chronic otitis media, or other factors, viewing these vestibular aqueducts as 'normal samples.' The results indicated that 95th percentile values for diameters of the vestibular aqueduct at its midpoint and at the opercular part where it opens into the posterior cranial fossa were 0.8 mm and 1.7 mm, respectively, with diameters of 0.9 mm or greater at the midpoint of the vestibular aqueduct and 1.8 mm or greater at the opercular part considered abnormal enlargement [4]. Other standards used, for example those in the paper by Colvin et al, define abnormal vestibular aqueduct enlargement as a diameter of 2.0 mm or greater at the midpoint of the vestibular aqueduct alone with enlargement of the ipsilateral endolymphatic sac, or a midpoint diameter of 1.4 mm or greater if the midpoint diameter on the contralateral side is 2.0 mm or more [5]. In actual clinical practice there is almost never a doubt as to whether or not enlarged vestibular aqueduct syndrome is present, but, as discussed below, since there is no single cause for this syndrome one would expect to find cases approaching the borderline between normal and abnormal. In such cases, it is necessary to take measurements using CT or MR images, compare them to standards such as those presented here, and make a quantitative decision.

Also, on a minor note concerning nomenclature used in this case, what was initially referred to here as "large vestibular aqueduct" or LVA, is recently more commonly referred to as "enlarged vestibular aqueduct" or EVA. Naturally, they refer to the same pathological condition and the terms can be used interchangeably.

Enlarged vestibular aqueduct is the most common inner ear malformation, and in addition to congenital hearing loss there are many cases of progressive hearing loss after birth. Gradual loss of hearing is more common, but in approx. ⅓ of cases the hearing loss is sudden. Of these, there are reports that nearly 80% are triggered by events such as a blow to the head, exercise, or common colds [5]. Some affected children, particularly those whose hearing is near the borderline for hearing aid effectiveness, are discouraged from participating in activities that involve strong head movements. As for vestibular symptoms, worsening hearing loss is frequently accompanied by vertigo, indicating that the condition is one that extends to the entire inner ear. In serious cases, simply inclining the head can sometimes give rise to rotary vertigo. Particularly in young children, care should be taken not to be distracted by attendant symptoms of nausea and vomiting, while overlooking the vertigo and nystagmus. From personal experience, I had a case which for many years was diagnosed as autointoxication. Hearing loss was essentially sensorineural, but on examination of the details one found mixed hearing loss with an air-bone gap of 20–30 dB in the low frequency range. One cause of this may have been that excessive endolymph volume increased inertial mass, limiting the mobility of the footplate of the stapes [6].

Based on MRI findings and the surgical findings described below, the content of the enlarged portion of the vestibular aqueduct and endolymphatic sac can be regarded as composed mainly of lymph from the endolymphatic space. When I have performed closure surgery on the vestibular aqueduct and endolymphatic sac in order to control vertigo in cases of enlarged vestibular aqueduct syndrome, fluid extracted from the endolymphatic sac was pale yellow and transparent. The electrolyte composition, which in endolymph would normally be high in potassium, had Na, K, and Cl densities of 140, 5.1, and 109 (mEq/l) respectively—the same low-potassium composition as normal perilymphatic fluid. On the other hand, when conducting a scala tympani fenestration of the basal turn of the cochlea during cochlear implantation in cases of enlarged vestibular aqueduct syndrome, the initial strong, pulsating discharge of labyrinthine fluid stops naturally after a while. In cases not involving enlarged vestibular aqueduct the volume of inner ear fluid (perilymph) discharged is minimal, with little or no pulsation. This finding indicates that in enlarged vestibular aqueduct syndrome intracranial pressure exerted on the endolymphatic sac from the posterior cranial fossa is directly transmitted to the cochlea, and the volume of discharge implies that the large quantity of endolymph in the endolymphatic sac and vestibular aqueduct is diverted from perilymphatic space in the cochlea and discharged from the scala tympani. However, as seen in Case 7, the fluid in the endolymphatic sac can sometimes be viscous fluid that is T2 hypointense or T1 isointense, and it is possible that this could work to impair the inner ear. On the other hand, there are reports that there is no relationship between the width (midpoint diameter) of the enlarged vestibular aqueduct and long-range deterioration of hearing—that is, it does not follow that the thicker the vestibular aqueduct the easier it is for hearing loss to worsen [5] —which suggests that the progression of hearing loss cannot be explained through the physical causes of pressure transmission from the vestibular aqueduct to the inner ear or reflux of high-density fluid alone.

Concerning the etiology of the case shown here, based on linkage analysis and genetic mutation screening, it is clear that a mutation of the responsible gene (SLC26A4/PDS) for Pendred syndrome (a syndrome accompanied by hearing loss and goiter) can give rise to non-syndromic

hearing loss different from the phenotype [3, 7], but reports vary widely on the frequency of enlarged vestibular aqueduct syndrome with recognized SLC26A4 genetic mutation, from around 30–90% [4, 8]. With SLC26A4 genetic mutation, it has been reported that enlargement of the vestibular aqueduct is greater when two alleles are affected than just one allele and that the hearing loss is more severe [4, 8]. Considering both that the SLC26A4 gene is expressed in the stria vascularis of the inner ear, the endolymphatic sac and endolymphatic duct, the vicinity of the vestibular macula and lateral scala media of the cochlea and that there is no correlation between the degree of hearing loss and the anatomical enlargement of the vestibular aqueduct alone, it can be surmised that the mechanism through which the SLC26A4 gene directly influences inner ear function by maintaining endolymph homeostasis and endocochlear potential [9] also plays an important role in the onset of hearing loss. On the other hand, even in clear cases of enlarged vestibular aqueduct syndrome, in many cases the SLC26A4 mutation is negative, and there are also reports of enlarged vestibular aqueduct syndrome with combined mutations in SLC26A4 and GJB2 [4]. These observations indicate that not one, but several factors bring about the common morphological abnormality of vestibular aqueduct enlargement, and this can be assumed to be one of the reasons for the variety of clinical manifestations.

■ Cochlear Implant Surgical Indication in Cases of Enlarged Vestibular Aqueduct Syndrome

When conducting cochlear implantation for conditions such as in Case 7, there are two approaches in determining on which side to perform the surgery. With the first approach, considering the fact that during the course of treatment to date hearing has been quite consistently favorable in the right ear, there is a possibility that if hearing improves a hearing aid can be used effectively on this side, so cochlear implant surgery should be performed on the opposite, left ear. With the other approach, on the assumption that since hearing is relatively better in the right ear the condition of the auditory nerve must also be favorable, cochlear implant surgery should be performed on the right ear where conditions are slightly better. Taking into consideration that, in the long term, hearing in the right ear may be lost completely with no chance of improvement, the second option may seem more rational, but if right ear hearing does improve and a hearing aid can be effectively used, there is a possibility of attaining binaural hearing even if only for a limited time. Also, given that on average the effectiveness of cochlear implants in cases of enlarged vestibular aqueduct syndrome is favorable [10], it is possible that there will be no significant difference in the postoperative effectiveness of the cochlear implant. It is up to the patient and parents to determine the timing and side of the surgery among themselves after receiving a complete explanation from the attending physician concerning the factors described above. With this disease, cochlear implantation often becomes necessary at school age, and considering the isolation and effect on studies experienced by a child with severe hearing loss, a more positive principle on the surgical indication may be appropriate.

References

1 Sugiura M, Naganawa S, Sato E, Nakashima T: Visualization of a high protein concentration in the cochlea of a patient with a large endolymphatic duct and sac, using three-dimensional fluid-attenuated inversion recovery magnetic resonance imaging. J Laryngol Otol 2006; 120:1084–1086.

2 Ogura Y, Clemis JD: A study of the gross anatomy of the human vestibular aqueduct. Ann Otol Rhinol Laryngol 1971;80:813–825.

3 Valvassori GE, Clemis JD: The large vestibular aqueduct syndrome. Laryngoscope 1978;88:723–728.

4 Madden C, Halsted M, Meinzen-Derr J, et al: The influence of mutation in the SLC26A4 gene on the temporal bone in a population with enlarged vestibular aqueduct. Arch Otolaryngol Head Neck Surg 2007;133:162–168.

5 Colvin IB, Beale T, Harrop-Griffiths K: Long-term follow-up of hearing loss in children and young adults with enlarged vestibular aqueducts: Relationship to radiologic findings and Pendred syndrome diagnosis. Laryngoscope 2006;116:2027–2036.

6 Sato E, Nakashima T, Lilly DJ, et al: Tympanometric findings in patients with enlarged vestibular aqueducts. Laryngoscope 2002; 112:1642–1646.

7 Usami S, Abe S, Weston MD, et al: Non-syndromic hearing loss associated with enlarged vestibular aqueduct is caused by PDS mutations. Hum Genet 1999;104:188–192.

8 Okamoto Y, Matsunaga T, Taiji H, et al: Mutation of SLC26A4 are associated with the clinical features in patients with bilateral enlargement of the vestibular aqueduct. Audiology Japan 2010;53:164–170.

9 Royaux IE, Belyantseva IA, Wu T, et al: Localization and functional studies of pendrin in the mouse inner ear provide insight about the etiology of deafness in pendred syndrome. J Assoc Res Otolaryngol 2003;4:394–404.

10 Buchman CA, Copeland BJ, Yu KK, et al: Cochlear implantation in children with congenital inner ear malformations. Laryngoscope 2004;114:309–316.

Points

❶ In cases of sensorineural hearing loss that progresses in childhood, suspect enlarged vestibular aqueduct syndrome.

❷ Enlarged vestibular aqueduct syndrome is sometimes accompanied by other inner ear malformations and sometimes arises independently.

❸ With this condition the vestibular aqueduct can be observed leading directly from the vestibule, which is not possible in normal images.

❹ SLC26A4 genetic mutation is an important causative factor.

Case 8 — Incomplete Partition Type III (IP-III)

Subject: male, 2 years, 11 months

■ History and Clinical Findings

The parents first took the subject to the ENT department of a local hospital after noticing that he did not respond clearly to sound. The child exhibited speech retardation and the ABR thresholds were 60 to 70 dB SPL in both ears. He had been using hearing aids bilaterally since confirmation of severe hearing loss, but speech development was unsatisfactory and he was referred to our department for further examination and possible surgical treatment.

The ASSR thresholds as examined in our department were approx. 90 dB in both ears, which were approx. 20 dB higher than previous ABR thresholds, suggesting progressive hearing deterioration. Hearing thresholds examined with conditioned orientation reflex audiometry were approx. 85 dB, and aided thresholds were between 45 and 65 dB. Developmental testing showed normal Cognitive-Adaptive development (developmental quotient: DQ 100), while Language-Social development was apparently delayed (DQ 50). The subject understood around 50 spoken words and could speak several meaningful words, but the phonation was excessively nasalized. Genetic testing for hearing loss has not yet been performed. There is no history of hearing loss among the subject's parents or relatives, and he is an only child. Temporal bone CT and MRI examinations were performed to search for the etiology of the patient's hearing loss.

■ Patient CT Findings

CT and MRI findings are the same in both ears. The images for the left ear are shown. The mastoid air cells are well developed and no abnormal soft tissue density is observed in the middle ear in the temporal bone CT. No anomalies can be identified in the middle ear, including the ossicular chains. In the inner ear, the interscalar septa of the cochlea are partially present, but the bony modiolus is completely absent, along with the septum between the cochlea and the internal auditory canal (fig. 43:1). The internal auditory canal directly communicates with the cochlea at its lateral end (fig. 43:1). The vestibule and semicircular canals appear normal, but the bony canal for the superior vestibular nerve is larger than normal (fig. 43:2). In addition, the labyrinthine segment of the facial nerve is located superior to the cochlea (fig. 43:3), which may be due to the abnormally inferior and posterior location of the cochlea in this patient.

■ Patient MRI Findings

Three-dimensional reconstructed MRI of the inner ear shows a poorly separated cochlear duct (fig. 44:1) and enlarged internal auditory canal (fig. 44:1). T2 weighted high resolution MRI reveals the cochlea as a high intensity area, and the low intensity structure corresponding to the cochlear nerve in the modiolus can also be identified (fig. 45:1). The bifurcation between the cochlear nerve and the vestibular nerve can be identified in the internal auditory canal (fig. 45:2) in the same way as in the normal control (fig. 45:n2). The diameter of the superior

Patient CT Findings

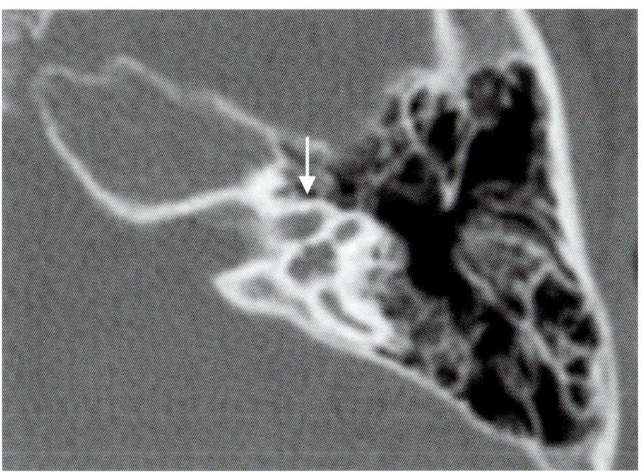

1. axial image

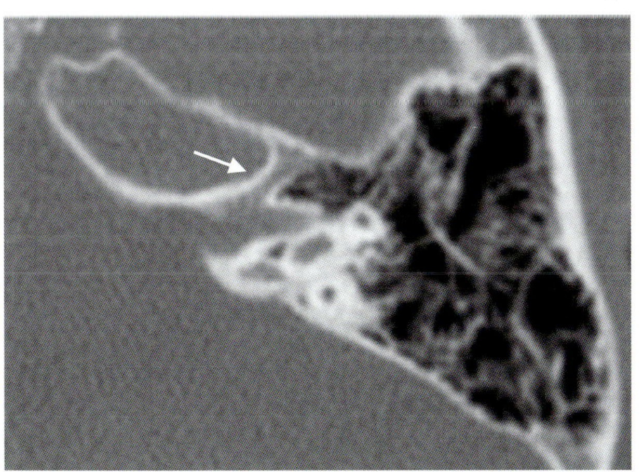

2. axial image

3. axial image

Normal Control CT Findings

n1. axial image

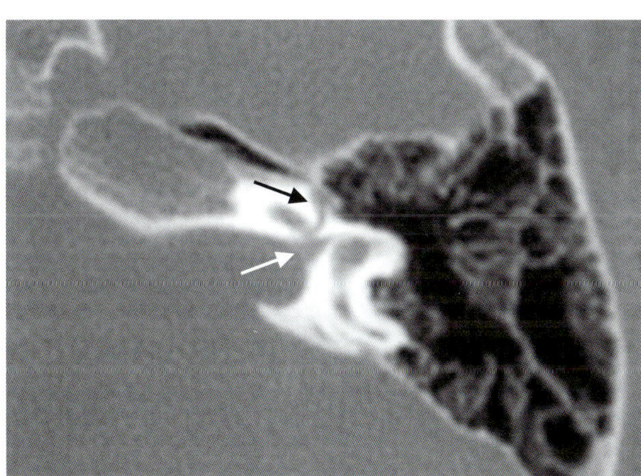

n2. axial image

Fig. 43. (Case 8) CT

[Patient CT Findings]

The mastoid air cells are well developed and no abnormal soft tissue density is observed in the middle ear in the temporal bone CT. No anomalies can be identified in the middle ear, including the ossicular chains. In the inner ear, the interscalar septa of the cochlea are partially present, but the bony modiolus is completely absent, along with the septum between the cochlea and the internal auditory canal (1: ↗). In the normal control, the modiolus and the bony septum at the base of the modiolus are clearly depicted (n1: ↗). The internal auditory canal directly communicates with the cochlea at its lateral end (1: ↗). The vestibule and semicircular canals appear normal, but the bony canal for the superior vestibular nerve is larger than normal (2: ⇓). In addition, the labyrinthine segment of the facial nerve is located superior to the cochlea (3: ↘), which may be due to the abnormally inferior and posterior location of the cochlea in this patient. In contrast, in the normal control image, the labyrinthine segment of the facial nerve is observed in the same section as the most superior part of the cochlear basal turn (n2: ↘), and the bony canal for the superior vestibular nerve (n2: ↗) is smaller than that of this patient.

vestibular nerve canal is large, inside of which the superior vestibular nerve can be observed as a low-intensity line (fig. 45:3). The hypointense septum between the cochlea and the internal auditory canal, however, is not visible.

■ Clinical Course

The patient is being followed up in our department, and his hearing, speech perception, and expression skills are being checked continuously to find out whether the hearing aids are effectively helping the child with his spoken language development. Cochlear implantation will be indicated if the progress of his speech development is too slow, or if pure tone hearing deteriorates further.

■ Incomplete Partition Type III (IP-III) Anomaly of the Inner Ear

IP-III is an X-linked inner ear anomaly that is marked by the absence of the bony modiolus and of the septum between the base of the cochlea and the internal auditory canal [1, 2]. The bony interscalar septa are partially present and the external dimensions of the cochlea do not differ from normal [1, 2]. In contrast, no anomalies are identified in the vestibular part of the inner ear. The soft tissue structures such as the cochlear nerve, vestibular nerve, and facial nerves appear normal in MR images. Cochlear implantation in a patient with this anomaly is possible and may show good postoperative performance, but requires utmost attention since a cerebrospinal fluid (CSF) gusher is inevitable [3] and there is a risk of aberrant electrode array insertion into the internal auditory canal. For details, see the following special article on IP-III by Professor Sennaroglu (Please see p.106).

References

1 Sennaroglu L, Sarac S, Ergin T: Surgical results of cochlear implantation in malformed cochlea. Otol Neurotol 2006;27:615–623.
2 Sennaroglu L: Cochlear implantation in inner ear malformations—a review article. Cochlear Implants Int 2010;11:4–41.
3 Incesulu A, Adapinar B, Kecik C: Cochlear implantation in cases with incomplete partition type III (X-linked anomaly). Eur Arch Otorhinolaryngol 2008;265:1425–1430.

<table>
<tr>
<td align="center">Patient 3-Dimensional
Reconstructed MRI Findings</td>
<td align="center">Normal Control 3-Dimensional
Reconstructed MRI Findings</td>
</tr>
<tr>
<td>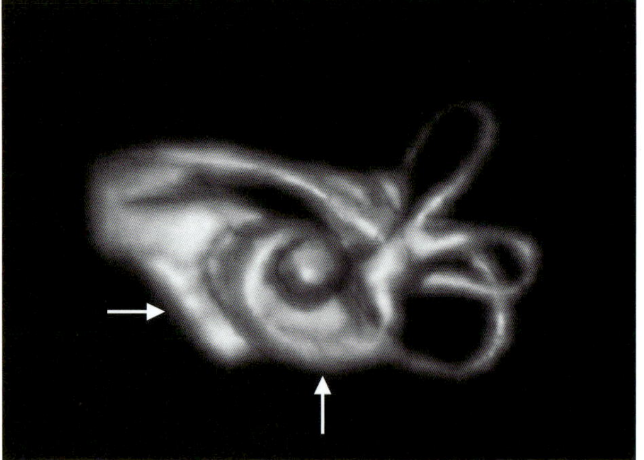</td>
<td>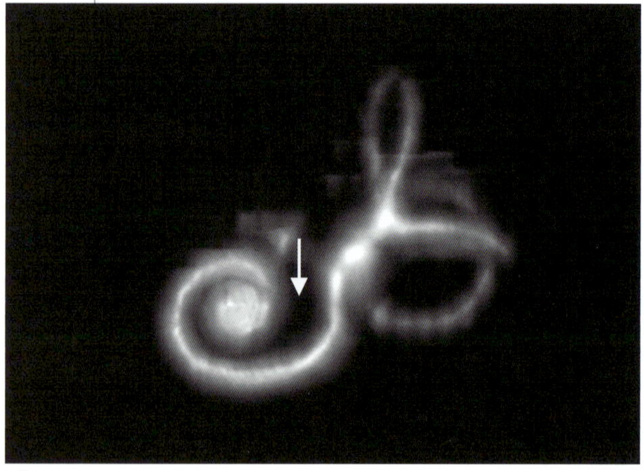</td>
</tr>
</table>

Fig. 44. (Case 8) 3-dimensional reconstructed MRI

[Patient 3-Dimensional Reconstructed MRI Findings]

Three-dimensional reconstructed MRI of the inner ear shows a poorly separated cochlear duct (1: ⇑) and enlarged internal auditory canal (1: ⇨). In a normal cochlea, the upper turn is clearly separated from the basal turn (n1: ⇓).

Patient MRI Findings	**Normal Control MRI Findings**

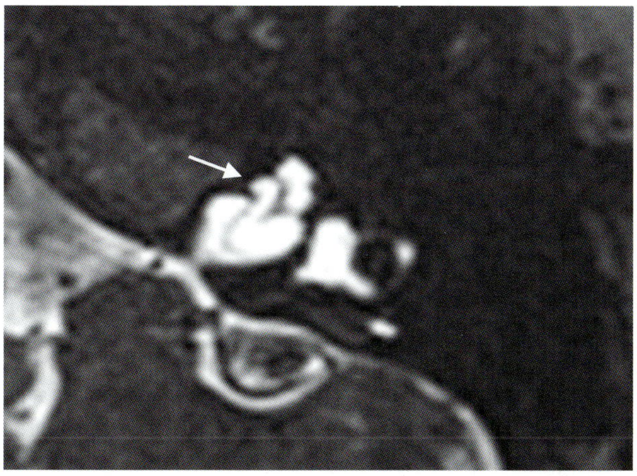

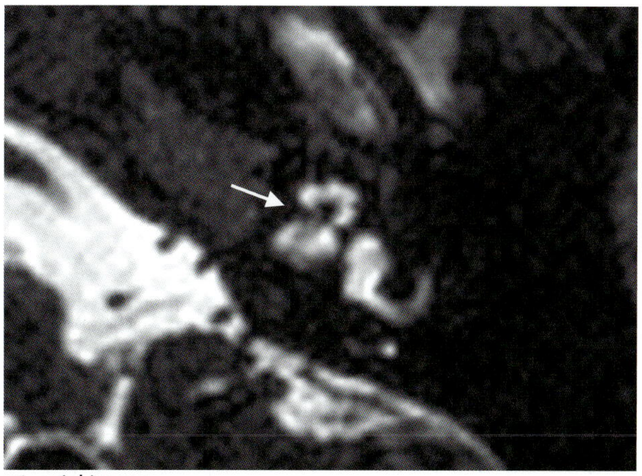

1. axial image

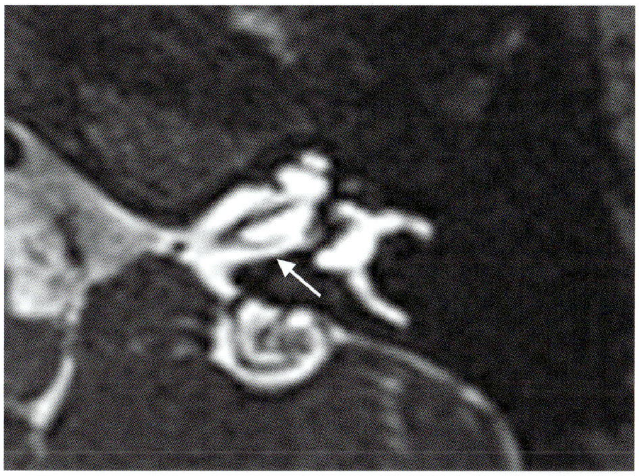

n1. axial image

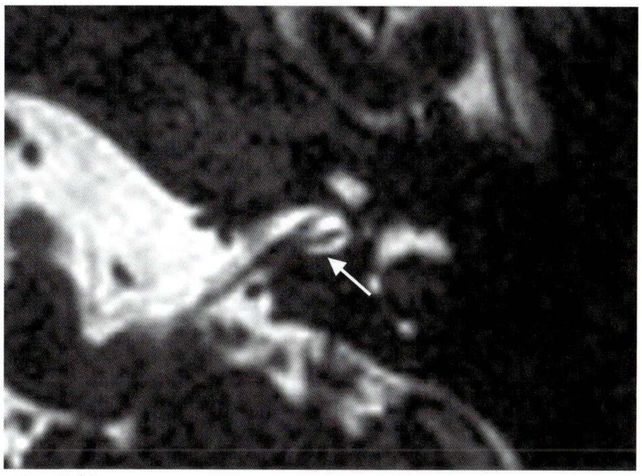

2. axial image

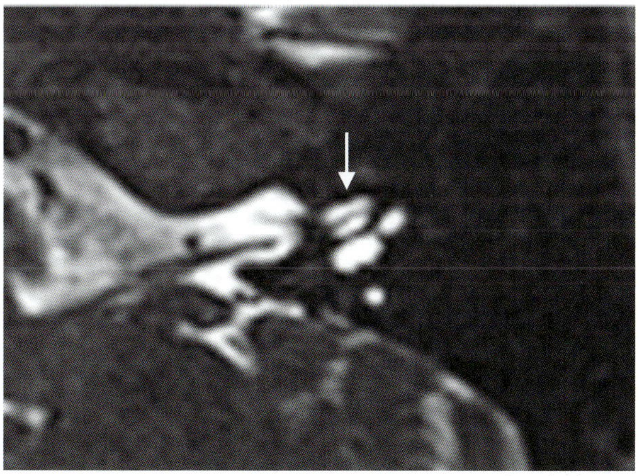

n2. axial image

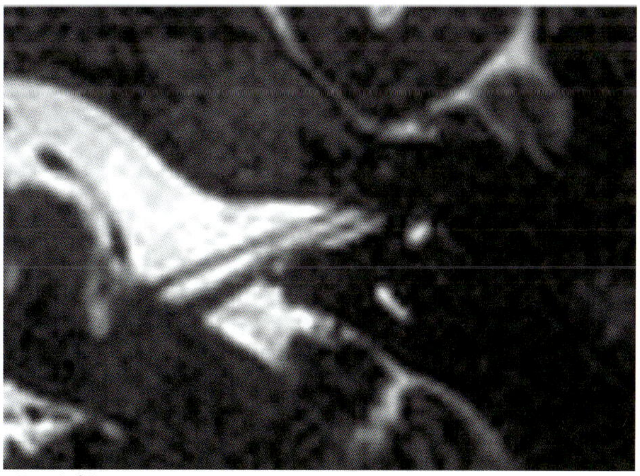

3. axial image

n3. axial image

Fig. 45. (Case 8) MRI

[Patient MRI Findings]

T2 weighted high resolution MRI reveals the cochlea as a high intensity area, and the low intensity structure corresponding to the cochlear nerve in the modiolus can also be identified (1: ↘). The bifurcation between the cochlear nerve and the vestibular nerve can be identified in the internal auditory canal (2: ↘) in the same way as in the normal control (n2 ↘). The diameter of the superior vestibular nerve canal is large, inside of which the superior vestibular nerve can be observed as a low-intensity line (3: ↓). The hypointense septum between the cochlea and the internal auditory canal, which can be identified in normal control (n1: ↘), however, is not visible (1).

Incomplete Partition Type III

Levent Sennaroglu, M.D.

Professor of Otolaryngology, Department of Otolaryngology
Hacettepe University Medical Faculty
Ankara, Turkey

Incomplete partition type III cochlear malformation is the type of anomaly present in X-linked deafness which was described by Nance et al [1] for the first time in 1971. They reported that the X-linked transmission of congenital mixed hearing loss is associated with a fixed stapes footplate and perilymph gusher during attempted stapedectomy. Although mainly seen in males they indicated that female heterozygotes had similar but milder audiological abnormalities. Later Papadaki et al [2] reported two cases of X-linked deafness with stapes gusher in females with normal male relatives. Bulbous dilatation of the fundus of the internal auditory canals (IAC), incomplete separation of the IAC from the base of the cochlea, and widened facial nerve canals were seen in both female patients.

There may be different ways of clinical presentation: sensorineural hearing loss (SNHL) or mixed type hearing loss. It is not infrequent to see air-bone gap in these patients. Bento and Miniti [3] reported four cases where hearing aid use was impossible. One of them was explored for stapedectomy. During the removal of the footplate there was severe gusher where a piston placement was impossible. Similar cases who had severe gusher during stapedetomy were reported in the literature [4, 5]. In those cases either the piston could not be placed or there were further SNHL. It appears from the experience of these authors that stapedectomy is to be avoided in this group of patients.

■ Genetics

According to de Kok et al [6] the underlying DFN3 gene (deafness with congenital stapes footplate fixation) has been mapped to the Xq21 region, and is caused by mutations in or around the POU3F4 gene. Female obligate carriers may be normal, or have a milder form of the same anomaly associated with milder hearing loss [7].

■ Audiological Features

The patients usually apply with hearing loss. There may be two different forms of presentation:

1-Mixed Type Hearing Loss:

SNHL component is most probably due to the modiolar defect. The air-bone gap observed in our patients usually involves high frequencies as well as low frequencies. Conductive component is due to stapedial fixation. Snik et al. [8] reported that if the degree of hearing loss was not too much, stapedius reflex could be obtained in this group of patients.

Tang et al [9] have a different explanation for the conductive hearing loss. They are in the opinion that the intracranial pressure is transmitted into the perilymphatic space, and the raised perilymphatic pressure that is exerted on the cochlear duct and the stapes footplate results in a mixed pattern of sensorineural and conductive hearing loss respectively.

Snik et al [8] explained the air-bone gap with the third window phenomenon. They reported that because of the congenital malformation audiovestibular system functioned more effective than normal system leading to better bone conduction levels. Their study revealed that audiological studies were in accordance with pure sensorineural hearing loss and air-bone gap in the audiogram did not have the significance of conductive hearing loss component.

2-The other common form of presentation is profound SNHL, where the severity may vary. This is most probably due to the absence of the modiolus and in this situation cochlear implant (CI) surgery is the option for restoring hearing. All three patients followed in our department had severe to profound SNHL and underwent CI surgery.

■ Radiology

The cochlea in incomplete partition type III has interscalar septa but the modiolus is completely absent (fig. 46:a, b).

This anomaly is the rarest form of incomplete partition cases. According to the radiological database in Hacettepe University Department of Otolaryngology incomplete partition cases are 41% of the whole inner ear malformations. IP-III constitutes 2% of the inner ear malformation group. So far only three patients received CI in Hacettepe University and one patient is being followed with hearing aid.

Radiological appearance of a cochlea with incomplete partition type III is very characteristic. HRCT findings were described elegantly by Phelps et al [7] for the first time, but this characteristic deformity was included under the category of incomplete partition deformities for the first time by Sennaroglu et al [10] in 2006.

Phelps et al [7] reported three main features of this rare disorder:
(1) bulbous internal auditory canal,
(2) incomplete separation of the coils of the cochlea from the internal auditory canal and
(3) wide first and second parts of the intratemporal facial nerve canal with a less acute angle between them.

Talbot and Wilson [5] later added that modiolus is absent in these patients. Later papers confirmed the existence of these deformities in other patient groups as well. Chee et al [11] mentioned bilateral and symmetric bulbous dilatation of the internal auditory canals. Kumar et al [4] reported that the labyrinthine segments of the facial nerve canals also appeared enlarged bilaterally.

Apart from these three features a more medial origin of the vestibular aqueduct with varying degree of dilatation was described by Talbot and Wilson [5]. Kumar et al [4] recently reported that this was not seen in their patient and has not been reported in any other patients. This feature is also seen bilaterally in one of our patients too.

In addition to these features the present author noticed

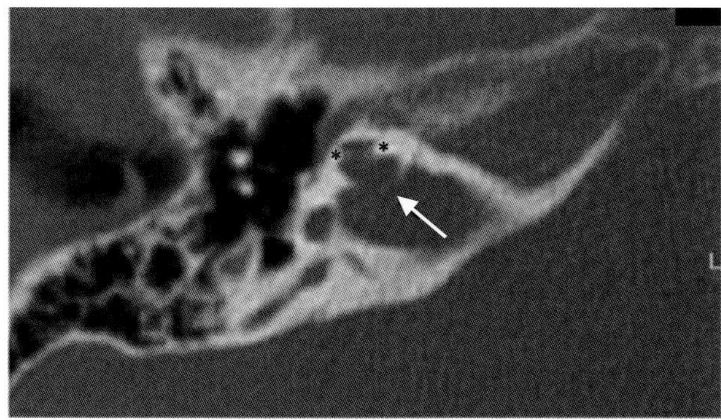

a. Axial section showing cochlea with incomplete partition type III deformity. It is possible to visualize interscalar septa (*), however there is a large defect at the base of the cochlea (✎).

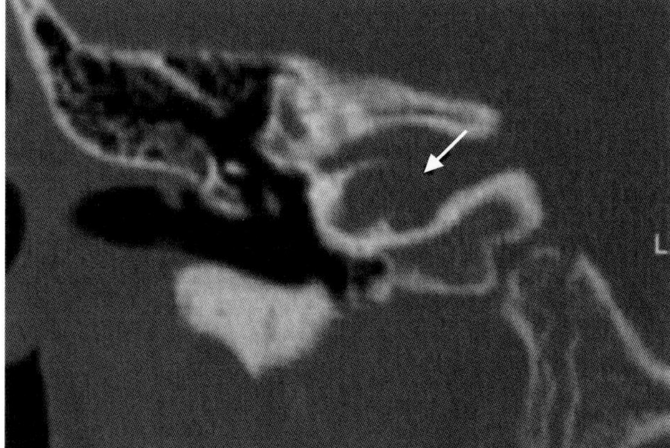

b. Coronal section with a defect at the base of the cochlea (✎).

Fig. 46

that in this deformity the interscalar septa are present but the modiolus is completely absent [12] (fig. 46:a, b). The cochlea was placed directly at the lateral end of the internal auditory canal instead of its usual anterolateral position. This gives the cochlea a characteristic appearance. From an earlier study the external dimensions of the cochlea (height and diameter) were found to be similar to normal cochlea [10]. Apart from these features the present author noticed that labyrinthine segment of the facial nerve has a more superior position in relation to cochlea; labyrinthine segment is located almost above the cochlea. If the axial sections are followed from top to bottom, the first structure is the labyrinthine segment of the facial nerve. In addition there is a very thin otic capsule around the cochlea and vestibule.

Talbot and Wilson [5] suggested that young males with congenital mixed type hearing loss should be studied with high resolution CT of the temporal bone. This is a very important suggestion that should be done.

■ Surgical Treatment

Incomplete Partition (IP) malformations have normal external dimensions but internal architecture is defective with variable degrees. The external dimensions of the cochlea (height and diameter) are not different from a normal cochlea. IP-I and IP-III have a defect at the base and this creates a route for cerebrospinal fluid (CSF) to fill the cochlea. Modiolus is partially present in IP-II and here the defect is less compared to IP-I and IP-III. Therefore,

during surgery of IP-I and IP-III there is a high likelihood of severe CSF gusher. In IP-II gusher is rare but oozing is more common. Therefore, during the surgery of IP-III two serious problems may occur:

1-gusher during cochleostomy
2-electrode misplacement into the IAC

The surgeon must be ready to cope with these problems. During electrode choice these factors should be kept in mind. Because of the defective modiolus electrodes with complete rings or contact surface on both sides may provide better stimulation. The probability of the longer electrodes entering the IAC is more than the shorter electrodes. Therefore, an electrode with full rings or contact surfaces on both sides that will make only one turn around the cochlea appears to be sufficient.

Modiolar hugging electrodes may have a tendency going towards the center of the cochlea. In IP-III this may result in misplacement into the IAC. Because of its length, Med El standard electrode may also go into the IAC. Therefore, Med El compressed array, and Nucleus 24 K appear to be options. The author developed an electrode with a "cork" type stopper (standard electrode 25 mm) appears to be ideal for these cases by properly sealing the cochleostomy (to prevent CSF fistula postoperatively) and also making one full turn around the cochlea,

A-Gusher:
These patients have severe gusher during surgery. If it is not properly sealed the postoperative CSF leakage may lead to recurrent meningitis. Ideally the size of the cochleostomy should be slightly larger than the electrode allowing a soft tissue to be placed around the electrode. Passing the electrode through a tiny piece of fascia and inserting this together with the electrode may have even a better seal at the cochleostomy.

The electrode with "Cork" type stopper has the following features: It has a "cork" like stopper instead of the usual silicon ring at the end of the intracochlear electrode to prevent CSF fistula after CI insertion. This was designed to close the cochleostomy more efficiently to stop the escape of CSF around the electrode. The diameter of the "cork" stopper is 1.9 mm. The diameter of the active electrode is 1 mm. A cochleostomy should be created with a burr size of 1.2 mm. This allows the active electrode to pass through without resistance, without letting the stopper with a diameter of 1.9 mm to pass through; thereby effectively closing the cochleostomy. The length of the electrode is 25 mm, to make one full turn around the cochlea. This is the standard "cork" (fig. 47a) electrode where contact spacing between active electrodes is 1.7 mm. It also has contact surfaces on both sides of the electrode for more effective stimulation rather than electrodes with half banded contacts facing the modiolus. Intraoperative radiology should be obtained in order to check the position of the electrode which is expected to be round shape following the contour of the cochlea (fig. 47b).

It is important to use the tissue glue after each layer of soft tissue added. After the first layer of soft tissue is placed, a little amount of tissue glue is added to fix this

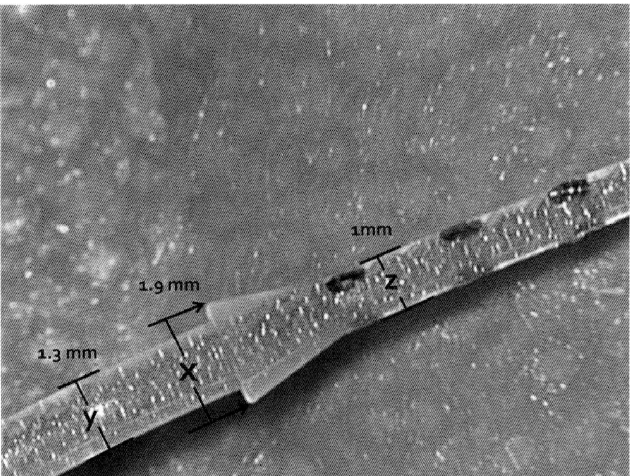

a. Electrode with cork stopper.

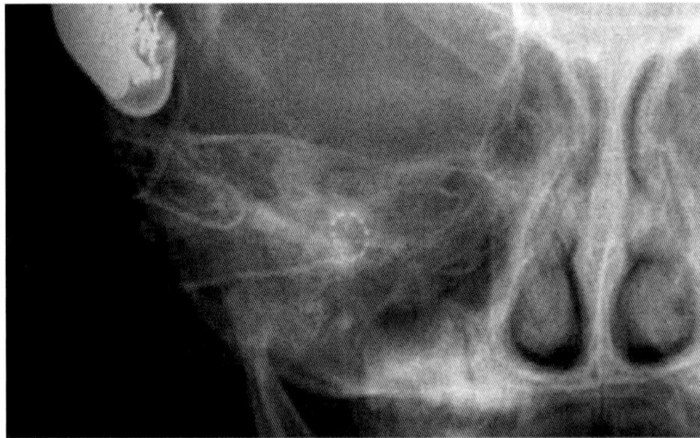

b. Transorbital view showing cork electrode in a case of IP-III

Fig. 47

part. Then a thin layer of fascia is added again and then a tiny amount of glue is added. This is continued until the opening around the electrode is properly closed and no CSF leakage is witnessed.

As a principle the surgeon should not leave the surgery without completely controlling the CSF leakage around the electrode. If there is a severe gusher postoperative continuous lumbar drainage may divert the CSF away from the cochleostomy area allowing the healing of the cochleostomy area. This is kept in place for 4–5 days. In case of difficult control of CSF gusher subtotal petrosectomy can be an additional precaution to eliminate the connection between the nasopharynx and the middle ear to prevent meningitis. However it should never be forgotten that subtotal petrosectomy is an additional measure and the first line of defense of proper control of the cochleostomy is mandatory.

B-Misplacement into the IAC:

Because of the wide connection between the IAC and the cochlea the electrode may go into the IAC inadvertently. Intraoperative radiology is advisable to check the position of the electrode. Modiolar hugging electrodes tend to turn towards the center of the cochlea where the defect is greatest. These type electrodes may go into the IAC more than the straight ones. If the postoperative X-ray shows a straight electrode revision should be planned as soon as possible.

Conclusion

IP-III is the rarest form of inner ear malformations and is observed in X-linked deafness. Because of the conductive component a stapedectomy is usually planned. In patients with congenital hearing loss a HRCT will demonstrate this pathology and a stapedectomy which may result in further hearing loss can be avoided. Hearing aid or cochlear implant can be offered according to the degree of hearing loss. In CI surgery a gusher and misplacement into the IAC may complicate the surgery. Every effort should be shown to fully control the CSF leakage.

References

1 Nance WE, Setleff R, McLeod A, Sweeney A, Cooper C, McConnell F: X-linked mixed deafness with congenital fixation of the stapedial footplate and perilymphatic gusher. Birth Defects Orig Artic Ser [Research Support, U.S. Gov't, Non-P.H.S.] 1971;7:64–69.

2 Papadaki E, Prassopoulos P, Bizakis J, Karampekios S, Papadakis H, Gourtsoyiannis N: X-linked deafness with stapes gusher in females. Eur J Radiol [Case Reports] 1998;29:71–75.

3 Bento RF, Miniti A: X-linked mixed hearing loss: four case studies. The Laryngoscope 1985;95:462–468.

4 Kumar G, Castillo M, Buchman CA: X-linked stapes gusher: CT findings in one patient. AJNR American journal of neuroradiology [Case Reports] 2003;24:1130–1132.

5 Talbot JM, Wilson DF: Computed tomographic diagnosis of X-linked congenital mixed deafness, fixation of the stapedial footplate, and perilymphatic gusher. The American journal of otology [Case Reports Comparative Study] 1994;15:177–182.

6 de Kok YJ, van der Maarel SM, Bitner-Glindzicz M, Huber I, Monaco AP, Malcolm S, et al: Association between X-linked mixed deafness and mutations in the POU domain gene POU3F4. Science [Research Support, Non-U.S. Gov't] 1995;267:685–688.

7 Phelps PD, Reardon W, Pembrey M, Bellman S, Luxom L: X-linked deafness, stapes gushers and a distinctive defect of the inner ear. Neuroradiology 1991;33:326–330.

8 Snik AF, Hombergen GC, Mylanus EA, Cremers CW: Air-bone gap in patients with X-linked stapes gusher syndrome. The American journal of otology [Case Reports] 1995;16:241–246.

9 Tang A, Parnes LS: X-linked progressive mixed hearing loss: computed tomography findings. Ann Otol Rhinol Laryngol [Case Reports] 1994;103:655–657.

10 Sennaroglu L, Sarac S, Ergin T: Surgical results of cochlear implantation in malformed cochlea. Otology & neurotology : official publication of the American Otological Society, American Neurotology Society [and] European Academy of Otology and Neurotology [Case Reports] 2006;27:615–623.

11 Chee NW, Suhailee S, Goh J: Clinics in diagnostic imaging (111): X-linked congenital mixed deafness syndrome. Singapore Med J 2006;47:822–824; quiz 5.

12 Sennaroglu L: Cochlear implantation in inner ear malformations —a review article. Cochlear implants international 2009 Apr 8.

④ Internal Auditory Canal

IAC Stenosis

The morphology (diameter and length) of the internal auditory canal (IAC) has previously been described based on measurements either of the temporal bone itself or using tomography, but recently many reports are emerging based on measurements taken using high-resolution CT images. Among these, a report by McClay et al [1] divides test subjects into two groups based on presence or absence of sensorineural hearing loss and measures and examines a large number of samples of IAC morphology. The results show that the IAC's anteroposterior diameter (as measured in an axial image, 2 mm lateral to the medial margin of the IAC's posterior wall) was 5.02 ± 1.22 mm in the group with no sensorineural hearing loss (307 samples) and 4.85 ± 1.07 mm in the group with sensorineural hearing loss (181 samples), with no significant difference between the two. Even the superoinferior diameter (as measured at the point of maximum vertical breadth at the IAC's midpoint) was 4.62 ± 1.16 mm in the group with no sensorineural hearing loss (292 samples) and 4.39 ± 1.18 mm in the group with sensorineural hearing loss (175 samples), again with no significant difference between the two. Consequently, it is difficult to determine a normal range for IAC diameter based simply on presence or absence of hearing loss alone. IAC length was also about the same in both groups, at around 11 mm. However, on examination of samples accompanied by malformation of the inner ear, one finds many cases of sensorineural hearing loss in which anteroposterior or superoinferior IAC diameter is 2 mm or less. On the other hand, enlargement of the internal auditory canal (defined in McClay's paper as an anteroposterior or superoinferior diameter of 8 mm or greater) is unrelated to hearing loss.

According to Lang's measurements [2], IAC diameter in newborns is approx. 3 mm, and approx. 4.5 mm in two years old, whereas in adults is it 6–7 mm, suggesting that it expands with age. The internal auditory canal also lengthens from around 5–7 mm at birth to 10–15 mm in adulthood. However, according to measurements using 3-dimensional computer reconstructions based on temporal bone histopathological samples by Sakashita and Sando [3], while the internal auditory canal clearly does grow longer, its increase in diameter with age is minimal or, at most, very slight. For example, if we measure the internal auditory canals in the pediatric standard temporal bone CT images at four months, one year, three years, and 16 years shown in this book according to McClay's method described above, IAC length increases with age, with a length of 5.8 mm at four months, 7.7 mm at one year, 10.6 mm at three years, and 12.9 mm at 16 years. The anteroposterior diameters, on the other hand, are 3.5 mm, 3.8 mm, 6.7 mm, and 4.8 mm respectively, indicating a somewhat narrower diameter in early years, although the individual differences are considerable, and it lacks the same clear enlargement trend seen with length. Consequently, the pattern of development for the internal auditory canal can be understood as one of lengthening with almost no change in diameter.

Development of the internal auditory canal is related to the formation and development of cranial nerve VIII, and cranial nerve VIII hypoplasty is accompanied by aplasia and stenosis of the internal auditory canal [4]. The indication of cochlear implants must be considered in cases of profound bilateral hearing loss, and the presence of IAC stenosis is an important factor to consider at this time. Generally, the success rate of cochlear implants in cases of IAC stenosis is lower than in those in which stenosis is not a factor [5].

On the other hand, the condition of the facial nerve, another nerve which traverses the internal auditory canal, does not necessarily correlate to IAC diameter, and even in the following cases containing IAC stenosis with cranial nerve VIII hypoplasia, there are no facial nerve abnormalities.

References

1   McClay JE, Tandy R, Grundfast K, et al: Major and minor temporal bone abnormalities in children with and without congenital sensorineural hearing loss. Arch Otolaryngol Head Neck Surg 2002; 128:664–671.
2   Lang J: Neuroanatomie der Nn. Opticus, Trigeminus, Facialis, Glossopharyngeus, Vagus, Accessorius und Hypoglossus. Arch Otorhinolaryngol 1981;231:1–69.
3   Sakashita T, Sando I: Postnatal development of the internal auditory canal studied by computer-aided three-dimansional reconstruction and measurement. Ann Otol Rhinol Laryngol 1995;104:469–475.
4   McPhee JR, Van de Water TR: Epithelial-mesenchymal tissue interactions guiding otic capsule formation: the role of the otocyst. J Embryol Exp Morphol 1986; 97:1 24.
5   Papsin BC: Cochlear implantation in children with anomalous cochleovestibular anatomy. Laryngoscope 2005; 115 (Suppl. 106):1–26.

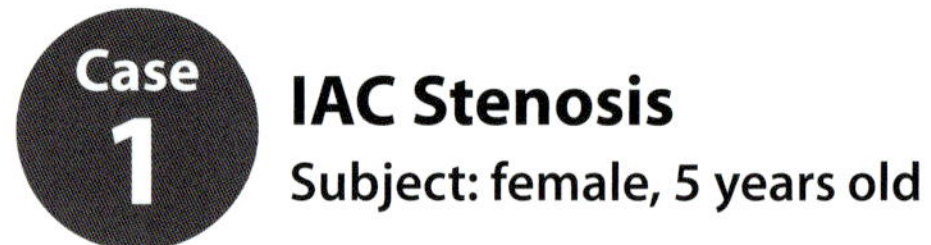

Case 1

IAC Stenosis

Subject: female, 5 years old

History and Clinical Findings

The subject had been healthy since birth and her parents were not aware of any particular problems, but recently when her parents held the phone up to her right ear she said she couldn't hear anything so they became worried and took her to the doctor. Pure tone audiometry (fig. 48) indicated average hearing level of 93.3 dB right and 13.3 dB left, for a finding of unilateral profound hearing loss in the right ear. For objective audiometry, ASSR testing was carried out, with right ear thresholds of from 100 dB (500 Hz) to 110 dB scale-out (4,000 Hz), whereas left ear thresholds were all less than 20 dB from 500 Hz to 4,000 Hz, confirming the finding of unilateral deafness in the right ear (fig. 49). In DPOAE testing as well, the right ear showed no response, while in the left ear response was normal. Temporal bone CT and MRI exams were conducted to further determine the cause. Image findings for the subject's affected (right) and healthy (left) ears are shown below.

Patient CT Findings

No abnormalities were found in the middle ear or ossicles in either side. In the inner ear as well, no clear morphological abnormalities were discovered in the cochlea or vestibule. However, the right internal auditory canal is clearly narrower, with an anteroposterior diameter at the opening to the posterior cranial fossa of 3.5 mm, just 60% the size of the healthy left side diameter of 5.7 mm (fig. 50:3R, 3L). Observing the lateral end of the internal auditory canal at its border with the modiolus, diameter of the opening at the base of the modiolus is less than 1 mm on the affected side, compared to 2.7 mm on the healthy side (fig. 50:1R, 1L). On the other hand, the facial nerve shows no bilateral discrepancies in either its path or thickness in the labyrinthine segment (fig. 50:2R, 2L). The singular foramen (through which the posterior ampullary nerve passes) on the affected side is more medial than normal and is separated from the internal auditory canal as it approaches the posterior ampulla (fig. 50:2R).

Examining the coronal images, there is a thin, tubular structure between the modiolus and the fundus of the internal auditory canal (fig. 51:1). This tunnel-like structure is not normally present (fig. 51:n1).

Patient MRI Findings

Almost no differences can be ascertained in cochlea itself between the affected and the healthy side, but the modiolus is somewhat narrower on the affected (right) side. In particular, the part corresponding to the cochlear area of the fundus of the internal auditory canal is clearly

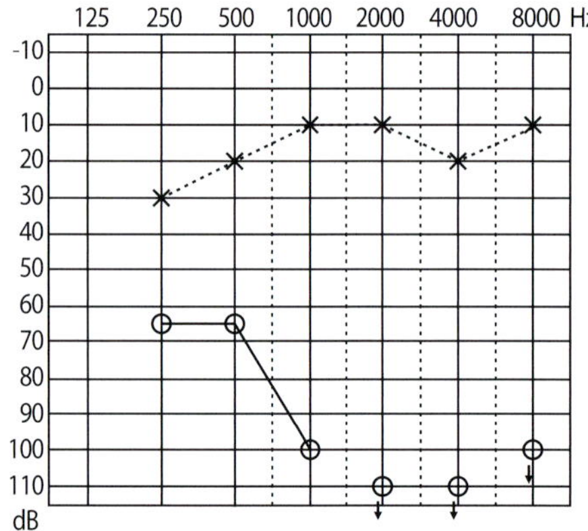

Fig. 48. (Case 1) Audiogram

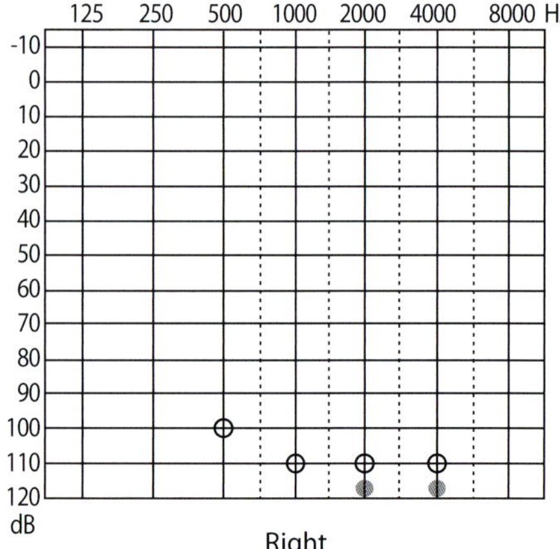

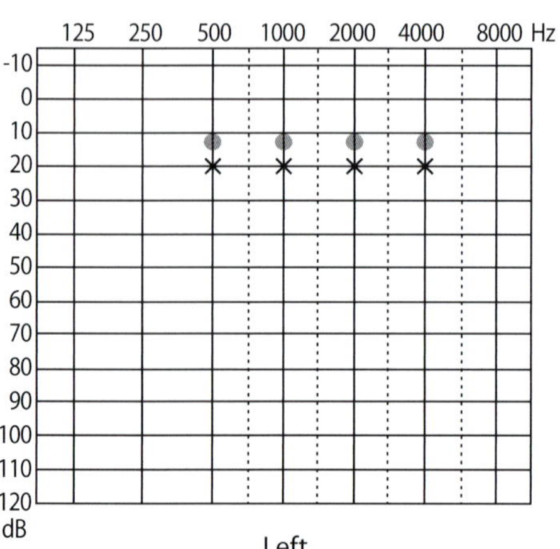

Fig. 49. (Case 1) ASSR test

Patient CT Findings

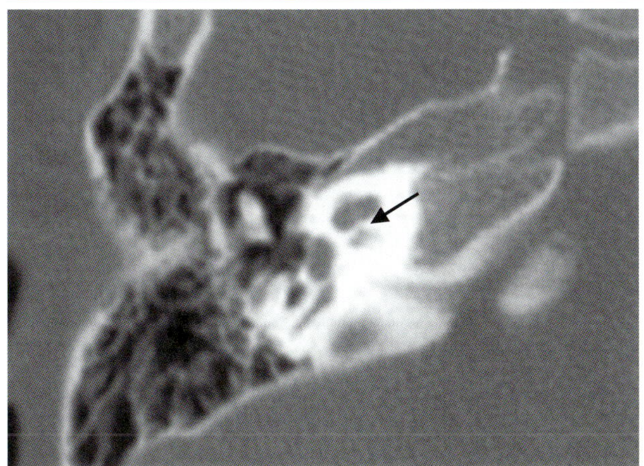

1R. axial image

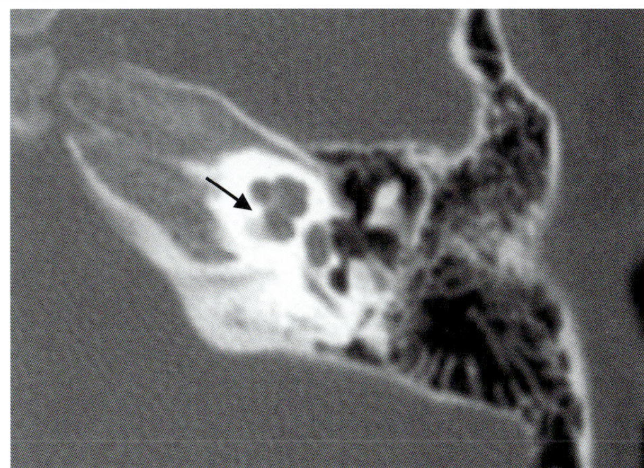

1L. axial image

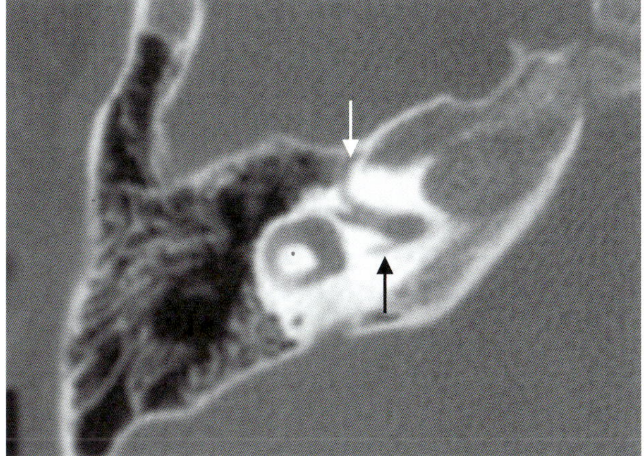

2R. axial image

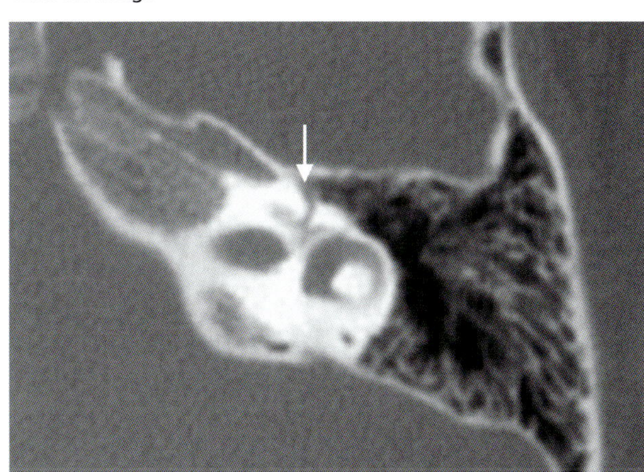

2L. axial image

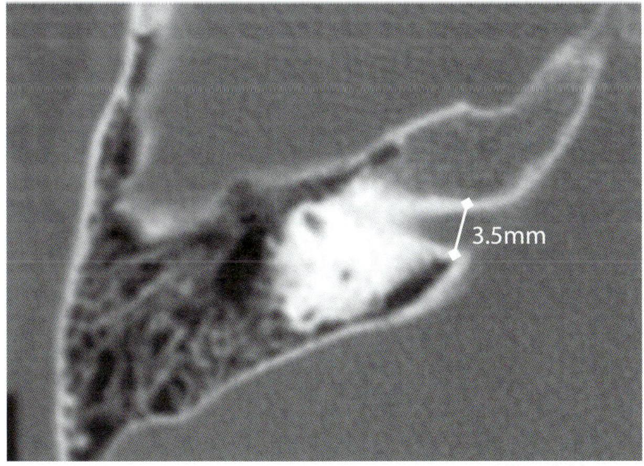

3R. axial image

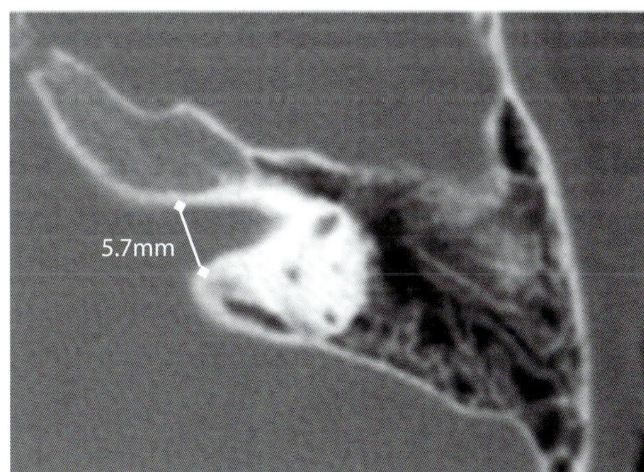

3L. axial image

Fig. 50. (Case 1) CT: R=affected side, L=healthy side

[Patient CT Findings]

No abnormalities were found in the middle ear or ossicles in either side. In the inner ear as well, no clear morphological abnormalities were discovered in the cochlea or vestibule. However, the right internal auditory canal is clearly narrower, with an anteroposterior diameter at the opening to the posterior cranial fossa of 3.5 mm, just 60% the size of the healthy left side diameter of 5.7 mm (3R, 3L). Observing the lateral end of the internal auditory canal at its border with the modiolus, the diameter of the opening at the base of the modiolus is less than 1 mm on the affected side, compared to 2.7 mm on the healthy side (1R : ↙ ; 1L: ↘). On the other hand, the facial nerve shows no bilateral discrepancies in either its path or thickness in the labyrinthine segment (2R & 2L: ⇓). The singular foramen (through which the posterior ampullary nerve passes) on the affected side is more medial than normal and is separated from the internal auditory canal as it approaches the posterior ampulla (2R: ↑).

Patient CT Findings	**Normal Control CT Findings**

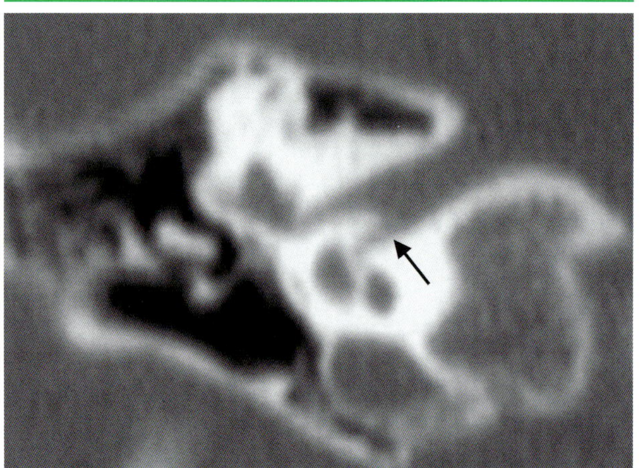 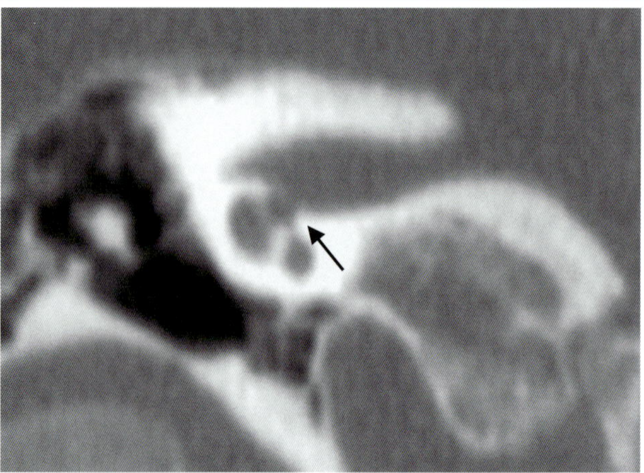

1. coronal image   n1. coronal image

Fig. 51. (Case 1) CT

[Patient CT Findings]
There is a thin, tubular structure between the modiolus and the fundus of the internal auditory canal (1:↖).

《Normal Control CT Findings》
Normally the base of the modiolus continues broadly into the internal auditory canal (n1:↖).

narrower on the affected side than the healthy side, and the cochlear nerve, which is plainly visible in the healthy side, cannot be ascertained on the affected side (fig. 52:1R, 1L). Normally, cranial nerve VIII can be observed bifurcating into the cochlear nerve (fig. 52:2L) and the vestibular nerve slightly medial to the fundus of the internal auditory canal, but in this case the narrowness of the internal auditory canal prevents observation of this bifurcation (fig. 52:2R). Cranial nerves VII and VIII are visible at the cerebellopontine angle. On the affected right side, both nerves are straddling the two slices (fig. 52:3R-a, b), but on careful comparison of the two, cranial nerve VIII on the affected side appears thinner than on the healthy side, even in cross-section b where it is easier to see. On the other hand, cranial nerve VII does not display the same bilateral disparity. From the above findings, one can surmise that in this case there is hypoplasia or atrophy of the cochlear nerve and cranial nerve VIII.

■ Post-diagnostic Course

As a case of unilateral profound hearing loss, it is not essentially indicated for treatment using a hearing aid or cochlear implant. The decision was made to periodically check to ensure that no problems with hearing arose on the healthy side.

Points

❶ Congenital IAC stenosis frequently accompanies sensorineural hearing loss, but enlargement does not correlate with hearing loss.

❷ The length of the internal auditory canal increases after birth, but its diameter shows little change.

❸ Internal auditory canal development is related to formation and development of cranial nerve VIII.

❹ The success rate of cochlear implants in cases of IAC stenosis is lower than in those in which stenosis is not a factor.

Patient MRI Findings

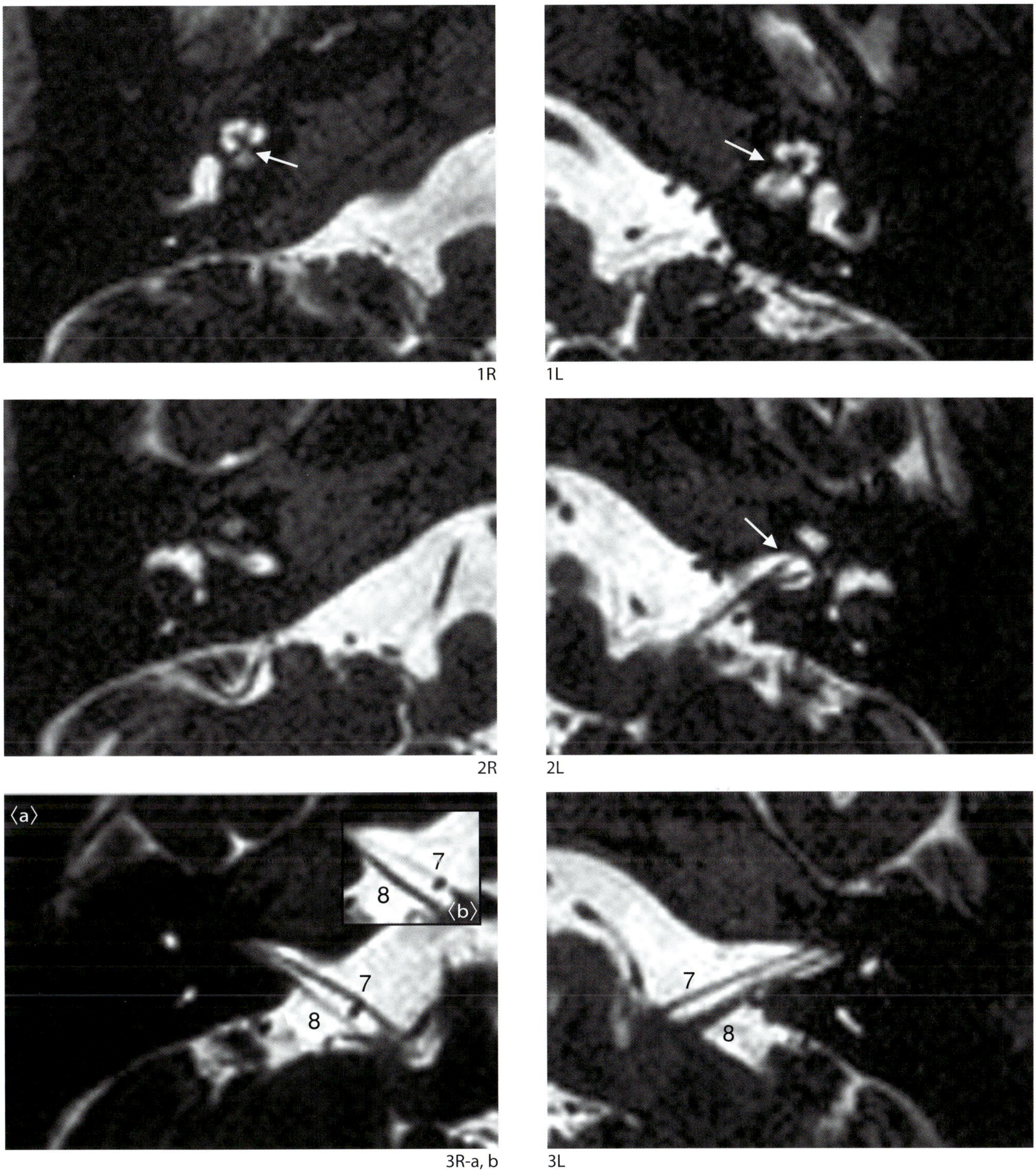

Fig. 52. (Case 1) MRI: R=affected side, L=healthy side

[Patient MRI Findings]

Almost no differences can be ascertained in cochlea itself between the affected and the healthy side, but the modiolus is somewhat narrower on the affected (right) side. In particular, the part corresponding to the cochlear area of the fundus of the internal auditory canal is clearly narrower on the affected side than the healthy side, and the cochlear nerve, which is plainly visible in the healthy side, cannot be ascertained on the affected side (1R: ↖ ; 1L: ↖). Normally, cranial nerve VIII can be observed bifurcating into the cochlear nerve (2L: ↖) and the vestibular nerve slightly medial to the fundus of the internal auditory canal, but in this case the narrowness of the internal auditory canal prevents observation of this bifurcation (2R). Cranial nerves VII and VIII can be observed at the cerebellopontine angle. On the affected right side, both nerves are straddling the two slices (3R-a, b), but on careful comparison of the two, cranial nerve VIII on the affected side is thinner than on the healthy side, even in cross-section b where it is easier to see. On the other hand, cranial nerve VII does not display the same bilateral disparity.

Case 2

Stenosis of Cochlear Nerve Canal
Subject: male, 1 year old

■ History and Clinical Findings

Four months previously (at eight months old), the subject was hospitalized at a pediatric hospital for bacterial meningitis. The meningitis was cured using antibiotics and steroid therapy but, when auditory brainstem response (ABR) testing was conducted before discharge from the hospital to check for inner ear dysfunction, no response was obtained in the right ear (fig. 53). The subject then was referred to our department for further testing.

ASSR testing conducted by our department returned near normal results for the left ear, but threshold values for the right ear were from 70 dB (500 Hz) to 110 dB (4,000 Hz) (fig. 54). However, DPOAE testing confirmed near normal response not only in the left ear, but in the right ear as well (fig. 55).

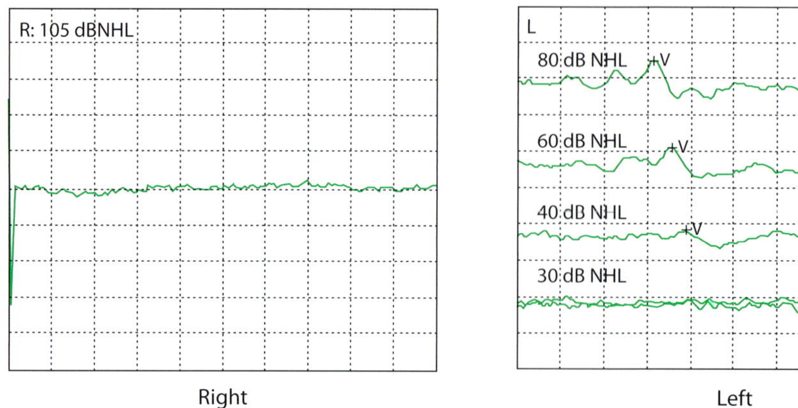

Fig. 53. (Case 2) Auditory brainstem response test (ABR)

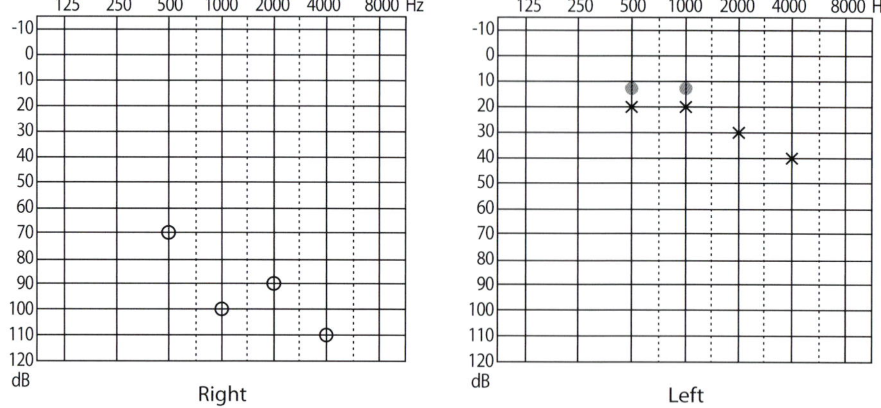

Fig. 54. (Case 2) ASSR test

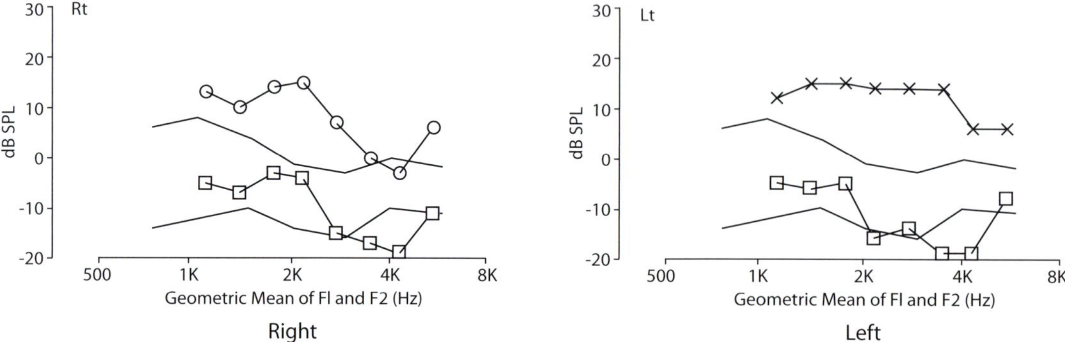

Fig. 55. (Case 2) DPOAE test

Patient 3-Dimensional Reconstructed MRI Findings

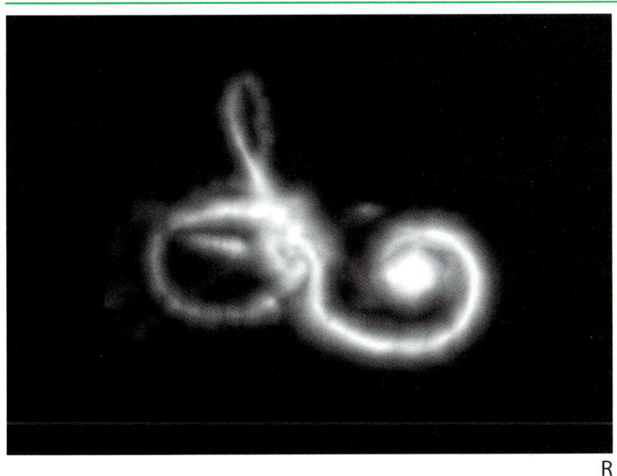

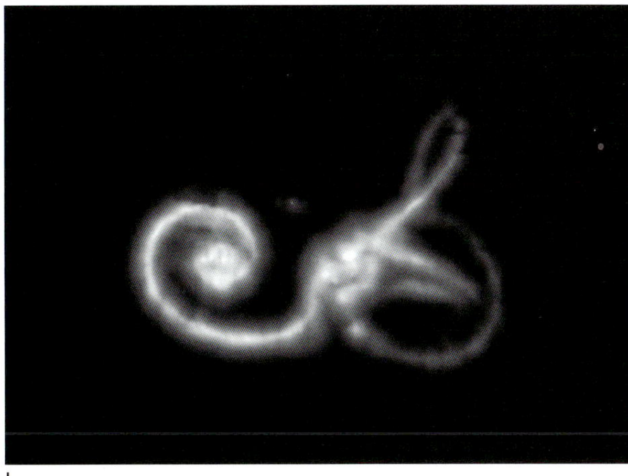

R   L

Fig. 56. (Case 2) 3-dimensional reconstructed MRI

[Patient 3-Dimensional Reconstructed MRI Findings]
No clear abnormalities or bilateral differences exist in either the affected side (R) or the normal side (L).

Patient CT Findings

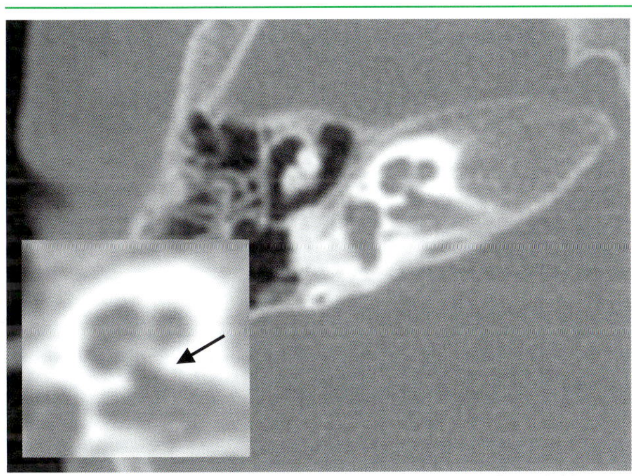

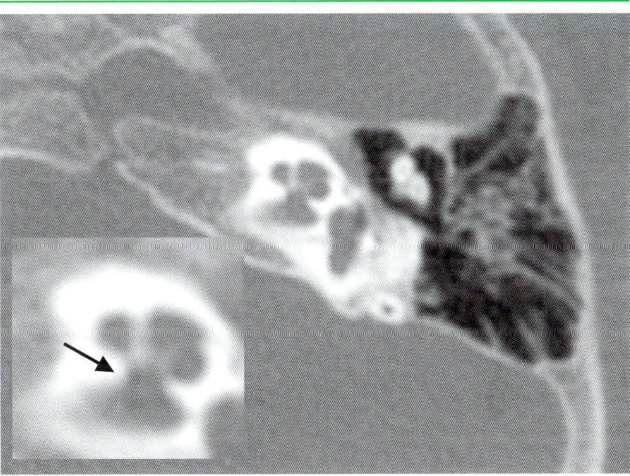

R. axial image   L. axial image

Fig. 57. (Case 2) CT

[Patient CT Findings]
In the right ear, the diameter of the transitional area between the fundus of the internal auditory canal and the modiolus— the so-called cochlear nerve canal (covered later in more detail)— is 1.7 mm. This is clearly narrower (R: ✔, L: ✔) than the left ear, which is 2.4 mm. There are no other abnormal findings in the right inner or middle ear. In the left ear there are no abnormal findings whatsoever, including the fundus of the internal auditory canal.

■ Patient 3-Dimensional Reconstructed MRI Findings

In observing the inner ear in 3-dimensional reconstructed MR images, there were no clear abnormalities or bilateral differences (fig. 56).

■ Patient CT Findings

In the right ear, the diameter of the transitional area between the fundus of the internal auditory canal and the modiolus—the so-called cochlear nerve canal (covered later in more detail)— is 1.7 mm. This is clearly narrower than the left ear, which is 2.4 mm. There are no other abnormal findings in the right inner or middle ear. In the left ear there are no abnormal findings whatsoever, including the fundus of the internal auditory canal (fig. 57).

■ Patient MRI Findings

Observing the nerves at the fundi of the left and right internal auditory canals, the respective difference is evident, with the right cochlear nerve depicted indistinctly (fig. 58:1R) and the left cochlear nerve clearly visible (fig. 58:1L). The right internal auditory canal is also somewhat narrower, with a diameter of 2.4 mm compared to the left's 3.7 mm. Cranial nerve VIII itself is also thinner on the right (fig. 58:2R) than on the left (fig. 58:2L).

Patient MRI Findings

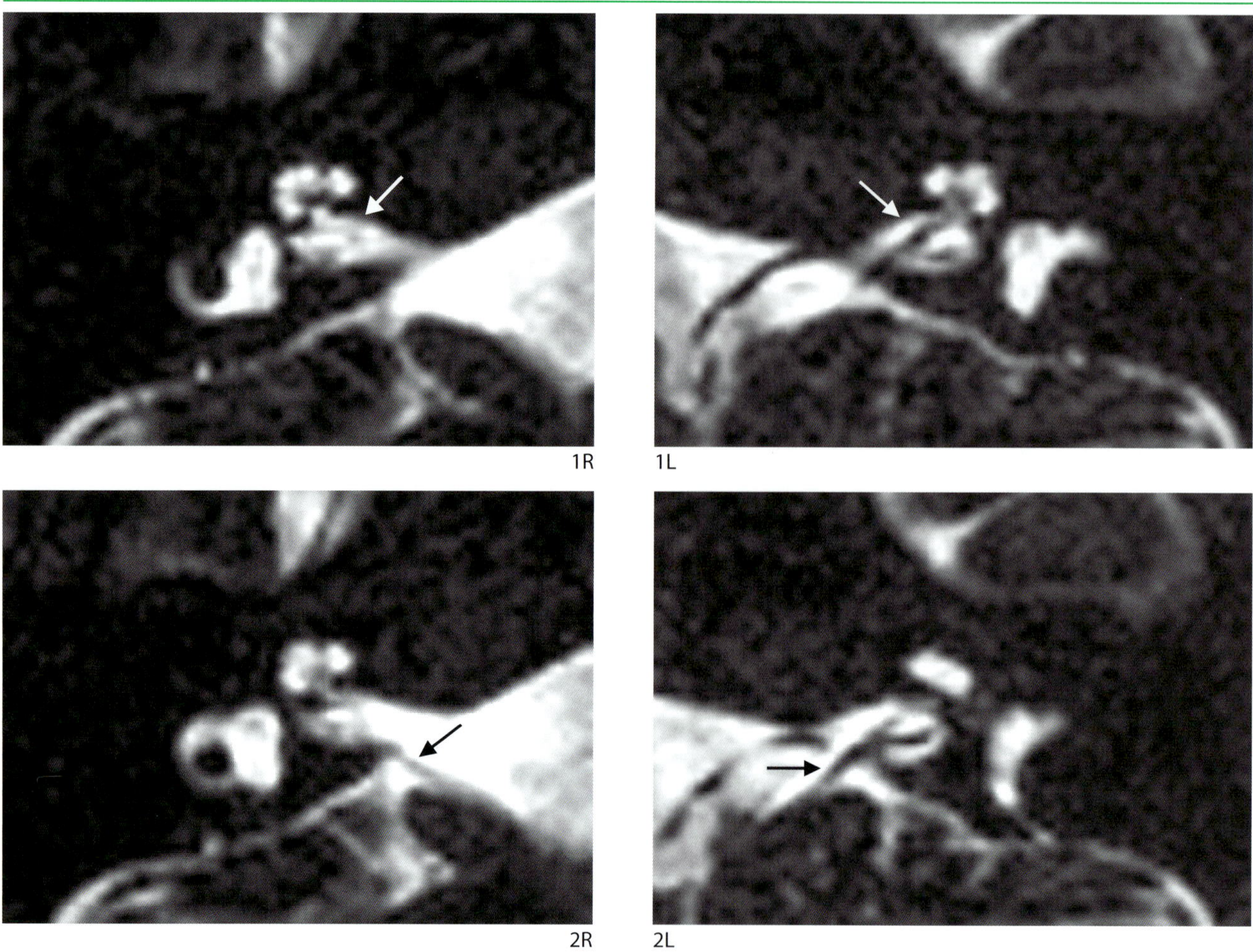

Fig. 58. (Case 2) MRI

[Patient MRI Findings]

Observing the nerves at the fundi of the left and right internal auditory canals, the respective difference is evident, with the right cochlear nerve depicted indistinctly (1R: ✎) and the left cochlear nerve clearly visible (1L: ↘). The right internal auditory canal is also somewhat narrower, with a diameter of 2.4 mm compared to the left's 3.7 mm. Cranial nerve VIII itself is also thinner on the right (2R: ✔) than on the left (2L: →).

■ Considerations and Diagnosis

In this case testing was conducted after the subject contracted meningitis and hearing loss was confirmed in the right ear, but as he was an infant and had not received newborn hearing screening, it was unclear as to whether or not the hearing loss existed prior to contracting meningitis. However, hearing loss due to bacterial meningitis normally arises through damage to both the sensory epithelium and the cochlear nerve due to inner ear infection and inflammation from the cochlear canaliculus or the internal auditory canal, so normal a DPOAE on the affected side, as is the case here, is exceptional. Also, ossification subsequent to labyrinthitis is thought to spread from the scala tympani or modiolus, at the basal turn of the cochlea where the cochlear canaliculus opens, to the cochlea and the entire inner ear, including the vestibule. It is very difficult to imagine that ossification would occur only in the cochlear nerve canal and make it narrower, as it has here. On the other hand, as we shall see later, there are many recent reports of congenital stenosis of the cochlear nerve canal at the fundus of the internal auditory canal, and this malformation is increasingly being recognized as a distinct disease entity. Based on the above considerations, we feel that this case, rather than being one of selective retrocochlear disturbance and ossification of the cochlear nerve canal caused by meningitis, is more likely one of retrocochlear hearing loss due to congenital hypoplasia of the cochlear nerve canal and cochlear nerve.

■ Cochlear Nerve Canal

The anteroinferior part of the internal auditory canal, referred to as the cochlear area, contains the tractus spiralis foraminosus through which the cochlear nerve bundles pass. While it forms a slight recess in the fundus of the internal auditory canal, no neural canal exists as a distinct anatomical structure. However, in some cases of sensorineural hearing loss, this area forms a narrow, tubular structure. As this tubular structure does not exist in normal anatomy and there is no official anatomical term for it, it was initially reported as the "bony canal for the cochlear nerve" [1], and later most often simply referred to as the "cochlear nerve canal" [2]. In cases of profound hearing loss accompanied by cochlear nerve canal stenosis observed in CT images, hypoplasia of the cochlear nerve is often confirmed through MRI observations [3, 4]. Clinically, there is low expectation for the effectiveness of cochlear implants when cochlear nerve canal stenosis with cochlear nerve hypoplasia is present [3, 4], making it an important point to focus on during clinical imaging diagnosis for cases of congenital sensorineural hearing loss.

References

1 Fatterpekar GM, Mukherji SK, Alley J, et al: Hypoplasia of the bony canal for the cochlear nerve in patients with congenital sensorineural hearing loss: initial observations. Radiology 2000;215:243–246.
2 Stjernholm C, Muren C: Dimensions of the cochlear nerve canal: a radioanatomic investigation. Acta Otolaryngol 2002;122:43–48.
3 Miyasaka M, Nosaka S, Morimoto N, et al: CT and MR imaging for pediatric cochlear implantation: emphasis on the relationship between the cochlear nerve canal and the cochlear nerve. Pediatr Radiol 2010 Mar 23 [Epub ahead of print].
4 Papsin BC: Cochlear implantation in children with anomalous cochleovestibular anatomy. Laryngoscope 2005;115 (Suppl. 106):1–26.

Points

❶ When the cause of sensorineural hearing loss is unclear, it is necessary to examine the cochlear nerve canal on the fundus of the internal auditory canal.

❷ Cases of cochlear nerve canal stenosis are frequently accompanied by cochlear nerve hypoplasia.

❸ Presence of cochlear nerve canal stenosis is an important factor when considering indication for cochlear implant surgery.

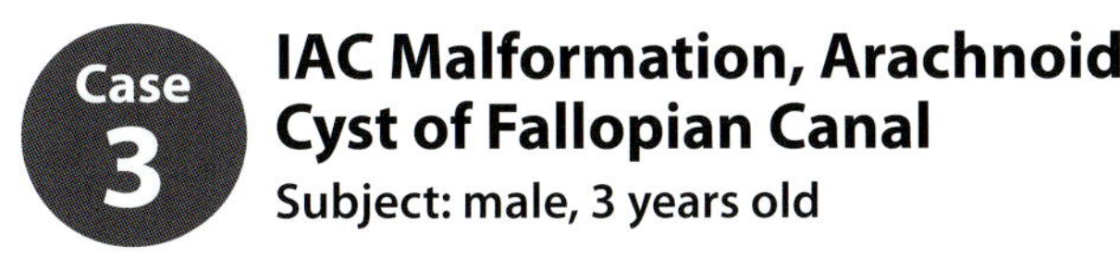

Case 3
IAC Malformation, Arachnoid Cyst of Fallopian Canal

Subject: male, 3 years old

■ History and Clinical Findings

Since around one year old the subject had experienced recurrent, bilateral acute otitis media along with repeated bouts of meningitis, and was referred to our department by a neighborhood otolaryngologist for testing to determine the cause of the meningitis. Another hospital had diagnosed right inner ear malformation and right-side deafness. Otitis media was recurring bilaterally, and our findings at time of initial exam indicated retraction of the tympanic membranes in both ears, along with effusion accumulation in the right ear. Hearing testing showed right-side deafness, with a hearing level of 30–40 dB in the left ear. Temporal bone CT and MRI exams were carried out.

■ Patient CT Findings

Mastoid air cell development is deficient on both sides and a soft tissue density (effusion) can be seen between the epitympanum and the mastoid segment, but no abnormalities can be ascertained in the ossicles. In the right inner ear, a portion of the basal turn of the cochlea, the vestibule, and the ampulla of the posterior semicircular canal are discernible, but other parts are ossified (fig. 59:1R, 2R, 3R). There is no clear stenosis or enlargement of the internal auditory canal, but starting at the fundus of the internal auditory canal the labyrinthine segment of the right facial nerve (fig. 59:3R) is enlarged compared to the normal control (fig. 59:n3), and in the part normally corresponding to the area between the geniculate ganglion and the tympanic segment of the facial nerve (fig. 59:n2), a soft tissue density of around 6.2 × 2.4 mm, longer anteroposteriorly, (fig. 59:2R, 3R) is visible. This continues posteriorly to become the tympanic and mastoid segments of the facial nerve, with no abnormalities in the peripheral fallopian canal.

Observing the coronal CT image, a thick neural canal can be identified running from the internal auditory canal directly to the geniculate ganglion (fig. 60:3R). Anterior to this, whereas in the normal control the area around and superior to the geniculate ganglion (fig. 60:n1) is composed of air cells, in this case it is occupied by a large, saccular structure with a superoinferior diameter of over 5 mm (fig. 60:1R, 2R). Please refer to the normal control images to confirm the proper path of the facial nerve's labyrinthine segment (fig. 60:n2, n3) and tympanic segment (fig. 60:n2, n3).

■ Patient MRI Findings

When observed in the MRI, it is apparent that the facial nerve (fig. 61:1R) actually passes inside the facial nerve labyrinthine segment on the fundus of the internal auditory canal that was observed in the CT images. The cystic area of the geniculate ganglion is hyperintense (fig. 61:1R, 2R) in T2 weighted imaging and is continuous with the internal auditory canal and may be filled with cerebrospinal fluid. Also, inside this area there is a slightly hypointense structure (fig. 61:2R) that is assumed to be either

Patient CT Findings

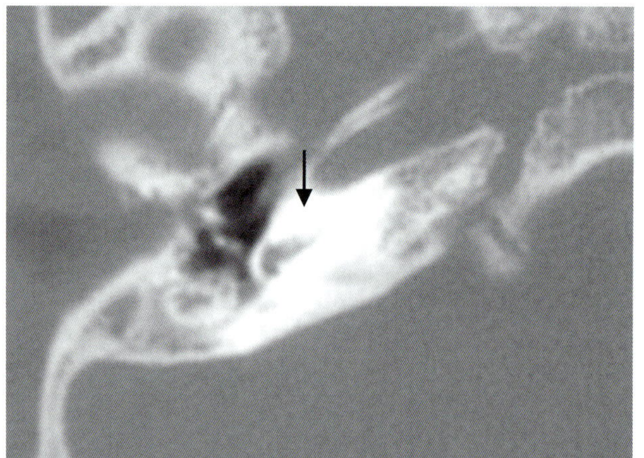

1R. axial image

Normal Control CT Findings

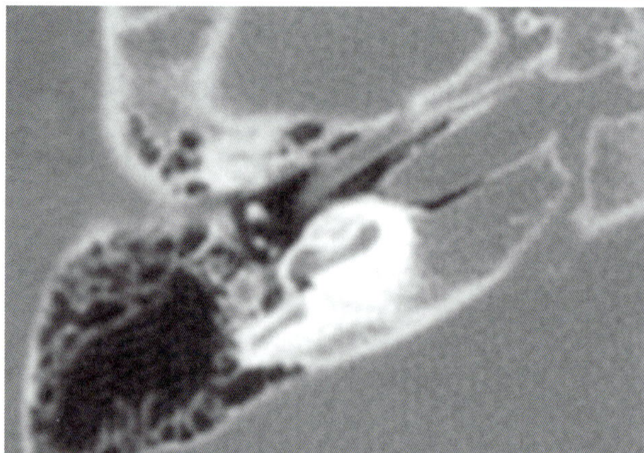

n1. axial image

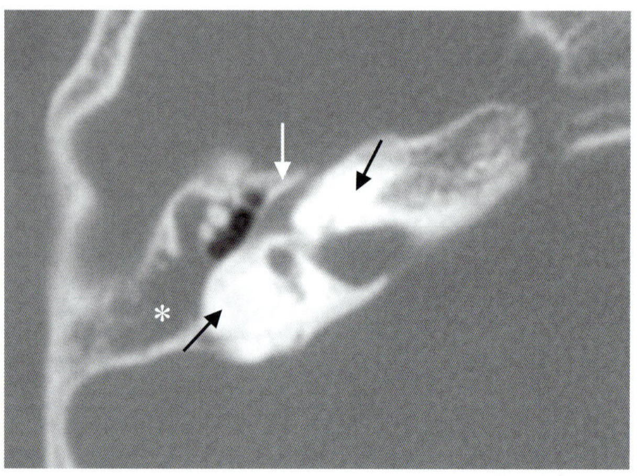

2R. axial image

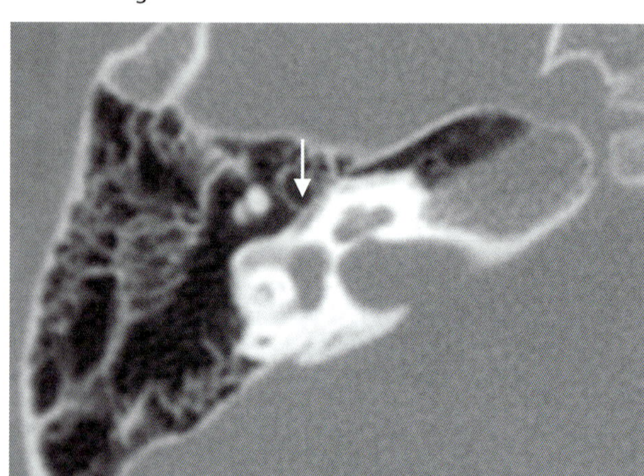

n2. axial image

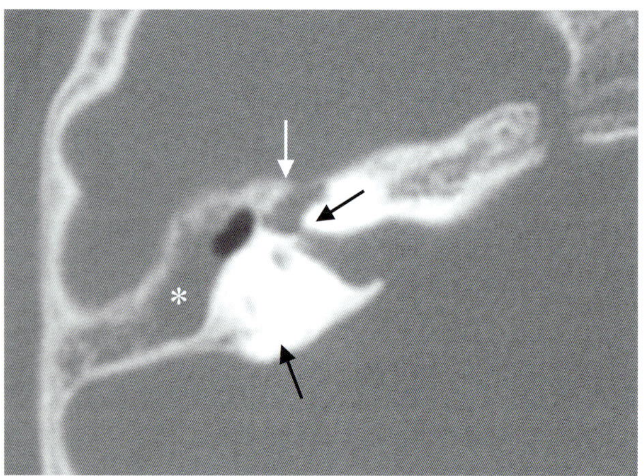

3R. axial image

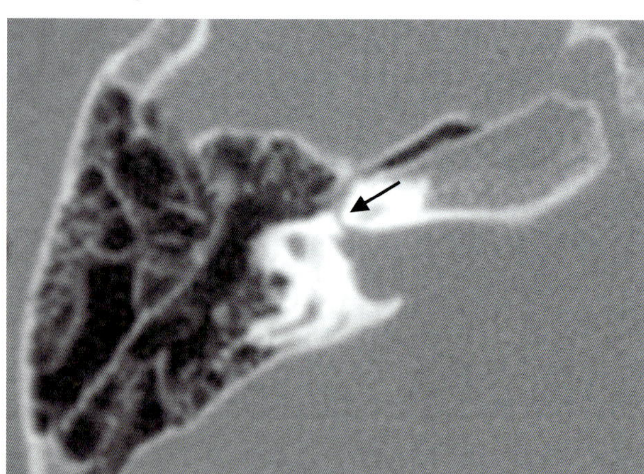

n3. axial image

Fig. 59. (Case 3) CT

[Patient CT Findings]

Mastoid air cell development is deficient and a soft tissue density (effusion) can be seen between the epitympanum and the mastoid segment, but no abnormalities can be ascertained in the ossicles. In the right inner ear, a portion of the basal turn of the cochlea, the vestibule, and the ampulla of the posterior semicircular canal are discernible, but other parts are ossified (1R ↓, 2R ↙ ↗, 3R ↖). There is no clear stenosis or enlargement of the internal auditory canal, but starting at the fundus of the internal auditory canal the labyrinthine segment of the right facial nerve (3R: ↙) is enlarged, and in the part normally corresponding to the area between the geniculate ganglion and the tympanic segment of the facial nerve, a soft tissue density of around 6.2 × 2.4 mm, longer anteroposteriorly, (2R: ⇓ , 3R: ⇓) is visible. No abnormalities were found in the peripheral fallopian canal.

《Normal Control CT Findings》

n1: cross-section enabling examination of the basal turn of the cochlea. n2: ⇓ tympanic segment of the facial nerve. n3: ↙ labyrinthine segment of the facial nerve.

Patient CT Findings

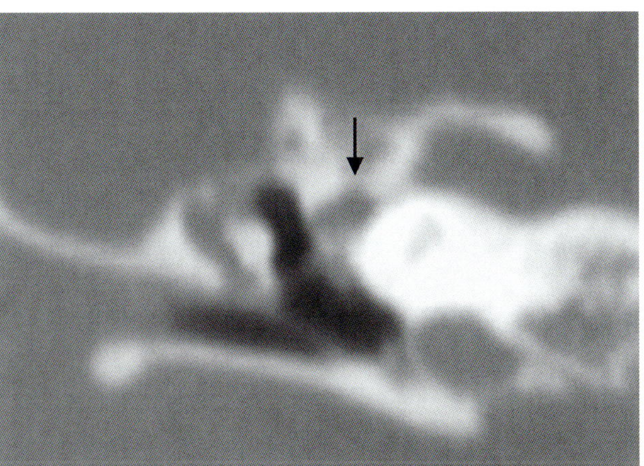

1R. coronal image

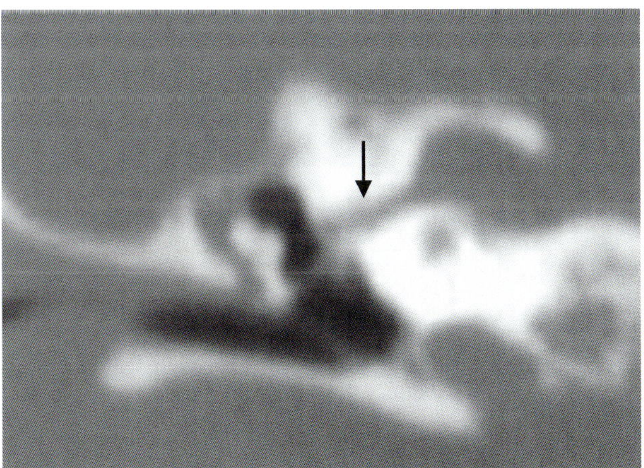

2R. coronal image

3R. coronal image

Normal Control CT Findings

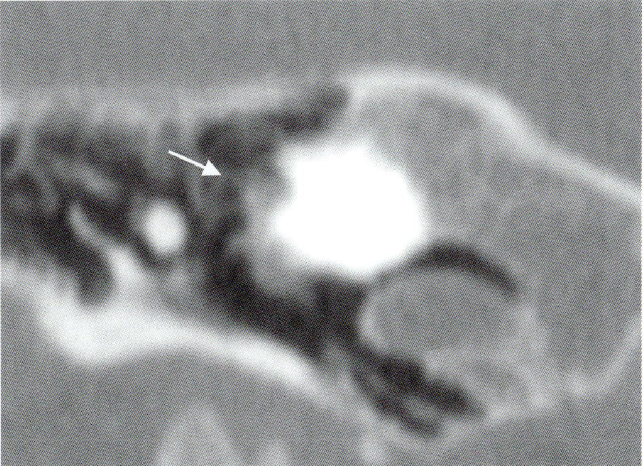

n1. coronal image

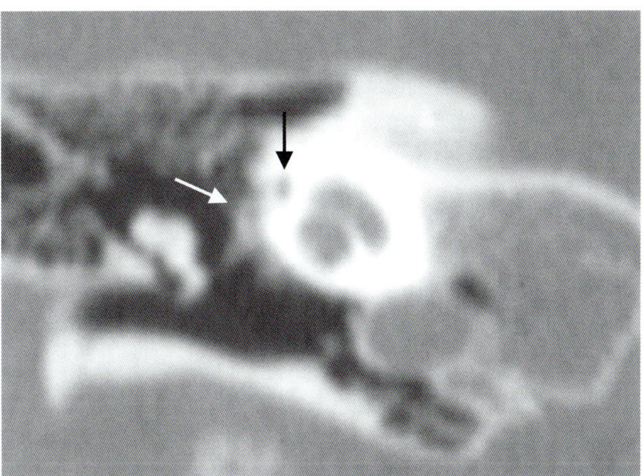

n2. coronal image

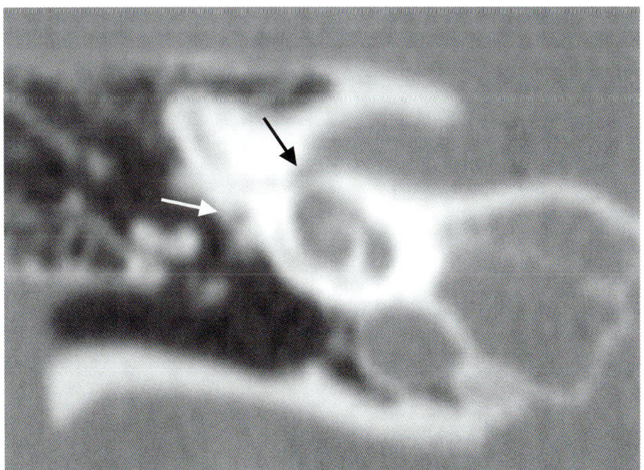

n3. coronal image

Fig. 60. (Case 3) CT

[Patient CT Findings]

A thick neural canal can be identified running from the internal auditory canal directly to the geniculate ganglion (3R: ↓). Anterior to this, a large, saccular structure can be observed (1R: ⇣, 2R: ↓). Please refer to the normal control images to confirm the proper path of the facial nerve's labyrinthine segment (n2:↓, n3:↘) and tympanic segment (n2: ↝, n3: ↝).

《Normal Control CT Findings》

n1: ↝ geniculate ganglion. n2: ↓ labyrinthine segment of facial nerve; ↝ tympanic segment of facial nerve. n3: ↘ labyrinthine segment of facial nerve; ↝ tympanic segment of facial nerve.

Patient MRI Findings

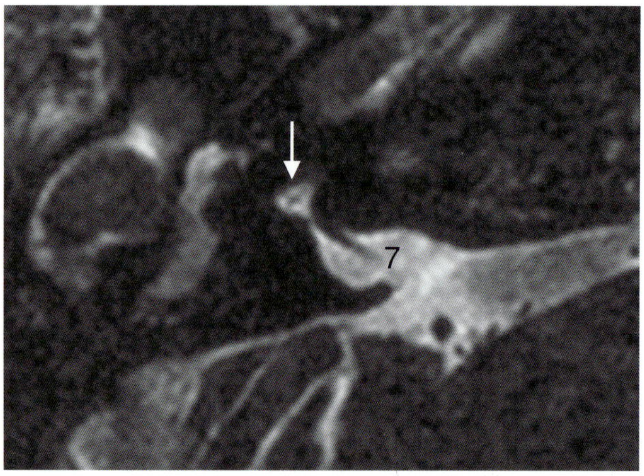

Normal Control MRI Findings

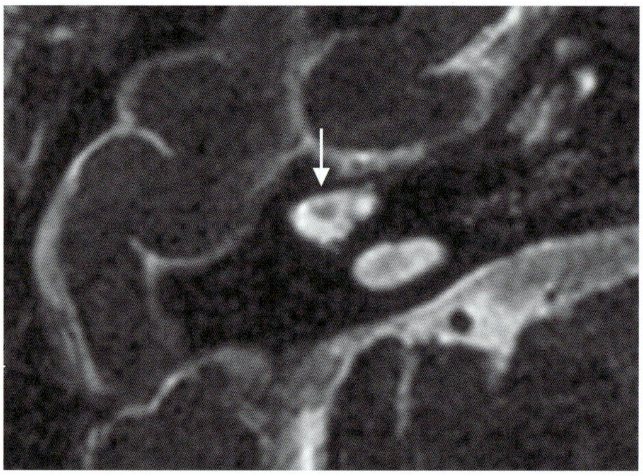

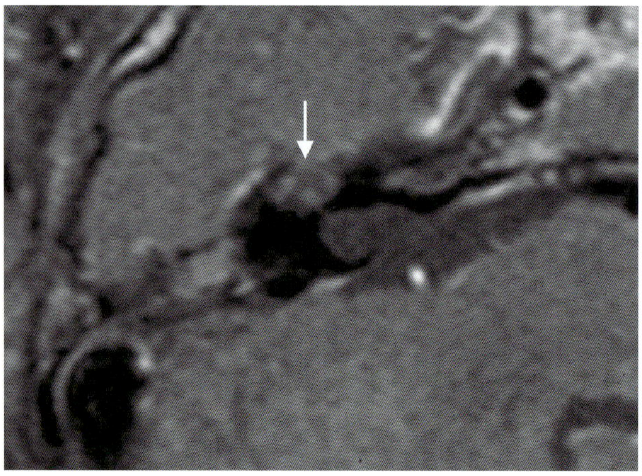

Fig. 61. (Case 3) MRI

[Patient MRI Findings]

It is apparent that the facial nerve (1R: **7**) actually passes inside the facial nerve labyrinthine segment on the fundus of the internal auditory canal. The cystic area of the geniculate ganglion is hyperintense (1R & 2R: ⇓) in T2 weighted imaging and is continuous with the internal auditory canal and may be filled with cerebrospinal fluid. Also, inside this area there is a slightly hypointense structure (2R: ⇓) that is assumed to be either nerve fibre or some kind of soft tissue. In T1 weighted Gd enhanced MRI performed later, neither the interior nor the margins of this cystic structure revealed contrast enhancement (3R: ⇓), contraindicating a tumor, granulation, cholesteatoma, or other lesion.

《Normal Control MRI Findings》

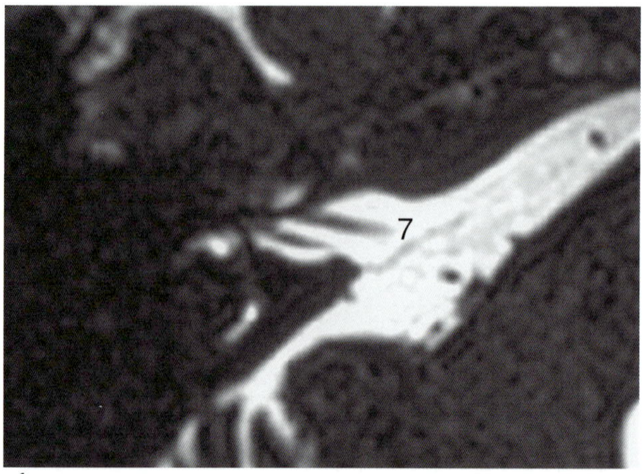

n1: **7** indicates the facial nerve inside the internal auditory canal. n2: In a hyperintense T2 weighted image such as this, the geniculate ganglion located lateroanterior to the fundus of the internal auditory canal is barely discernible.

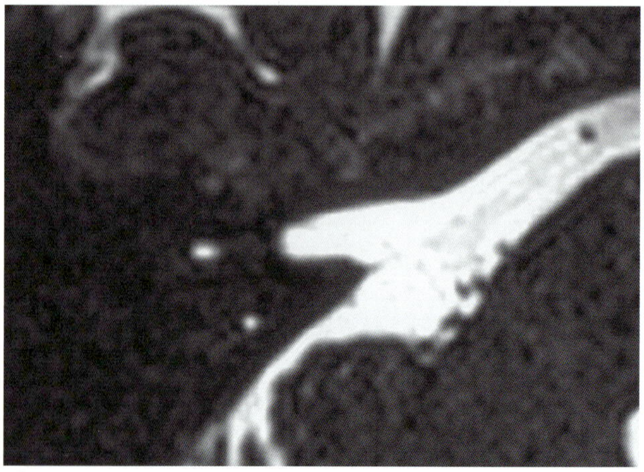

nerve fibre or some kind of soft tissue. In T1 weighted Gd enhanced MRI performed later, neither the interior nor the margins of this cystic structure exhibited contrast enhancement (fig. 61:3), contraindicating a tumor, granulation, cholesteatoma, or other lesion.

Also, on close inspection of the simple T2 weighted cranial MRI (fig. 62), there is a T2 hyperintense area extending from the area posterior to the right ear subcutaneously below the ear, which may be accumulation of cerebrospinal fluid leaked from the fallopian canal.

■ Clinical Course and Surgical Findings

Initially, based on the CT findings in this case, I assumed that the bony defect in the geniculate ganglion area was either a cyst or a congenital cholesteatoma, but in the MRI there was no contrast enhancement around the margin and it was continuous with the internal auditory canal, so I concluded there was a high probability that it was an arachnoid cyst that had herniated and enlarged into the fallopian canal. I hypothesized that this had led to effusion of cerebrospinal fluid into the fallopian canal, with retrograde infection from the area communicating with the middle ear, which gave rise to recurrent meningitis. Later the subject again contracted severe meningitis, which caused paresis of the right facial nerve around one year after our initial consultation, so we inspected the

geniculate ganglion using a temporal craniotomy/middle cranial fossa approach with the objective of arresting the cerebrospinal fluid leak by opening, confirming, and obliterating the lesion site. As suggested from the MR images, the area consisted of a cyst covered in a thin membrane, the incision of which resulted in a strong outflow of spinal fluid. Inside was a cobweb-like fibrous structure, possibly the facial nerve. The area where the cyst flowed in from the fundus of the internal auditory canal was patched with several layers of periosteum fragments and glued in place. The inside of the cyst was also filled with bone putty, but in order to avoid permanent facial paralysis we were careful not to pack the space too firmly.

Postoperatively the facial paralysis worsened slightly, but there was no recurrence of the meningitis. Middle ear ventilation tube insertion and other therapies to prevent recurrence of middle ear infection were also pursued concurrently. However, one year later there was a reoccurrence of severe meningitis, so after consultation with the parents it was decided to completely obliterate and close the cyst area, even though it may not be possible to preserve facial nerve function.

Two years six months after initial examination in our department, a right temporal craniotomy was once again performed and the cyst in the geniculate ganglion opened up via the middle cranial fossa. This time the area was opened broadly all the way to the internal auditory canal and the labyrinthine segment of the fallopian canal packed firmly with periosteum fragments. The interior of the cyst was filled with bone putty that was strongly compacted without regard for facial nerve damage. Histopathological examination of the specimen collected at this time confirmed that the wall of the cyst was arachnoid membrane. Postoperatively, the facial nerve score fell temporarily, but then gradually recovered, and currently has improved to partial paresis. Also, there has been no recurrence of meningitis up to this time, two years six months after revision surgery.

■ Arachnoid Cyst of Fallopian Canal

It is common to observe the arachnoid membrane forming a cyst and enlarging intracranially, but these cysts are often asymptomatic and require no particular treatment. However, on rare occasions the arachnoid cyst may herniate outside the cranium and present a variety of pathological findings, including meningitis. In particular, there are cases of cysts developing peripherally within the fallopian canal of the temporal bone along the path of the facial nerve, with recurring meningitis. Aside from this case, we have also experienced a similar case in an adult.

There have been several reports to date concerning cases of cerebrospinal fluid leak via along the fallopian canal due to congenital defects, in which retrograde infection caused recurring meningitis [1–3]. The area surrounding the geniculate ganglion is one route along which cholesteatomas develop from the epitympanum to the petrous apex, and in a differential diagnosis cholesteatoma is

Patient MRI Findings

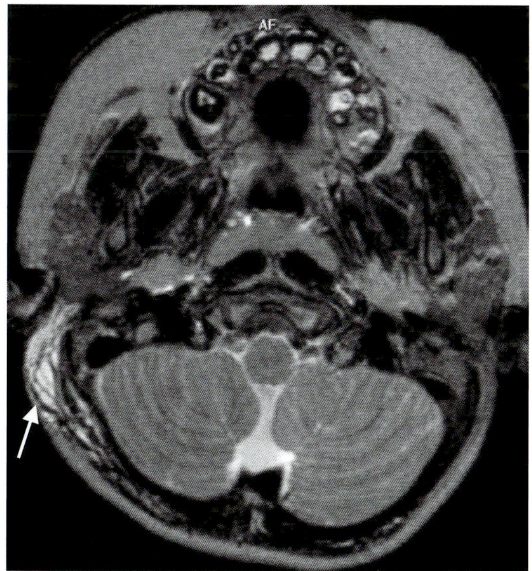

T2 weighted image

Fig. 62. (Case 3) MRI

[Patient MRI Findings]

There is a T2 hyperintense area extending from the area posterior to the right ear subcutaneously below the ear (↑), which may be accumulation of cerebrospinal fluid leaked via the fallopian canal.

what first comes to mind. In this case, however, the MRI signal characteristics differed from that of a cholesteatoma, and the finding of cerebrospinal fluid emanating subcutaneously from the stylomastoid foramen would not occur with cholesteatoma, so knowledge of this disease facilitates correct diagnosis. In our surgical findings, the nerve inside the cyst did not form a simple bundle as usual, but instead, except for the main nerve bundle, spread out like a cobweb of fine fibers. The poorly defined hypointense area observed inside the cyst in the T2 weighted MRI is how the separated nerve bundles or fibers within the cyst are depicted.

Concerning treatment, in all previously reported cases it has been difficult to find a balance between the need to completely block cerebrospinal fluid leak and concern for damage to the facial nerve as a result of surgery, as failure to firmly block the fallopian canal will result in recurrence of meningitis. In this case also, the area around the facial nerve was initially sealed lightly to avoid nerve damage, but due to the later recurrence of possibly life-threatening meningitis, in the second operation the parents were fully consulted and the cyst cavity firmly obliterated without regard to preservation of facial nerve function, finally preventing the meningitis from reoccurring. However, because we avoided removing the facial nerve before obliterating the cavity, there has been considerable long-term recovery of facial nerve function. A trans-mastoid approach has been attempted for a case of cerebrospinal fluid leakage and meningitis similar to this one [2], but control of leakage was difficult and in the end required subtotal extirpation of the temporal bone. Approaching via the middle cranial fossa is comparatively minimally invasive and effective and should be considered one of the surgical options in treatment of cerebrospinal fluid leak via the fallopian canal.

References

1 Foyt D, Brackmann DE: Cerebrospinal fluid otorrhea through a congenitally patent fallopian canal. Arch Otolaryngol 2000;126:540–542.
2 Isaacson JE, Linder TE, Fisch U: Arachnoid cyst of the fallopian canal: a surgical challenge. Otol Neurotol 2002;23:589–593.
3 Mong S, Goldberg AN, Lustig LR: Fallopian canal meningocele: report of two cases. Otol Neurotol 2009;30:525–528.

Points

❶ The fallopian canal is sometimes the causative route for infant meningitis.

❷ Herniation of an arachnoid cyst through the fallopian canal can cause facial paralysis, cerebrospinal fluid leak, and meningitis.

❸ Obliteration of the region of the geniculate ganglion and labyrinthine segment of the facial nerve via the middle cranial fossa was an effective treatment.

Pediatric Ear Diseases
Diagnostic Imaging Atlas and Case Reports

Inflammatory Diseases of the Middle Ear

Otitis media is the most common pediatric ear disease encountered in everyday clinical practice. Otitis media has two forms: acute otitis media, marked by sudden onset and short-term recovery; and chronic otitis media, in which symptoms including otorrhea and hearing loss continue over long periods without recovery. Chronic otitis media is further classified as narrowly defined chronic otitis media, which includes middle ear infection and tympanic membrane perforation, and cholesteatomatous otitis media, in which a portion of the tympanic membrane's epithelium invades and expands into the middle ear cavity.

There are also cases in which, even after recovery from acute otitis media, effusion is retained in the middle ear cavity for an extended period and develops into refractory otitis media with effusion. With ordinary acute otitis media, clinical symptoms and tympanic membrane findings are sufficient to enable a diagnosis and recovery is swift, so temporal bone CT or other advanced imaging is not required, but in cases of chronic otitis media or acute otitis media with complications, imaging diagnosis is required to investigate the cause of impaired recovery, observe the condition of the auditory ossicles, and determine a treatment policy including whether or not surgery is required. Also, in cases in which tympanoplasty or other surgical procedures are performed, imaging diagnosis plays a major role not only in surgical planning, but in postoperative follow-up as well.

Chapter 4

❶ Otitis Media and Cholesteatoma
❷ Image Findings after Tympanoplasty

❶ Otitis Media and Cholesteatoma

Eustachian Tube Function and Mastoid Air Cell Development

The most difficult problem with acute otitis media in young children is its persistent recurrence [1]. Over half of children will have contracted acute otitis media at least once by the age of three, with peak infection occurring between six and eleven months after birth. Moreover, 10–20% of children contract acute otitis media three times or more by the time they reach one year old. The source of infection for acute otitis media is the nasopharynx, with infection spreading to the middle ear via the eustachian tube. Consequently, prolonged exposure to daycare and other group settings, in which children frequently exchange upper respiratory infections, exacerbates the recurrence of otitis media. There are many factors influencing the recurrence of otitis media, including individual eustachian tube function, immunocompetence, the presence of siblings, and environmental factors in the home such as whether or not the parents smoke [2].

Otitis media recurs easily between the ages of one and ten years old, after which it abates and the child enters a stable condition with no clinically significant inflammation. However, in cases that have experienced recurrent otitis media during childhood, latent problems continue and sometimes develop in later years into middle ear cholesteatoma, adhesive otitis media, or other intractable diseases requiring surgical intervention, so caution is required. The causes for inflammatory diseases of the middle ear becoming protracted or intractable are complex rather than singular, and there is no doubt that contraction of otitis media before one year old or its later recurrence forms an important background for later difficulties [3].

As mentioned in Chapter 1, the tympanic cavity, epitympanum (attic), aditus ad antrum, and mastoid antrum are already formed in the newborn's middle ear and pneumatization is present. However, the surrounding air cells are only marginally formed, developing and enlarging after birth to finally form extensive pneumatic cavities. More specifically, mastoid air cell development begins with extremely rapid expansion between birth and one year old, with rapid expansion continuing from one year to five years old. Expansion after that is comparatively slower, ceasing in adolescence between 15 and 18 years old when middle ear development is complete [4].

Mastoid air cell development is suppressed by inflammation in the middle ear [5]. Consequently, examination of the degree of mastoid air cell development in temporal bone CT images of older children or adults allows one to estimate the degree of middle ear inflammation experienced by the patient during early childhood years when the mastoid air cells were developing. If mastoid air cell development is favorable and middle ear cavity volume large, the pneumatic cavities serve to buffer sudden changes in external air pressure and mitigate changes in middle ear pressure [6]. Also, with negative pressurization of the middle ear, even if a fixed amount of air is aspirated from the middle ear via the eustachian tube due to the 'sniffing' that is a factor in middle ear cholesteatoma formation, the

larger the middle ear cavity the more the relative negative pressurization can be reduced. Middle ear pressure is controlled by two mechanisms, the eustachian tube and gas exchange through the middle ear mucosa [7, 8], and if the mastoid air cells are well developed the surface area of the middle ear mucosa covering their surface is larger, increasing gas exchange capacity in the middle ear cavity. Middle ear cavity pressure regulation and ventilation via the eustachian tube and mastoid air cells is vitally important for maintaining healthy conditions in the middle ear [9, 10], and its impairment is believed to play a major role in the development of intractable middle ear diseases such as middle ear cholesteatoma [11]. Also, the success rate for tympanoplasties used in the treatment of chronic middle ear infections is higher in cases in which middle ear ventilation via the eustachian tube and mastoid air cells is favorable [12].

Therefore, in order to grasp the condition of a middle ear disease, it is important both to observe the morphologies of the tympanic membrane and temporal bone and to evaluate functional aspects such as eustachian tube functioning. In particular, assessment of the mastoid air cells should not be limited to simple morphological evaluation, but also take into account that, as a site of gas exchange, they can provide extremely valuable information for functional evaluation of middle ear ventilation capacity.

Points

❶ When interpreting temporal bone CT images for middle ear disease, first observe mastoid air cell development.

❷ Mastoid air cell development is inhibited by recurrent otitis media during infancy.

❸ Middle ear cavity pressure regulation and ventilation via the mastoid air cells is important for maintaining healthy conditions in the middle ear.

❹ Impaired mastoid air cell development forms the background for the development of intractable middle ear diseases and reduces the success rate of surgical treatment.

References

1 Brouwer CN, Rovers MM, Maill AR, et al: The impact of recurrent acute otitis media on the quality of life of children and their caregivers. Clin Otolaryngol 2005;30:258–265.

2 Gultekin E, Develioglu ON, Yener M, et al: Prevalence and risk factors for persistent otitis media with effusion in primary school children in Istanbul, Turkey. Auris Nasus Larynx 2010;37:145–149.

3 van der Veen EL, Schilder AG, van Heerbeek N, et al: Predictors of chronic suppurative otitis media in children. Arch Otolaryngol Head Neck Surg 2006;132:1115–1118.

4 Cinamon Udi: The growth rate and size of the air cell system and mastoid bone: a review and reference. Eur Arch Otorhinolaryngol 2009; 266:781–786.

5 Valtonen HJ, Dietz A, Qvarnberg YH, et al: Development of mastoid air cell system in children treated with ventilation tubes for early-onset otitis media: a Prospective radiographic 5-year follow-up study. Laryngoscope 2005;115:268–273.

6 Doyle WJ: The mastoid as a functional rate-limiter of middle ear pressure change. Int J Pediatr Otorhinolaryngol 2007;71:393–402.

7 Takahashi H, Sugimaru T, Honjo I, et al: Assessment of the gas exchange function of the middle ear using nitrous oxide. A preliminary study. Acta Otolaryngol 1994;114:643–646.

8 Gaihede M, Dirckx JJJ, Jacobsen J, et al: Middle ear pressure regulation —Complementary active actions of the mastoid and the Eustachian tube. Otol Neurotol 2010;31:603–611.

9 Takahashi H, Honjo I, Naito Y, et al: Gas exchange function through the mastoid mucosa in ears after surgery. Laryngoscope 1997;107:1117–1121.

10 Honjo I, Takahashi H, Sudo M, et al: Pathophysiological and therapeutic considerations of otitis media with effusion from viewpoint of middle ear ventilation. Int J Pediatr Otorhinolaryngol 1998;43:105–113.

11 Miura M, Takahashi H, Honjo I, et al: Influence of the gas exchange function through the middle ear mucosa on the development of sniff-induced middle ear diseases. Laryngoscope 1998;108:683–686.

12 Takahashi H, Sato H, Nakamura H, et al: Correlation between middle-ear pressure-regulation function and outcome of type-I tympanoplasty. Auris Nasus Larynx 2007;34:173–176.

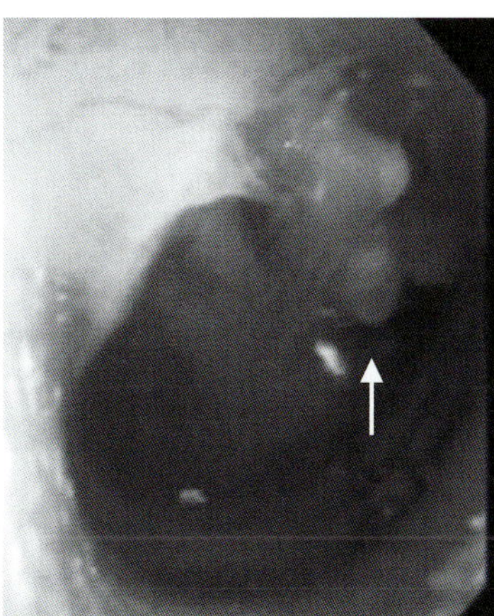

Fig. 1. (Case 1) Tympanic membrane finding for this case prior to surgery. A spherical, white mass (⇡) is visible medial to the intact tympanic membrane and anterior to the handle of the malleus, in the anterosuperior quadrant of the tympanic membrane.

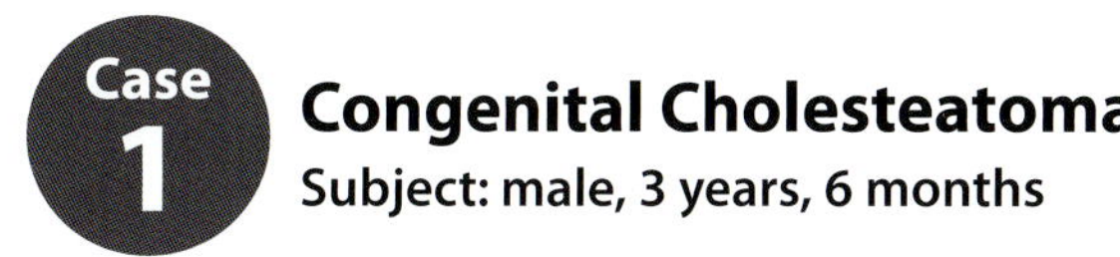

Congenital Cholesteatoma
Subject: male, 3 years, 6 months

■ History and Clinical Findings

The subject had contracted right acute otitis media on month previously, which had improved after treatment by a local physician at an ear-nose-and-throat clinic, but was referred to our department when the same doctor later discovered abnormal findings on examination of the tympanic membrane. Observation during our initial examination revealed a spherical, white mass in the anterosuperior quadrant of the right tympanic membrane (fig. 1). No abnormalities were ascertained on the left tympanic membrane. Average hearing level was 20.0 dB on the right and 22.5 dB on the left, which was normal on both sides.

■ Patient CT Findings

CT images are of the right ear. Mastoid air cell development is favorable, with no soft tissue density or other abnormal findings. However, on observation of the tympanic cavity, in the anterosuperior part a 2–3 mm diameter soft tissue density can be ascertained contacting the malleus from its handle to its neck (fig. 2:1, 2). It is apparent that this mass is also contacting the tensor tympani tendon (fig. 2:3). There are no findings of destruction of the ossicles or surrounding bone. Also, though not shown here, no abnormal findings whatsoever were ascertained in the left ear.

■ Surgical Findings and Postoperative Course

Arriving at the tympanic cavity via postauricular incision with a transcanal approach, we secured field of view posteriorly and from the direction of the epitympanum. The tympanic membrane was detached along the handle of the malleus to reveal the cholesteatoma in the anterosuperior area of the tympanic cavity. The cholesteatoma was a closed type and was adhered to the malleus from its neck to its handle, but was not continuous with or adhered to the tympanic membrane, so could be detached and extracted in a single mass without damaging the matrix. The surgery was concluded in the same manner as a type I tympanoplasty. Because there was an area anterior to the neck of the malleus and tensor tympani tendon that could not be observed from any angle during the removal of the cholesteatoma, caution was exercised and one year later a CT examination was performed but no residual cholesteatoma was found. Postoperative hearing was normal and unchanged from its preoperative level.

■ Postoperative CT Findings

In the one-year postoperative CT images, the cholesteatoma mass has been removed without a trace, and the soft tissue density anterior to the neck of the malleus (fig. 2: p1, p2) and in the vicinity of the tensor tympani tendon is gone, allowing a diagnosis of no findings of residual cholesteatoma on the images. The condition of the mastoidectomy (fig. 2:p1, p2, p3) and posterior tympanotomy can be observed (fig. 2:p2)

Patient CT Findings: Preoperative

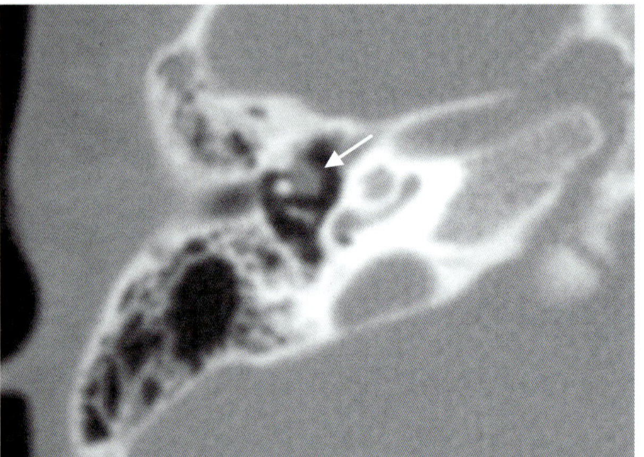

1. axial image

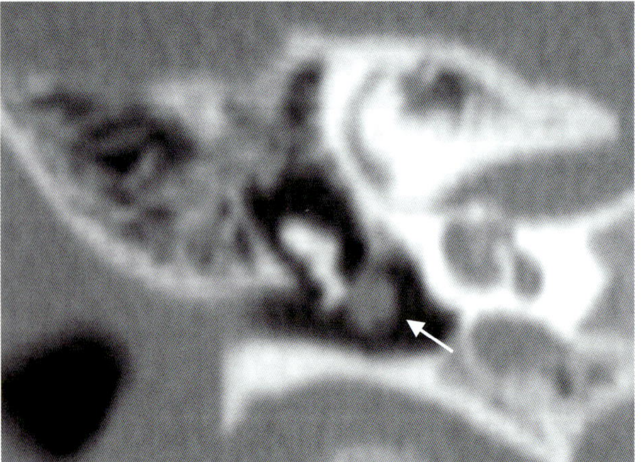

2. axial image

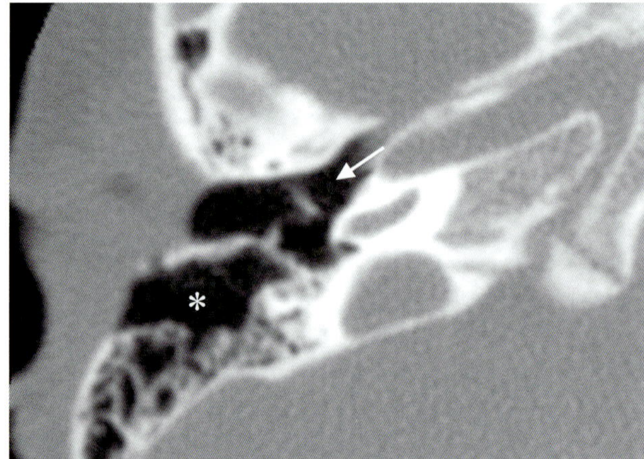

3. coronal image

Patient CT Findings: Postoperative

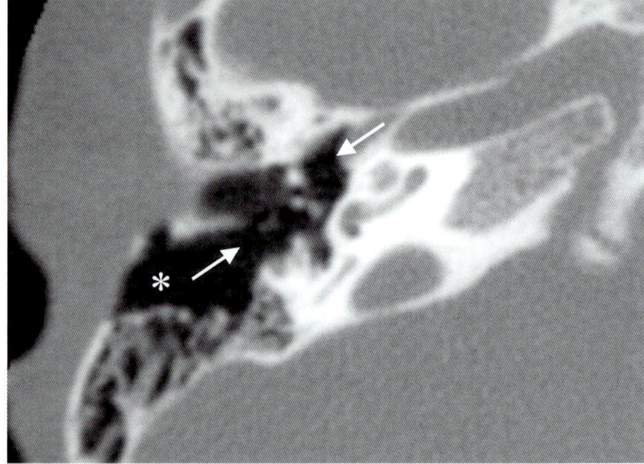

p1. axial image

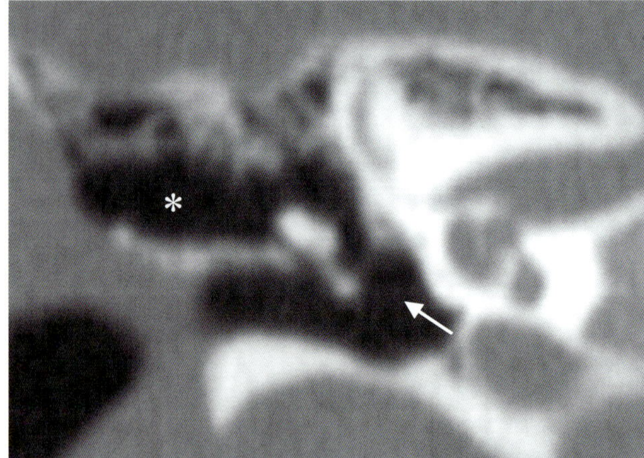

p2. axial image

p3. coronal image

Fig. 2. (Case 1) Right ear CT: preoperative, postoperative

[Patient CT Findings]

In preoperative CT images, mastoid air cell development is favorable, with no soft tissue density or other abnormal findings. However, in the anterosuperior part of the tympanic cavity a 2–3 mm diameter soft tissue density can be ascertained contacting the malleus from its handle to its neck (1, 2: ✐). This mass is also contacting the tensor tympani tendon (3: ✎). There are no findings of destruction of the ossicles or surrounding bone.

In the one-year postoperative CT images (p1–p3), the cholesteatoma mass has been removed without a trace, and the soft tissue density anterior to the neck of the malleus (p1, p2: ✐) and in the vicinity of the tensor tympani tendon (p3: ✎) is gone, allowing a diagnosis of no findings of residual cholesteatoma on the images. The condition of the mastoidectomy (p1, p2, p3: ✿) and posterior tympanotomy can be observed (p2: ✐).

■ Congenital Cholesteatoma

When skin (keratinized stratified squamous epithelium) invades the middle ear, an agglomeration of keratinized tissue accumulates in the sealed cavity and forms a cholesteatoma; when skin diverges or persists in the middle ear cavity during embryonic development, it forms a congenital middle-ear cholesteatoma. However, in clinical cases confirmation that skin was congenitally present in the middle ear cavity is effectively impossible, and is diagnosed through postulation based on the location of the cholesteatoma and its clinical course. If there is no history of otitis media and the tympanic membrane is completely normal and the cholesteatoma is fully separated from it, it is safe to assume that it is congenital, but in practice such cases are rare. In cases such as this one in which there is a history of otitis media and the cholesteatoma is contacting the tympanic membrane, strictly speaking one cannot deny the possibility that squamous epithelium may have invaded the cavity through the margin of a tympanic membrane perforation as a secondary development of otitis media, but since there was no partial retraction of the tympanic membrane connected to a perforation or cholesteatoma and the cholesteatoma was smooth and spherical, it is highly probable that it was congenital. Also, mastoid air cell development was favorable, allowing the presumption that at least there was not recurrent or chronic inflammation, further supporting the argument that the lesion was congenital.

The favorite sites for congenital cholesteatomas are in the neighborhood of the neck of the malleus and cochleariform process in the anterosuperior part of the tympanic cavity, and in the vicinity of the incudostapedial joint in the posterosuperior part. In reports from the U.S. and South Korea, the former is listed as more common [1, 2], while in Japan the latter is reported as more common [3], with rare occurrences at the petrous apex [3, 4]. Cholesteatomas originating at individual sites within the tympanic cavity may enlarge and develop to occupy multiple sites and even reach the mastoid if they grow sufficiently large. With respect to morphology, most cholesteatomas are cystic (closed type), but there are also cases in which the matrix is open and the cholesteatoma spreads in a sheet over the middle ear membrane (open type) [1]. The former appears on CT images as a round soft tissue density with a smooth border, but the latter is poorly featured in images, the only finding being of a partial thickening of the middle ear membrane, making further diagnosis difficult. Open type cholesteatomas are also prone to persistent recurrence after surgical resection [1].

References

1 McGill TJ, Merchant S, Healy GB, et al: Congenital cholesteatoma of the middle ear in children: a clinical and histopathological report. Laryngoscope 1991;101:123.
2 Choi HG, Park KH, Park SN, et al: Clinical experience of 71 cases of congenital middle ear cholesteatoma. Acta Otolaryngol. 2010;130:62–67.
3 Kojima H, Tanaka Y, Shiwa M, et al: Congenital cholesteatoma clinical features and surgical results. Am J Otolaryngol 2006;27:299–305.
4 DeSouza CE, Menezes CO, DeSouza RA, et al: Profile of congenital cholesteatomas of the petrous apex. J Postgrad Med 1989;35:93–97.

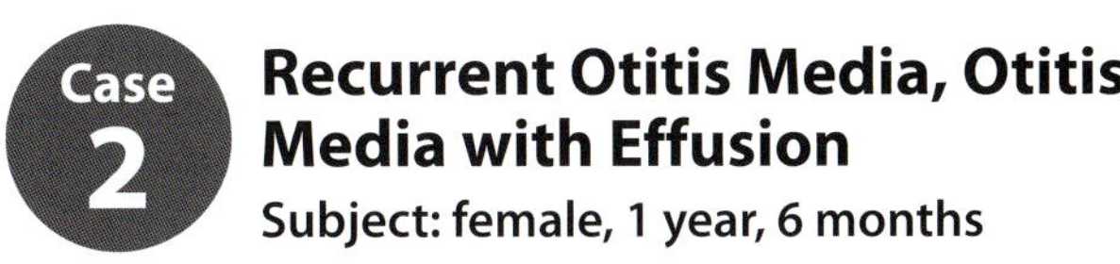

Case 2 Recurrent Otitis Media, Otitis Media with Effusion
Subject: female, 1 year, 6 months

■ History and Clinical Findings

The subject suffered from recurrent bilateral acute otitis media since around one year old. The disease was intractable, with antibiotic-resistant bacteria detected in bacteriological examination of otorrhea cultures. The effect of the myringotomy, however, was short lived and there were repeated relapses, so temporal bone CT examination was performed in order to obtain a detailed assessment of the condition of the middle ear.

■ Patient CT Findings Prior to Ventilation Tube Insertion

Findings were the same for both ears; the right ear is shown here. Mastoid air cell development is favorable, suggesting that there was no middle ear disease present for some time after birth. However, at the time the subject was introduced to our department the middle ear, including the tympanic cavity, was filled with soft tissue density (fig. 3:1, 2) and the tympanic membrane swollen (fig. 3:1, 3). The finding is basically otitis media with effusion, with no sign of bone destruction.

Bilateral myringotomy was performed under general anesthesia and the internal area inspected through the incision opening. No cholesteatomas were ascertained, so tympanic ventilation tubes were inserted bilaterally and the operation concluded.

■ Patient CT Findings Post Ventilation Tube Insertion

CT images (fig. 3:p1, p2, p3) show the right ear six months after ventilation tube insertion. The ventilation tube is observed to be properly positioned (fig. 3:p3) and the soft tissue density seen extending from the tympanic cavity to the mastoid air cells prior to surgery (fig. 3:1, 2) has disappeared (fig. 3:p1, p2). Mastoid air cell development is favorable, and has further expanded, though only slightly (fig. 3:p1, p2), since prior to surgery just six months previously (fig. 3:1, 2).

■ Image Findings and Clinical Features

Tympanic ventilation tube insertion is an effective treatment for recurrent otitis media and intractable otitis media with effusion. When, as in this case, effusion has accumulated throughout the entire middle ear, even after effusion has been aspirated from the tympanic cavity via myringotomy and a ventilation tube inserted, normally three months or more are required for the effusion to disappear completely from the mastoid air cells. The significance of conducting temporal bone CT examination on infants with recurrent otitis media is first to evaluate the state of mastoid air cell development, including the effect of the otitis media to date and to a certain extent predict the prognosis going forward, and second to check for the presence of complications such as cholesteatomas or tumors that may be a factor in the disease's intractability. If mastoid air cell development is deficient, this finding suggests that the otitis media has resisted healing over

Patient CT Findings: Preoperative   **Patient CT Findings: Postoperative**

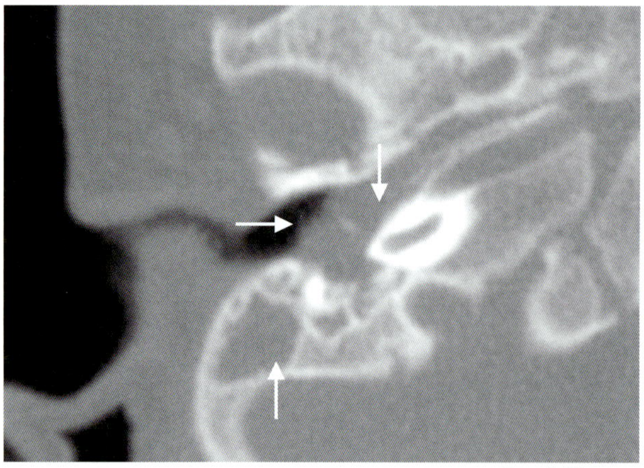

1. axial image 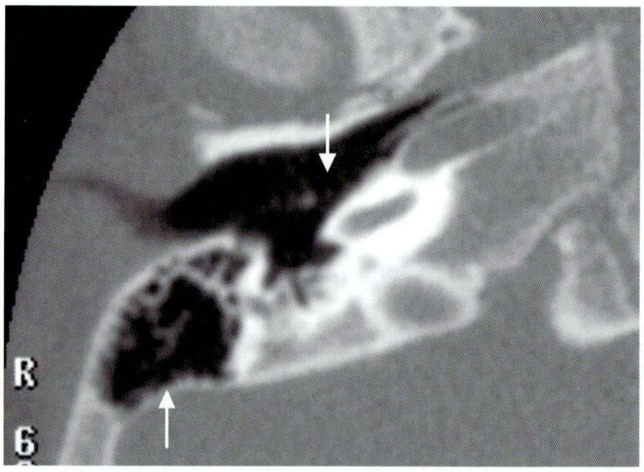   p1. axial image

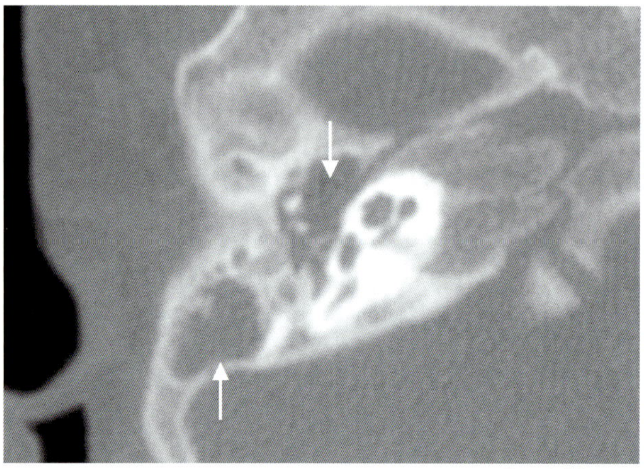

R
6

2. axial image 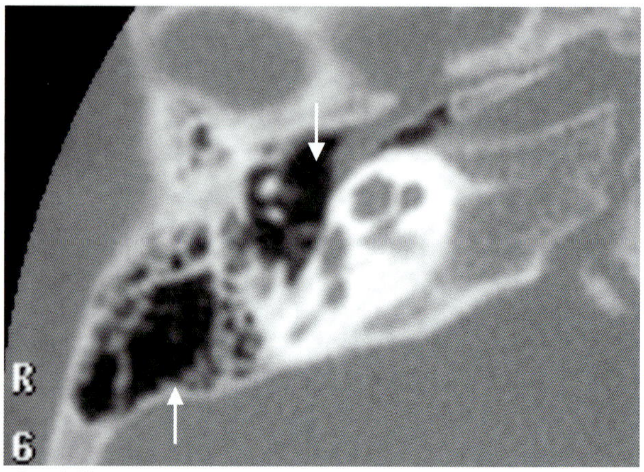   p2. axial image

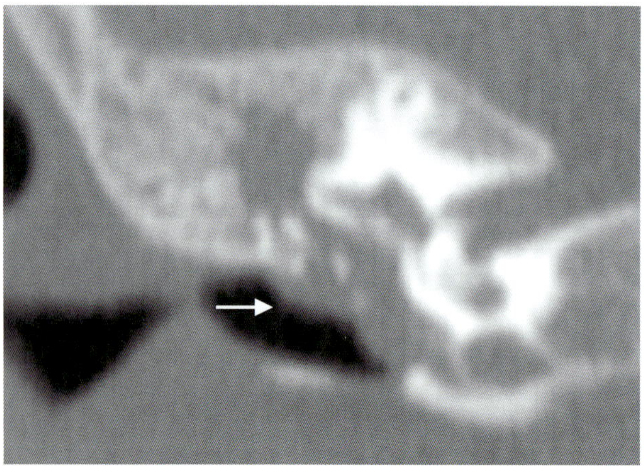

R
6

3. coronal image 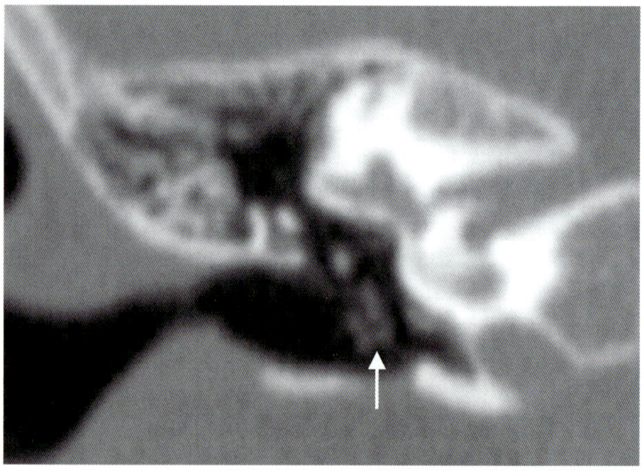   p3. coronal image

Fig. 3. (Case 2) Right ear CT: preoperative; p=post tympanic ventilation tube insertion

[Patient CT Findings]

Mastoid air cell development is favorable, suggesting that there was no middle ear disease present for some time after birth. However, at the time the subject was introduced to our department the middle ear, including the tympanic cavity, was filled with soft tissue density (1, 2: ⇩ ⇧) and the tympanic membrane swollen (1, 3: ⇨). The finding is basically otitis media with effusion, with no sign of bone destruction.

In CT images of the right ear six months after tympanic ventilation tube implantation (p1, p2, p3), the ventilation tube is observed to be properly positioned (p3: ⇧) and the soft tissue density seen extending from the tympanic cavity to the mastoid air cells prior to surgery has disappeared (p1, p2: ⇩ ⇧). Mastoid air cell development is favorable and has further expanded, though only slightly (p1, p2: ⇧), since prior to surgery just six months previously (1, 2: ⇧).

a protracted period of time and that a more aggressive surgical approach such as myringotomy and ventilation tube insertion should be considered. When otitis media is intractable, one should consider the possibility of factors other than simple infection, such as congenital cholesteatoma. However, when the middle ear is filled with effusion, it is the same density on a CT image as a cholesteatoma and cannot always be discerned through imaging, so careful inspection for osteolysis of the ossicles or other bone structure is required. No osteolysis was observed in this case.

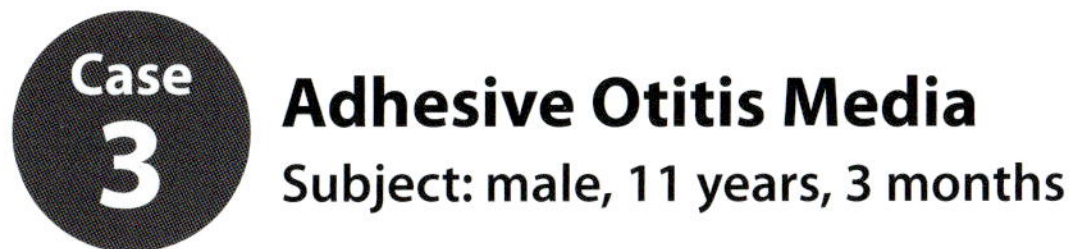

Adhesive Otitis Media

Case 3

Subject: male, 11 years, 3 months

History and Clinical Findings

The subject had experienced recurring otitis media since around three years old. He had first been examined by our department for right otitis media with effusion and left adhesive otitis media at five years, eight months old. The otitis media with effusion in the right ear healed after two operations to insert tympanic ventilation tubes. However, in the left ear, the adhesion in the posteroinferior quadrant of the tympanic membrane spread with age, with occasional otorrhea, so when the subject was eleven years old it was decided to perform a planned staged tympanoplasty. Preoperative average hearing level was 11.7 dB in the right ear and 28.3 dB in the left ear, with a 16.7 dB air-bone gap in the left ear.

Preoperative CT Findings

Temporal bone CT images for the left ear prior to tympanoplasty are shown (fig. 4:1–3). Mastoid air cell development is moderate and no soft tissue densities can be ascertained, but the inferior part of the tympanic membrane is retracted and in contact with the medial wall of the hypotympanum and the promontory (fig. 4:1, 2). There is a soft tissue density between the adhered tympanic membrane and the medial bony wall of the tympanic cavity (fig. 4:1, 2), with no pneumatization. No abnormalities have been ascertained in the ossicular chain, but the handle of the malleus is being pulled by the adhered tympanic membrane which has collapsed and is contacting the promontory (fig. 4:2). In the coronal section, it is apparent that the tympanic membrane is contacting the incudostapedial joint and is also clinging to the promontory (fig. 4:3). However, it is impossible to accurately determine from the image findings alone whether the tympanic membrane is actually adhered to the medial wall of the tympanic cavity, or is merely collapsed against it.

Surgical Findings and Postoperative Course

Observing the interior of the tympanic cavity, the tympanic membrane was clinging to the promontory and the medial wall of the hypotympanum from the incudostapedial joint, and was completely adhered to and could not be separated from the tympanic mucosa. Leaving the superior part of the tympanic membrane, we completely detached and removed the inferior half. Leaving the ossicular chain as it was, a silicon plate was implanted in the tympanic cavity and a type I tympanoplasty performed using temporalis fascia.

The second stage operation was performed one year later. The silicon plate was extracted and it was confirmed that there was pneumatization and there was no persistence of epithelium or cholesteatoma formation. Two years after the second stage operation, left ear hearing level was 15.0 dB, indicating favorable course.

Postoperative CT Findings

Temporal bone CT images shown here were taken one year following the second stage operation (fig. 4:p1–p3). Mastoid air cell development is favorable and has spread slightly but surely since one year previously, with no soft tissue density (fig. 4:p1, p2). The tympanic membrane shows mild thickening, but no retraction (fig. 4:p1–p3), and the soft tissue density noted preoperatively between the tympanic membrane and the wall of the tympanic cavity has disappeared (fig. 4:p1, p2). The handle of the malleus floats above the promontory (fig. 4:p2) and in the posterosuperior tympanic cavity the tympanic membrane is separated from the incudostapedial joint (fig. 4:p3).

Image Findings and Clinical Features

Adhesive otitis media is a form of chronic otitis media in which the tympanic membrane collapses and adheres to the medial wall of the tympanic cavity, and is difficult to treat using conservative therapy. Moreover, the result of tympanoplasty for this disease is worst among the various middle ear diseases, with a success rate of around 50–60% according to the success criteria of air-bone gap less than 20 dB. In unsuccessful cases, after surgery the tympanic cavity frequently is not pneumatized and the tympanic membrane re-retracts and forms an adhesion. It is hypothesized that eustachian tube function is insufficient to support pneumatization. One countermeasure for this is a cartilage palisade tympanoplasty, in which auricular cartilage is thinly sliced into narrow rectangles and lined up to form a tympanic membrane [1, 2, 3]. I use this method in cases of adhesive otitis media in which intractability is anticipated. Not only in adhesive otitis media, but in chronic otitis media in general, formation of a tympanic membrane using cartilage has been reported to deliver the same or superior results to the method using temporalis fascia [4], but formation of the tympanic membrane using cartilage is more involved than with temporalis fascia and has the drawback that the condition of the tympanic cavity's interior cannot be observed through the tympanic membrane postoperatively, so standard criteria for its indication need to be established. The state of pneumatization of the tympanic cavity and mastoid air cells are useful in this evaluation. As argued at the beginning of this chapter, mastoid air cell development and pneumatization affect long-term middle ear ventilation and inflammation, so a finding of insufficient air cell development and pneumatization would promote the selection of tympanic membrane formation using cartilage. Conversely, in this case mastoid air cell development was not complete but sufficient and pneumatization was good, so there was a high probability that the procedure could be performed with the usual method using temporalis fascia. The actual result was favorable and the postoperative hearing was good.

References

1 Caye-Thomasen P, Andersen J, Uzun C, et al: Ten-year results of cartilage palisades versus fascia in eardrum reconstruction after surgery for sinus or tensa retraction cholesteatoma in children. Laryngoscope 2009;119:944–952.
2 Neumann A, Kevenhoerster K, Gostian AO: Long-term results of palisade cartilage tympanoplasty. Otol Neurotol 2010;31:936–939.
3 Ozbek C, Ciftci O, Ozdem C: Long-term anatomic and functional results of cartilage tympanoplasty in atelectatic ears. Eur Arch Otorhinolaryngol 2010;267:507–513.
4 Cabra J, Monux A: Efficacy of cartilage palisade tympanoplasty: randomized controlled trial. Otol Neurotol 2010;31:589–595.

Patient CT Findings: Preoperative

Patient CT Findings: Postoperative

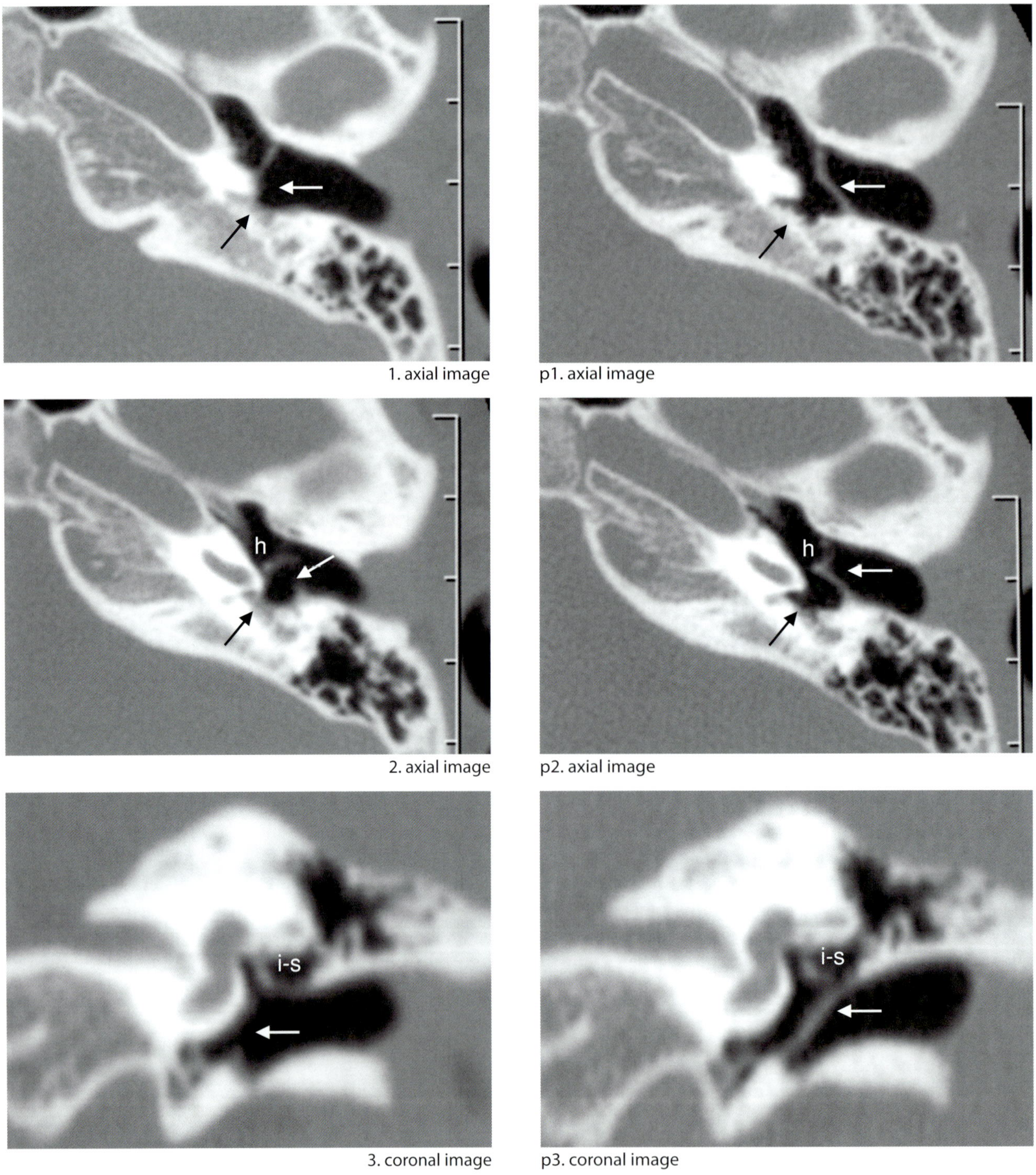

1. axial image

p1. axial image

2. axial image

p2. axial image

3. coronal image

p3. coronal image

Fig. 4. (Case 3) Left ear CT: preoperative; p=one year post planned staged tympanoplasty

〔Patient CT Findings〕

Temporal bone CT images for the left ear prior to tympanoplasty (1–3) and temporal bone CT images taken one year following the second stage operations of the staged tympanoplasty (p1–p3) are shown.

In the preoperative CT images, mastoid air cell development is moderate and no soft tissue densities can be ascertained, but the inferior part of the tympanic membrane is retracted and in contact with the medial wall of the hypotympanum and the promontory (1, 2: ⇐ ↗). There is a soft tissue density between the adhered tympanic membrane and the medial bony wall of the tympanic cavity (1, 2: ↗), with no pneumatization. The handle of the malleus is being pulled by the adhered tympanic membrane which has collapsed and is contacting the promontory (2: **h**). In the coronal section, it is apparent that the tympanic membrane is contacting the incudostapedial joint (3: **i-s**) and is also clinging to the promontory (3: ⇐).

Viewing the temporal bone CT images taken one year following the second stage operation (p1–p3), mastoid air cell development is favorable and has spread slightly but surely since one year previously, with no soft tissue density (p1, p2). The tympanic membrane shows mild thickening, but no retraction (p1–p3: ⇐), and the soft tissue density noted preoperatively between the tympanic membrane and the wall of the tympanic cavity has disappeared (p1, p2). The handle of the malleus floats above the promontory (p2: **h**) and in the posterosuperior tympanic cavity the tympanic membrane is separated from the incudostapedial joint (p3: **i-s**).

Case 4

Acute Otitis Media, Sigmoid Sinus Thrombosis

Subject: male, 5 years old

History and Clinical Findings

The subject was examined by a local otolaryngologist for a complaint of left otalgia. Acute otitis media was identified and a left myringotomy performed. However, the ear pain had not improved by the following day and two days after the onset of symptoms the subject was referred to us through a local community hospital. When he arrived at our emergency department he was still complaining strongly of left ear and head pain, but was fully conscious. A serous bloody discharge was present in the left external auditory canal, but there was no redness or swelling in the postauricular region so the clinical presentation differed from acute mastoiditis. Blood test findings indicated infection and severe inflammation, with a white blood cell count of 10,100/mm^3 and CRP of 21.1 mg/dl. Audiometry could not be conducted due to the pain.

Patient CT Findings

Mastoid air cell in the left is well developed, but the middle ear is filled with soft tissue density overall (fig. 5:a). There is no evidence of osteolysis in the ossicles or elsewhere. In the temporal bone target image there is no contrast in the soft tissue (fig. 5:a), but in the cranial contrast-enhanced CT taken with soft-tissue window (fig. 5:b) an enlargement is visible on the left sigmoid sinus. Its density is higher than the brain parenchyma, but lower than that of the contralateral sigmoid sinus or basilar artery. Based on this, it was hypothesized that there was a high probability the left sigmoid sinus was obstructed with a thrombus, restricting blood flow. MRI examination was added to more closely investigate the soft tissue of the left middle ear and sigmoid sinus.

Patient MRI Findings

The enlarged left sigmoid sinus is hypointense in T2 weighted imaging (fig. 6:a), but in T1 weighted imaging it is isointense (fig. 6:b), with no flow void due to blood flow and no contrast enhancement except at the margin on the dura side (fig. 6:c). Overall findings are compatible with a thrombus. On the other hand, the mastoid segment shows strong contrast enhancement (fig. 6:c), so the soft tissue density seen in the temporal bone CT is assumed to be, not effusion accumulation, but granulation tissue with abundant blood flow. In MR venography, blood flow from the superior sagittal sinus to the right transverse sinus and sigmoid sinus is cleanly seen, but on the left side there is no signal whatsoever of blood flow from the transverse sinus to the sigmoid sinus (fig. 7).

Surgical Findings

Four hours after the patient's arrival a left mastoidectomy was performed under general anesthesia. The mastoid air cells were filled with inflammatory granulation tissue, which exhibited much stronger bleeding than ordinary otitis media cases during the procedure. Hemorrhaging gradually abated as granulation tissue within the mastoid air cells was quickly and thoroughly removed, until at the conclusion of the mastoidectomy it had stopped almost completely. Leaving a thin layer of bone on the lateral part of the sigmoid sinus, its contour was exposed and a portion of the bony wall carefully fenestrated. Inside the sigmoid sinus was filled, not with pus, but with jelly-like coagulation. The fenestrated area was glued shut using fragments of temporalis fascia. Fibrous granulation tissue spread in particular from the aditus ad antrum to around the body of the incus and head of the malleus, completely obstructing communication between the tympanic cavity and the mastoid antrum. Assuming this to be the cause of the principal disease, the granulation tissue in this area was carefully removed to secure a broad ventilation route, and the operation was concluded.

Patient CT Findings

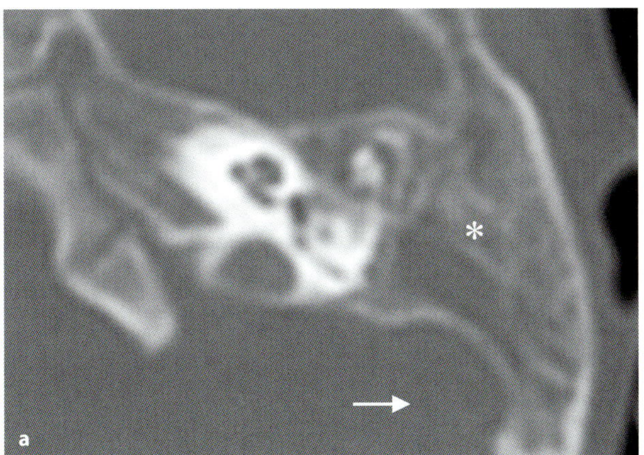
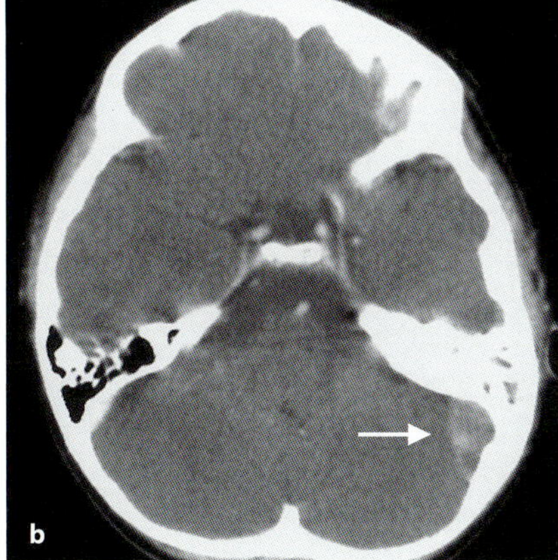

Fig. 5. (Case 4) CT: axial images

[Patient CT Findings]

Mastoid air cell development in the left ear is favorable, but the middle ear overall is filled with soft tissue density (a: ✳). There is no evidence of osteolysis in the ossicles or elsewhere. In the temporal bone target image there is no contrast in the soft tissue (a: ⇨), but in the cranial contrast-enhanced CT taken with soft-tissue window an enlargement is visible on the left sigmoid sinus (b: ⇨). Its density is higher than the brain parenchyma, but lower than that of the contralateral sigmoid sinus or basilar artery.

Patient MRI Findings: Preoperative

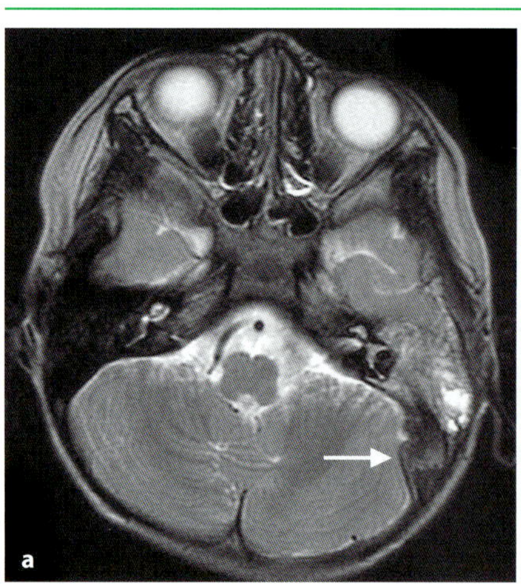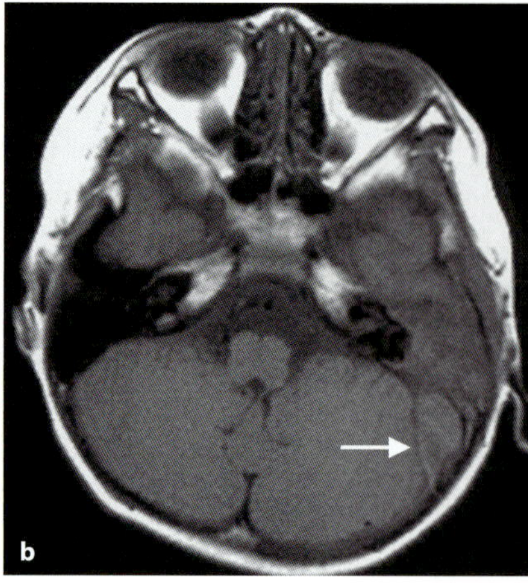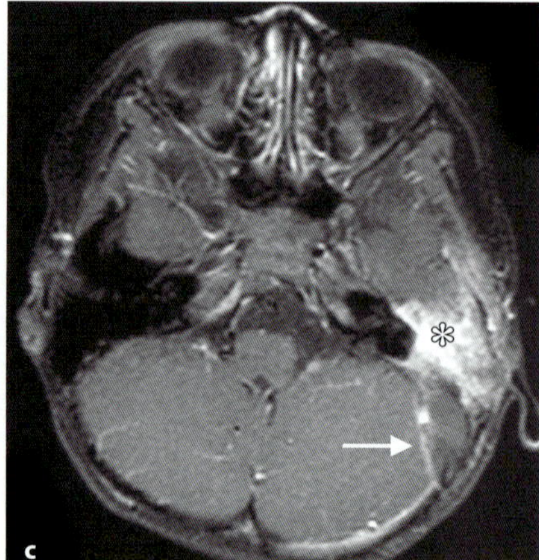

Fig. 6. (Case 4) MRI: a=T2 weighted imaging; b&c=T1 weighted imaging

■ Postoperative Course and Image Findings

Left ear pain vanished after surgery, and in a T2 weighted MRI taken seven days postoperatively a flow void was visible in a portion of the left sigmoid sinus (fig. 8:a), indicating possible recanalization of a portion of the blood vessel. The left sigmoid sinus had almost completely recanalized 110 days after surgery (fig. 8:b), with the area between the left transverse sinus and the sigmoid sinus depicted cleanly in MR venography (fig. 9). It is also apparent that the left side was originally dominant for venous drainage.

Patient MRV Findings: Preoperative

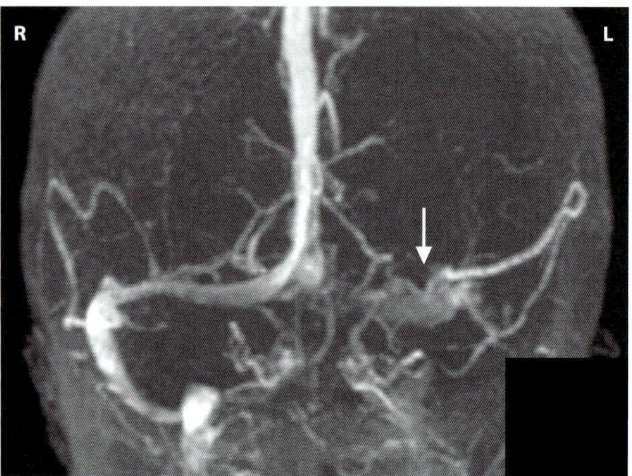

Fig. 7. (Case 4) MR venography imaging

■ Sigmoid Sinus Thrombosis

Sigmoid sinus thrombosis is a serious complication of acute and chronic otitis media or head injury [1], and may result in death if not treated in time. If the thrombus expands from the sigmoid sinus and blocks the superior sagittal sinus, spinal fluid absorption from the choroid plexus is obstructed causing hydrocephalus. If the thrombus progresses inferiorly it may cause thrombosis between the internal jugular vein and the superior vena cava or a pulmonary infarction due to bacteremia. Based on images, the pathogenic mechanism whereby otitis media not accompanied by bone destruction gives rise to a thrombus in the major intracranial veins is thought to begin with an occlusion caused by inflammation due to infection in the small veins of the mastoid segment, which then leads to clot formation in the venous sinus to which these smaller vessels feed [2].

This disease is diagnosed using clinical symptoms, along with CT and MRI. Clinical symptoms include strong ear pain and headache, while in CT images the key diagnostic factor is an enlargement of the sigmoid sinus without contrast enhancement, but with contrast enhancement in the dura mater surrounding the sigmoid sinus. The sigmoid sinus itself is slightly higher density due to the thrombus inside. Even with the same CT scan, when targeting the temporal bone the window width is set wide and, as can be seen in the target image in this case, one must exercise caution as there is no density contrast in the thrombus and surrounding cerebrospinal fluid or cerebellum. When intracranial complications are suspected with otitis media, observation using a soft tissue window is indispensable.

On the other hand, MRI is more useful for thrombosis imaging and produces more information, but when evaluating the MRI one must consider how much time has lapsed since thrombus formation, as the signal intensity

Patient MRI Findings: Postoperative

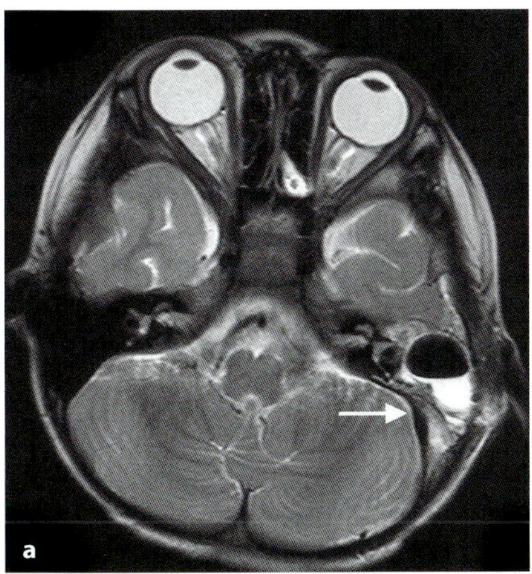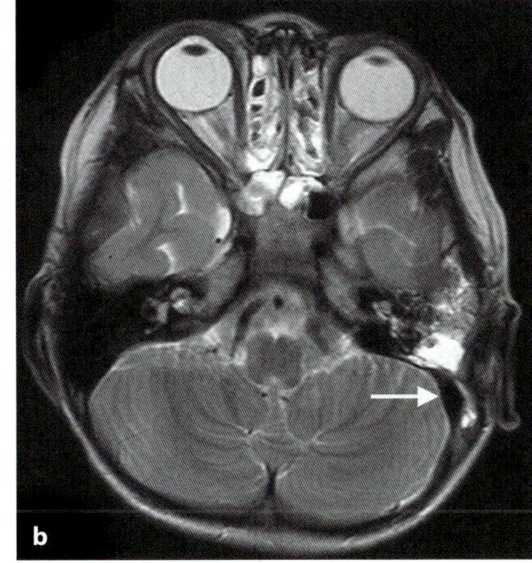

Fig. 8. (Case 4) MRI: T2 weighted imaging

pattern on T1 and T2 weighted imaging changes with time after the thrombus develops. In the hyperacute phase, within one day after formation of the hematoma, T1 weighted imaging is isointense and T2 weighted imaging is hyperintense, followed by the acute phase, up to around three days, in which the T1 weighted image shows no change, but the T2 weighted image becomes hypointense. (The case introduced here displays a signal pattern for a hematoma in the acute phase.) Next, in the subacute phase, up to around one week, T1 weighted image is hyperintense and T2 weighted image is hypointense, followed by a period in which both are hyperintense. In the chronic phase, after two weeks, both T1 and T2 weighted images are hypointense.

Also in MR imaging, blood flow through the arteries or veins can be selectively depicted by using movement of substances within the imaged cross-section as an indicator, but, as is apparent in the images for this case, for sigmoid sinus thrombosis the use of MR venography for observation of veins is particularly effective [3, 4].

Concerning treatment, there have been previous reports in which, in addition to mastoidectomy, ligature and lavage of the sigmoid sinus was also performed. Since the development of antibiotics, though, currently the more common approach is to suppress inflammation through mastoidectomy combined with powerful systemic administration of antibiotics, as was done in this case. It is currently being debated as to whether thrombolytic and anticoagulant therapies should also be implemented. There are reports of remission through aggressive treatment of the thrombus [1], but it is difficult to confirm whether or not selection of this treatment was responsible for the disease being cured. All approaches support the efficacy of surgical suppression of otitis media through early-stage mastoidectomy, and mastoidectomy is the basic treatment approach followed in this disease.

Patient MRV Findings: Postoperative

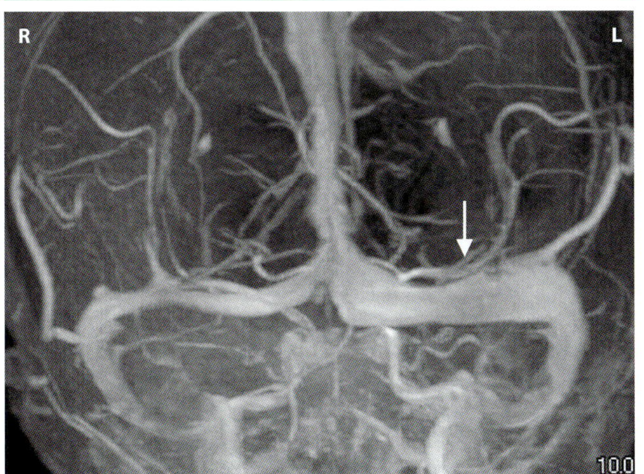

Fig. 9. (Case 4) MR venography imaging: 110 days postoperative

References

1 Zinis LOR, Gasparotti R, Campovecchi C, et al: Internal jugular vein thrombosis associated with acute mastoiditis in a pediatric age. Otol Neurotol 2006;27:937–944.
2 Kuczkowski J, Mikaszewski B: Intracranial complications of acute and chronic mastoiditis: report of two cases in children. Int J Pediatr Otorhinolaryngol 2001;60:227–237.
3 van den Bosch MA, Vos JA, de Letter MA, et al: MRI findings in a child with sigmoid sinus thrombosis following mastoiditis. Pediatr Radiol 2003;33:877–879.
4 Vazquez E, Castellote A, Piqueras J, et al: Imaging of complications of acute mastoiditis in children. Radiographics 2003;23:359–372.

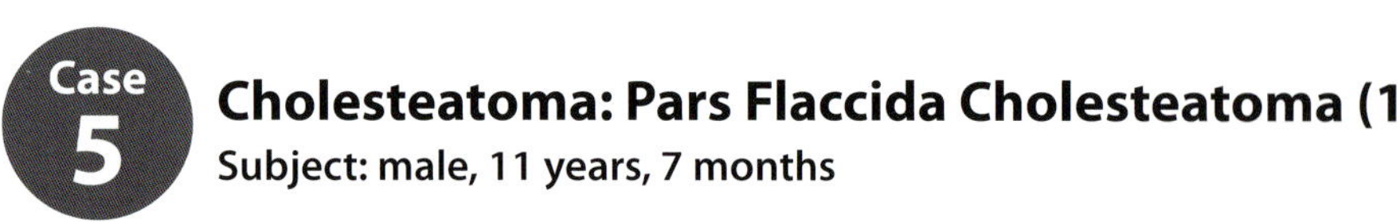

Case 5 — Cholesteatoma: Pars Flaccida Cholesteatoma (1)

Subject: male, 11 years, 7 months

■ History and Clinical Findings

The subject had contracted otitis media with effusion, having experienced recurring acute otitis media since infancy. He was receiving treatment from a local physician, particularly for ongoing otorrhea in the left ear, but the doctor referred him to our department due to the disease's intractability and suspected cholesteatoma formation. On our initial examination, we observed retraction and scabbing of the pars flaccida of the tympanic membrane, and diagnosed the subject with pars flaccida cholesteatoma. Average hearing level was 13.3 dB in the right ear and 16.7 dB in the left, indicating slight hearing loss.

■ Patient CT Findings

Left mastoid air cell development is deficient, with a striking difference between the patient (fig. 10:1–3) and the normal control (fig. 10:n1–n3). However, there is little soft tissue density within the mastoid antrum and the mastoid air cells, making active infection or inflammation unlikely. Soft tissue density is restricted to the lateral epitympanum, and osteolysis of the epitympanum's lateral wall (scutum) is visible (fig. 10:1–3; Fig. 11:1, 2). There is also an erosion of the head of the malleus and lateral half of the body of the incus (fig. 10:2, 3). The soft tissue density has progressed medially beyond the head of the malleus (fig. 11:2), but has not progressed to the tympanic cavity or the mastoid segment. Normally air cell pneumatization expands and develops laterally from the epitympanum (fig. 11:n1, n2), but in this case, there is no air cell development in the region lateral to the epitympanum and the middle cranial fossa is drooping (fig. 11:1, 2).

■ Surgical Findings and Postoperative Course

A staged tympanoplasty (primary) was performed. The posterior wall of the external auditory canal was slightly fenestrated through a postauricular incision and the incudostapedial joint confirmed and severed. From the external auditory canal the lateral wall of the epitympanum was fenestrated and the cholesteatoma matrix detached while maintaining a distinct view of the malleoincudal joint. The incus was then extracted and the head of the malleus severed and extracted to provide a clear view for total removal of the cholesteatoma. The defect in the pars flaccida of the tympanic membrane was reconstructed using temporalis fascia and the operation concluded. In second stage surgery, we plan to perform tympanoplasty using cartilage and partially obliterate the epitympanum if there is a tendency for the pars flaccida to re-retract.

■ Image Findings and Clinical Features

With regard to both history and image findings, this is a typical case of pars flaccida cholesteatoma. The diagnosis itself can be determined from tympanic membrane findings and CT images alone, but for surgical planning it is important to obtain more detailed findings. The most important findings are deficient mastoid air cell development lateral to the epitympanum and drooping of the middle cranial fossa. It can be assumed that the subject in this case suffered chronic otitis media during early childhood when mastoid air cell development is normally active, as the difference to the normal control is plainly evident. Drooping of the middle cranial fossa, as in this case, narrows the field of view when removing bone from the lateral side to extract the cholesteatoma, requiring careful drilling so as not to damage the dura of the middle cranial fossa. Another important finding to focus on is the continuity of the ossicular chain. Even if the cholesteatoma has disrupted the ossicles, so long as there is complete continuity of the conductive chain, the incudostapedial joint must be severed early in the operation and the efforts made to prevent inner ear damage through surgical manipulation.

Also, when mastoid air cell development is this deficient at this age, even if the middle ear inflammation is cured there is little hope of significant air cell development in the future. Consequently, because postoperative middle ear ventilation is expected to be poor, during the second stage surgery a plan will be required to prevent re-retraction of the tympanic membrane and external auditory canal in the long term.

Patient CT Findings

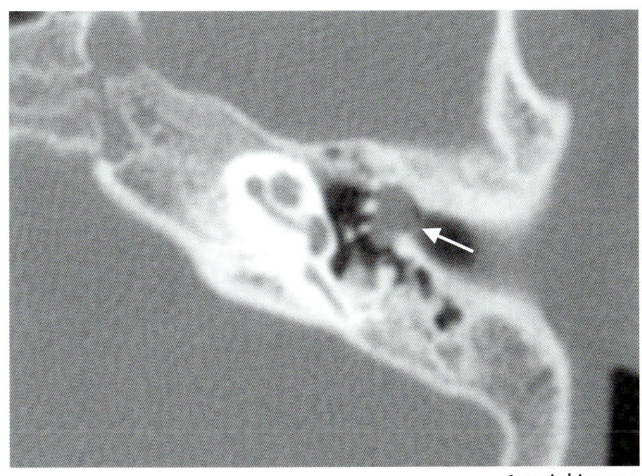

1. axial image

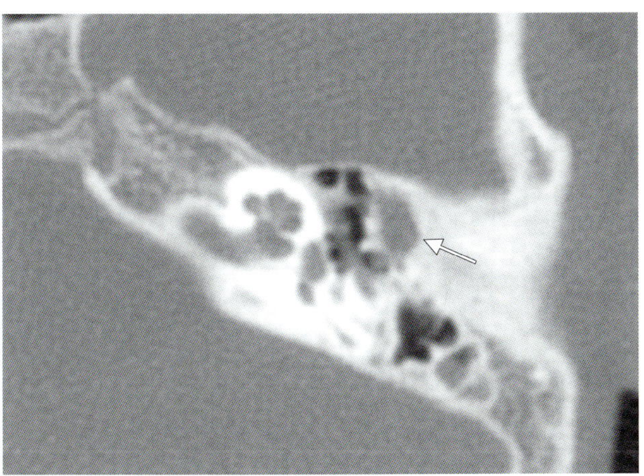

2. axial image

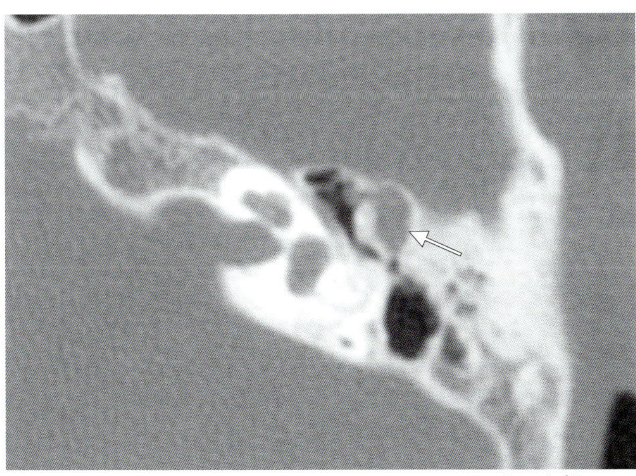

3. axial image

Normal Control CT Findings

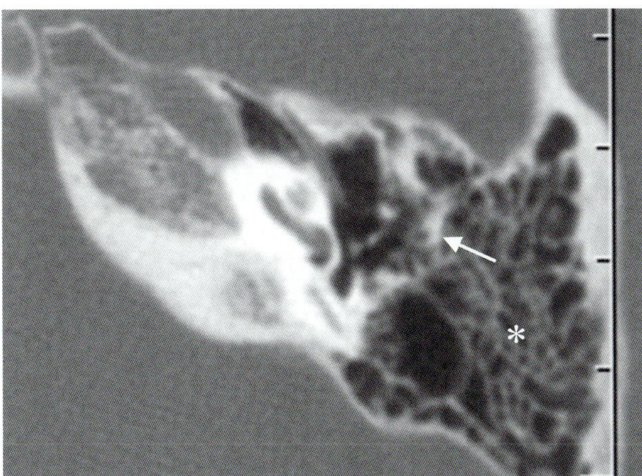

n1. axial image

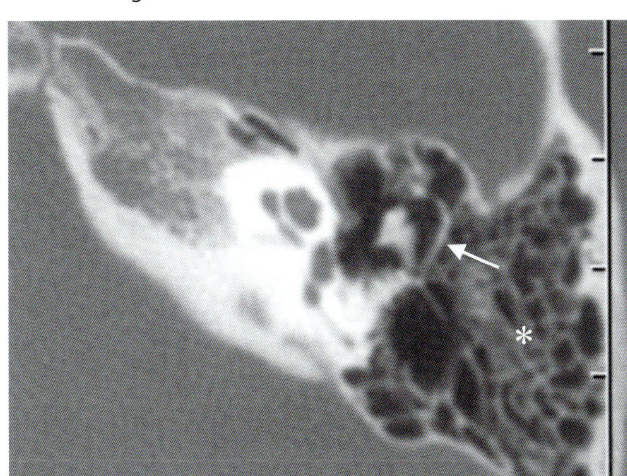

n2. axial image

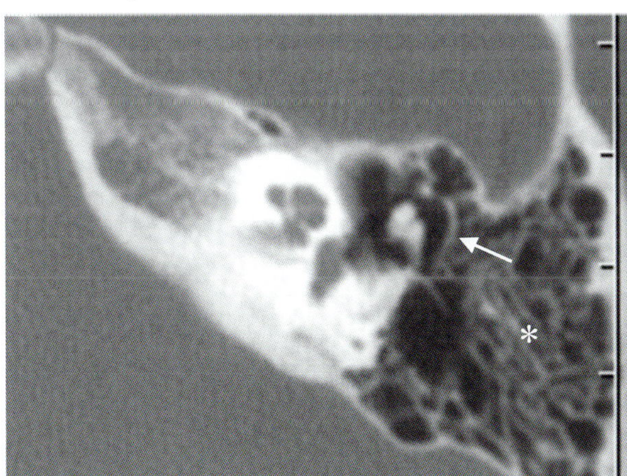

n3. axial image

Fig. 10. (Case 5) Left ear CT: preoperative

[Patient CT Findings]

Left mastoid air cell development is deficient, with a striking difference between the patient and the normal control (n1–n3: ✿). However, there is little soft tissue density within the mastoid antrum and the mastoid air cells. Soft tissue density is restricted to the lateral epitympanum, and destruction of the epitympanum's lateral wall (scutum) is visible (1–3: ✎). There is also an erosion of the head of the malleus and lateral half of the body of the incus (2, 3). In the normal control images the lateral wall of the epitympanum is present (n1–n3: ✎) and there is significant development of pneumatized air cells lateral to that (n1–n3: ✿).

Patient CT Findings	**Normal Control CT Findings**

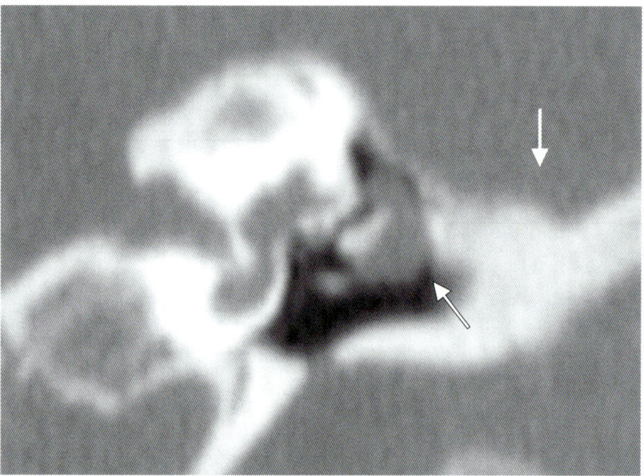

1. coronal image

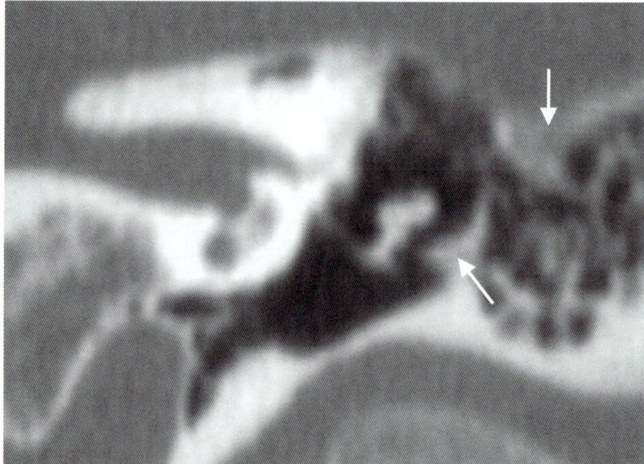

n1. coronal image

2. coronal image

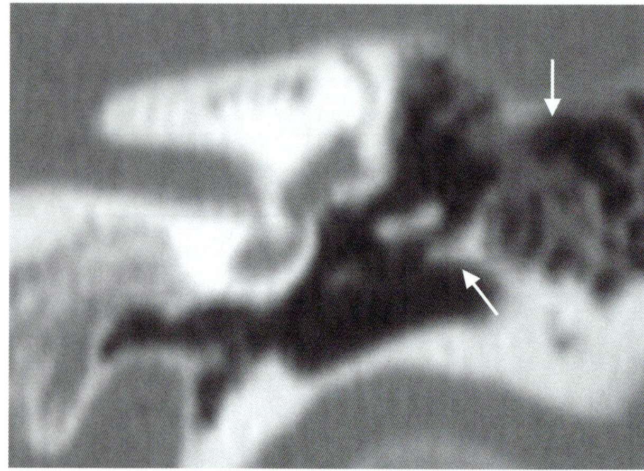

n2. coronal image

Fig. 11. (Case 5) Left ear CT: preoperative

〔Patient CT Findings〕

The lateral wall of the epitympanum (scutum) is destroyed (1, 2: ↖) and the cholesteatoma's soft tissue density has progressed medially beyond the head of the malleus (2). Normally air cell pneumatization expands and develops laterally from the epitympanum (n1, n2: ⇓), but in this case, there is no air cell development in the region lateral to the epitympanum and the middle cranial fossa is drooping (1, 2: ⇓).

In the normal control, the scutum projects sharply from the medial margin of the upper wall of the external auditory canal (n1, n2: ↖).

Points

❶ Recurrent otitis media in infancy is a factor in the formation of middle ear cholesteatoma in later years.

❷ Early-phase pars flaccida cholesteatoma causes only minor hearing loss.

❸ Signs of destruction of the scutum tip in coronal temporal bone CT images is key to imaging diagnosis.

❹ An accurate evaluation of the extent of the cholesteatoma's development and degree of destruction to the ossicles is important for surgical planning.

Case 6

Cholesteatoma: Pars Flaccida Cholesteatoma (2)

Subject: male, 15 years old

■ History and Clinical Findings

The subject contracted recurring bilateral otitis media in infancy, but the otitis media almost completely disappeared shortly after reaching school age and no particular medical treatment was required. However, two weeks previously the subject was treated by a local otolaryngologist for left ear pain and otorrhea, whereupon the possibility of cholesteatoma was identified and he was referred to our department. At time of our initial examination, the pars flaccida of the left tympanic membrane was retracted, with scabbing and pus accompanied by redness of the surrounding skin (fig. 12), resulting in a diagnosis of pars flaccida cholesteatoma. On careful observation of the pars tensa of the tympanic membrane, the central part was slightly swollen and a white mass was visible inside (fig. 12). The left ear displayed conductive hearing loss, with hearing level of approx. 30 dB. Mastoid air cell development was deficient on the right side as well, but middle ear pneumatization was favorable overall and no other abnormalities were ascertained.

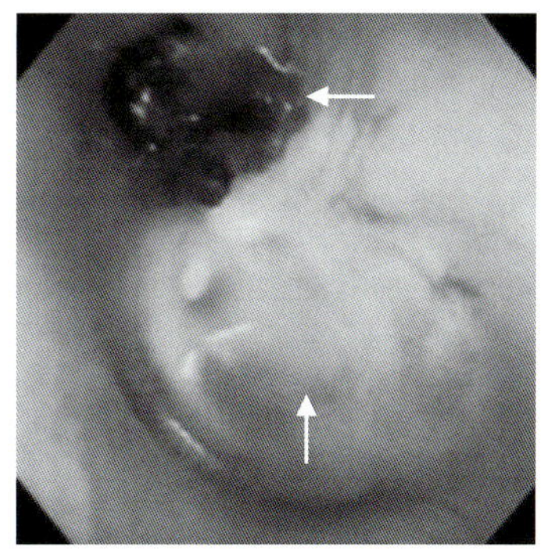

Fig. 12. (Case 6) Findings for left tympanic membrane. The pars flaccida is retracted with scabbing and pus, accompanied by redness of the surrounding skin (⇐). The central part of the pars tensa of the tympanic membrane is slightly swollen and a white mass is visible inside (⇑).

■ Patient CT Findings

Findings shown are for the left ear. Mastoid air cell development is deficient, with little air cell development visible other than in the epitympanum and the mastoid antrum (fig. 13:1, 2). The difference compared to favorable mastoid air cell development as seen in the normal control (fig. 13:n1, n2) is striking. The area from the epitympanum and mastoid antrum to the superior half of the mesotympanum is filled with soft tissue density (fig. 13:1, 2). Particularly in the mesotympanum, we see that the cholesteatoma has divided and extends anterior to the malleus and along the posterosuperior part of the tympanic

Patient CT Findings

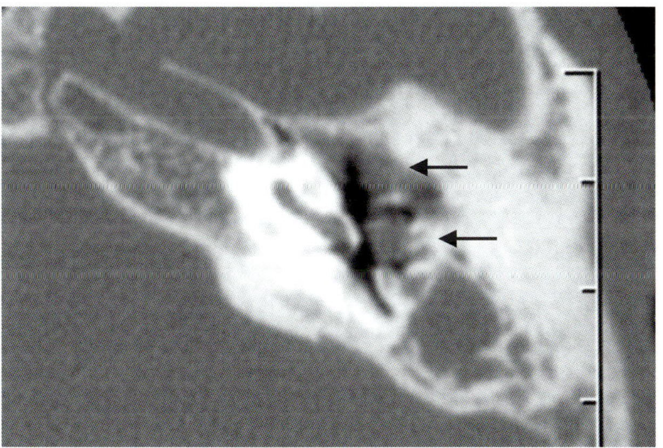

1. axial image

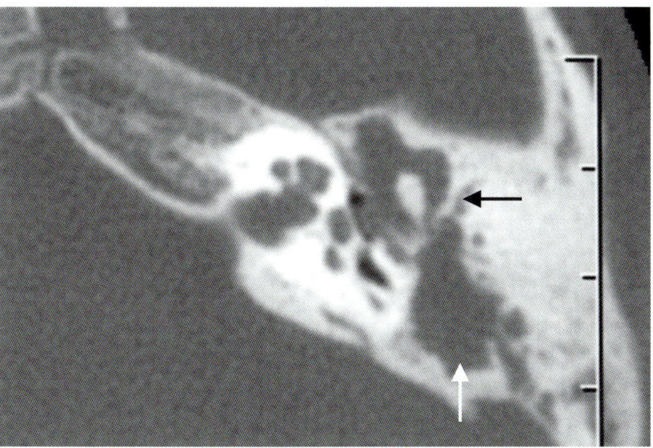

2. axial image

Normal Control CT Findings

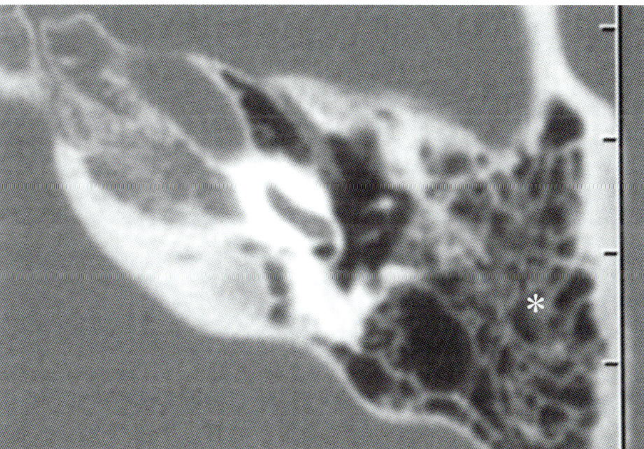

n1. axial image

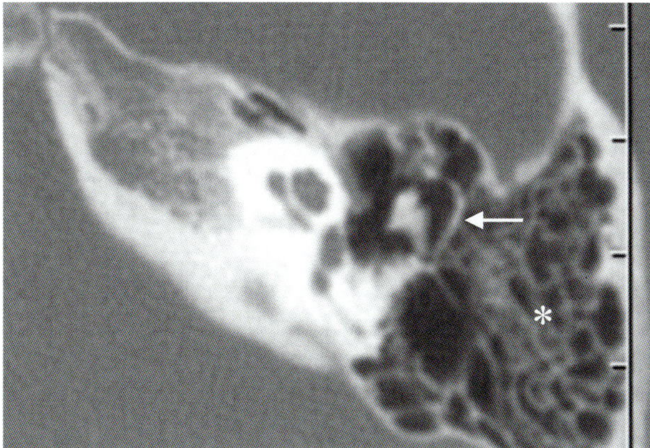

n2. axial image

Fig. 13. (Case 6) Left ear CT: preoperative

[Patient CT Findings]

Mastoid air cell development is deficient, with little air cell development visible other than in the epitympanum and the mastoid antrum (1, 2). The difference compared to the normal control (n1, n2: ✳) is striking. The area from the epitympanum and mastoid antrum (2: ⇑) to the superior half of the mesotympanum is filled with soft tissue density (1, 2). Particularly in the mesotympanum, we see that the cholesteatoma has divided and extends anterior to the malleus and along the posterosuperior part of the tympanic cavity (1: ←). However, insofar as can be observed in the axial section, the lateral wall of the epitympanum (2: ←) appears just as in the normal control (n2: ⇐).

cavity (fig. 13:1). However, insofar as can be observed in the axial section, the lateral wall of the epitympanum (fig. 13:2) appears just as in the normal control (fig. 13:n2). In the coronal section, the medial margin of the external auditory canal, which is the bony wall (scutum) continuous with the lateral wall of the epitympanum (see normal control, Fig. 14:n1), is eroded (fig. 14:1), and the epitympanum is filled with soft tissue density. In the medioinferior area this cholesteatoma has spread to the superior half of the mesotympanum (fig. 14:1, 2) and is positioned as if to cover the oval window (fig. 14:2), but it is unclear if the head of the malleus and body of the incus are eroded. Mastoid air cell development lateral to the epitympanum is deficient (fig. 14:1, 2) and the area that would normally be pneumatized (fig. 14:n1, n2) is composed of thick, bony tissue (fig. 14:1, 2). The floor of the middle cranial fossa is drooping slightly.

■ Surgical Findings

A staged tympanoplasty (primary) was performed in the form of a canal wall down tympanoplasty with soft wall reconstruction. The incudostapedial joint was confirmed and severed, then the cholesteatoma was extracted. The incus and head of the malleus were extracted and preserved for use as columella in the second stage surgery. The cholesteatoma had spread from the epitympanum to fill the mesotympanum, mastoid antrum and mastoid air cells, and a cholesterol granuloma was ascertained in its distal end in the mastoid segment and extracted along with the cholesteatoma epithelium. A silicon plate was inserted and embedded in the mesotympanum and the anterior and posterior tympanic isthmi, and the defect in the tympanic membrane was reconstructed using temporalis fascia.

■ Image Findings and Clinical Features

The cholesteatoma in this case extended from the epitympanum to the mastoid antrum, swelling inferiorly into the mesotympanum so as to straddle the cochleariform process. Compared to the first example of pars flaccida cholesteatoma, the cholesteatoma fills the area from the epitympanum to the mastoid segment and furthermore mastoid air cell development is deficient with no pneumatization, making conditions less favorable for tympanoplasty. If pneumatization is not acquired prior to second stage surgery, considerable ingenuity will be required to prevent long-term re-formation of the cholesteatoma.

Patient CT Findings   Normal Control CT Findings

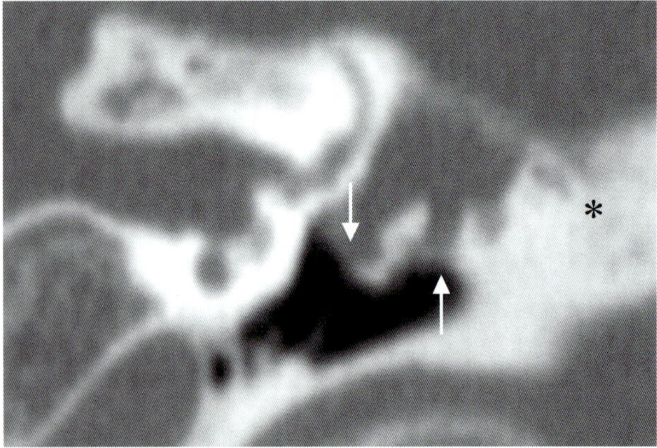

1. coronal image

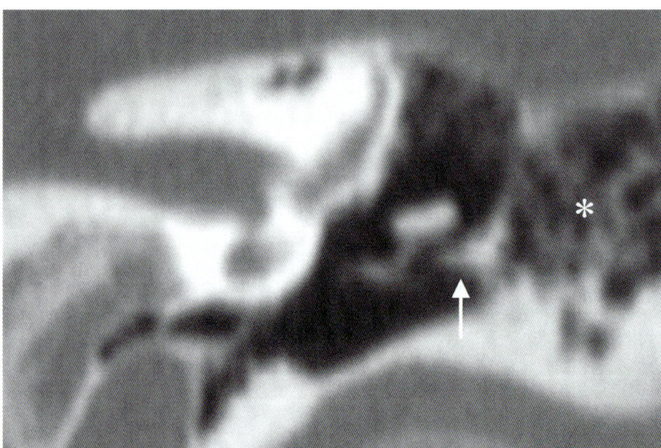

n1. coronal image

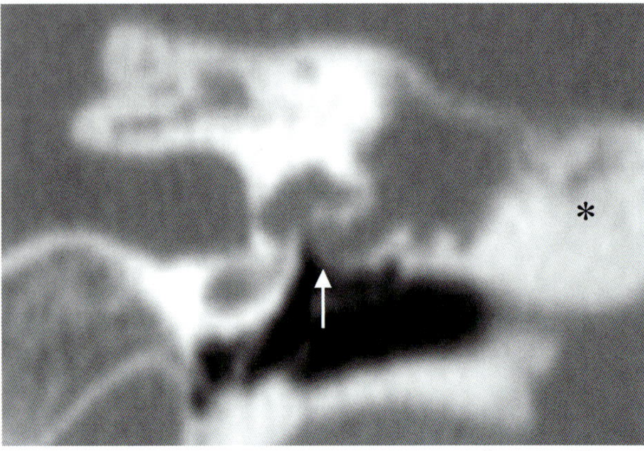

2. coronal image

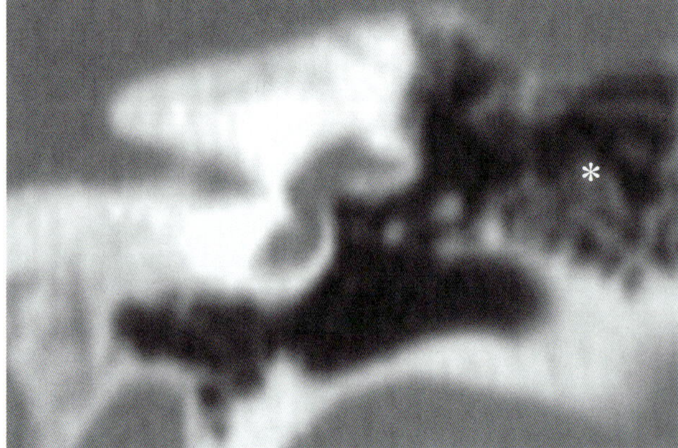

n2. coronal image

Fig. 14. (Case 6) Left ear CT: preoperative

[Patient CT Findings]

In the coronal section, the medial margin of the external auditory canal, which is the bony wall (scutum) continuous with the lateral wall of the epitympanum (n1: ⇧), is eroded (1: ⇧), and the epitympanum is filled with soft tissue density. In the medioinferior area this cholesteatoma has spread to the superior half of the mesotympanum (1: ⇩) and is positioned as if to cover the oval window (2: ⇧), but it is unclear if the head of the malleus and body of the incus are eroded. Mastoid air cell development lateral to the epitympanum is deficient, and the area that would normally be pneumatized (n1, n2: ✿) is composed of thick, bony tissue (1, 2: ✱). The floor of the middle cranial fossa is drooping slightly.

Case 7: Cholesterol Granuloma
Subject: male, 20 years old

■ History and Clinical Findings

The subject has previously undergone operations for right middle ear cholesteatoma at around 11–12 years old, and for left middle ear cholesteatoma at around 15 years old. Since that time he had been under observation by a local physician, who referred him to our department when swelling developed in the right external auditory canal. No subjective symptoms were present. Pure tone average was 22.3 dB right and 17.5 dB left, with no air-bone gap.

■ Patient CT Findings

The posterior and superior walls of the bony part of the external auditory canal are partially eroded and a soft tissue density is continuous from the mastoid antrum to the epitympanum and external auditory canal (fig. 15:1, 2). Particularly in the coronal section, is it readily apparent that the swelling originating in the middle ear cavity is occupying and obstructing the external auditory canal from above (fig. 15:3). The tympanic membrane is properly preserved (fig. 15:3) and there is pneumatization from the mesotympanum to the eustachian tube. There is no bone destruction in the floor of the middle cranial fossa.

■ Patient MRI Findings

A space-occupying lesion continuous from the mastoid antrum to the external auditory canal can be ascertained in the area coinciding with the soft tissue density observed in the CT image from the middle ear to the EAC. The lesion swelling in the external auditory canal is hyperintense in both T1 and T2 weighted imaging (fig. 16:1, 2), allowing a diagnosis of cholesterol granuloma cyst. On the other hand, a portion of the distal part of the mastoid air cells is slightly weaker than the EAC lesion in both T1 and T2 weighted imaging, which is assumed to be due to a difference in content characteristics.

■ Surgical Findings and Postoperative Course

A postauricular incision was made and the skin of the external auditory canal's posterosuperior wall was detached, revealing a cyst filled with dark brown fluid that continued into the mastoid antrum. The cyst was detached from the skin of the external auditory canal to free up the lumen and a mastoidectomy was performed. A compound cyst was present from the epitympanum to the mastoid antrum and the lumen was filled with a brown fluid that included sparkling cholesterol crystals, with granulation on a portion of the cyst wall. Leaving the ossicular chain, which had been previously reconstructed, as is, intercourse was widened and secured between the epitympanum and mesotympanum and between the epitympanum and anteriorly to the tympanic opening of the eustachian tube, which had become narrow with new bone and membranous tissue.

Postoperative hearing was favorable as before, but the posterior wall of the external auditory canal gradually expanded and retracted into the excised mastoid antrum. As of four years postoperatively, there are no clinical findings to indicate recurrence.

■ Cholesterol Granuloma

Cholesterol granuloma occurs as a result of seepage of blood or blood plasma into the closed cavity of the middle ear, where the cholesterol in the accumulated blood forms needle-shaped crystals that stimulate further granuloma formation. In the middle ear, cholesterol granulomas may either be primary or secondary, caused when the excretion route in the mastoid cavity becomes obstructed with granuloma, cholesteatoma, or other materials. With the latter, a cure can be effected by surgically cleaning the mastoid cavity and securing the excretion route, but with the former, even after removing the granuloma via a thorough mastoidectomy or other procedure the disease often returns without having made a full recovery. Research based on temporal bone histopathology in cases of cholesterol granulomas in children particularly identifies the importance of bone marrow bleeding and eustachian tube dysfunction [1]. When the granuloma occurs at the petrous apex, there are no abnormal findings for the tympanic membrane, the main complaint is of deep head pain, and it is discovered through CT or MRI examination. When it occurs in the epitympanum, it may disrupt the tegmen and advance into the middle cranial fossa, forming an enormous cyst that pushes up the temporal lobe.

In CT images, soft tissue density is seen in the mastoid segment, epitympanum, and petrous apex. When a mass or swelling of the tympanic membrane can be observed from the external auditory canal, the cyst frequently contains dark brown fluid [2]. In MRI, a characteristic finding is hyperintense signal in both T1 and T2 weighted images.

References

1 Miura M, Sando I, Orita Y, et al: Histopathologic study of the temporal bones and Eustachian tubes of children with cholesterol granuloma. Ann Otol Rhinol Laryngol 2002;111:609–615.
2 Nikolaidis V, Malliari H, Psifidis D, et al: Cholesterol granuloma presenting as a mass obstructing the external ear canal. BMC Ear Nose Throat Disord 2010;10:4.

Patient CT Findings

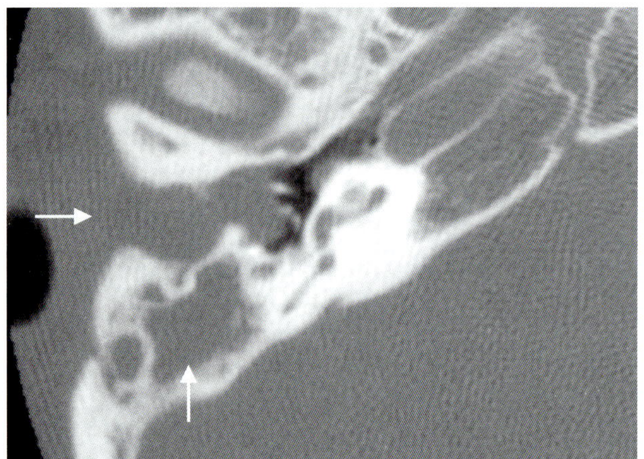

1. axial image

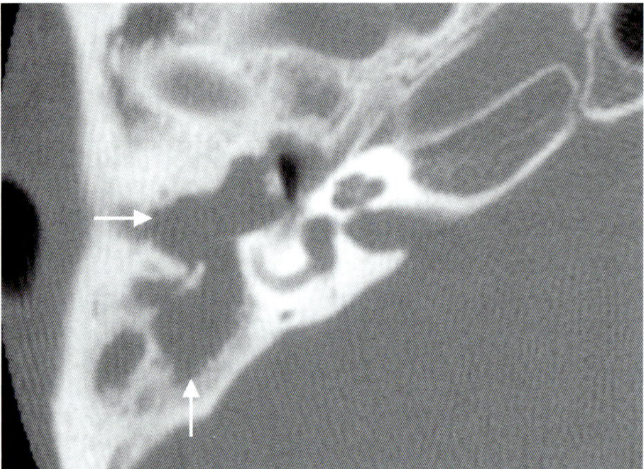

2. axial image

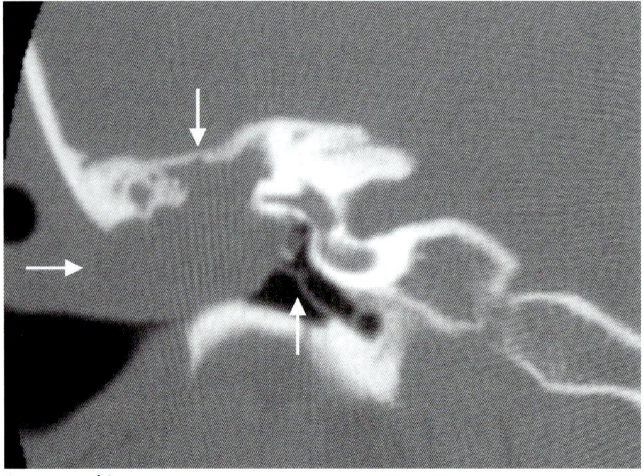

3. coronal image

Fig. 15. (Case 7) Right ear CT: preoperative

〔Patient CT Findings〕

The posterior and superior walls of the bony part of the external auditory canal are partially deficient and a soft tissue density is continuous from the mastoid antrum (1, 2: ⇑) to the epitympanum and the external auditory canal (1, 2: ⇨). Particularly in the coronal section, it is readily apparent that the swelling originating in the middle ear cavity is occupying and obstructing the external auditory canal from above (3: ⇨). The tympanic membrane is properly preserved (3: ⇑), and there is pneumatization from the mesotympanum to the eustachian tube. There is no bone destruction in the floor of the middle cranial fossa (3: ⇓).

Patient MRI Findings

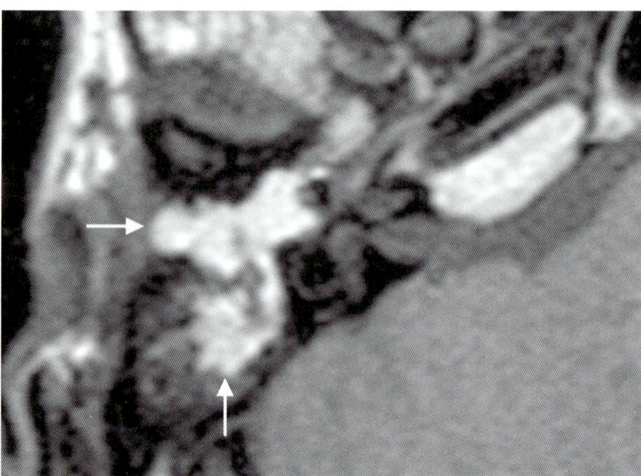

1. T1 weighted imaging

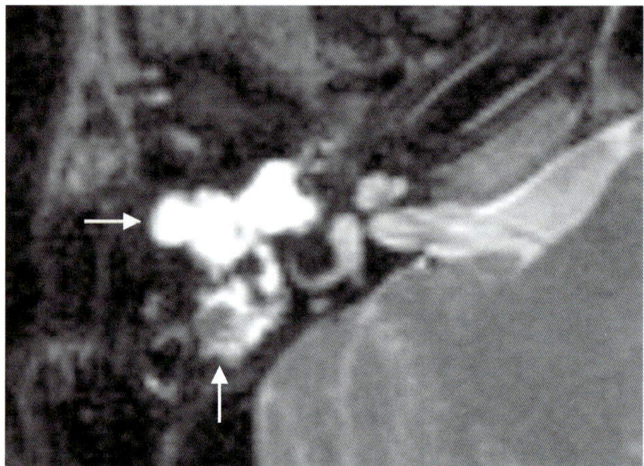

2. T2 weighted imaging

Fig. 16. (Case 7) Right ear MRI: preoperative

〔Patient MRI Findings〕

A space-occupying lesion continuous from the mastoid antrum to the external auditory canal can be ascertained in the area coinciding with the soft tissue density observed in the CT image from the middle ear to the EAC. The lesion swelling in the external auditory canal is hyperintense in both T1 and T2 weighted imaging (1, 2: ⇨), allowing a diagnosis of cholesterol granuloma cyst. On the other hand, a portion of the distal part of the mastoid air cells (1, 2: ⇑) is slightly weaker than the EAC lesion in both T1 and T2 weighted images, which is assumed to be due to a difference in content characteristics.

❷ Image Findings after Tympanoplasty

Classification of Tympanoplasty

The purposes of tympanoplasty are to eradicate disease in the middle ear and to reconstruct the hearing mechanism. Tympanic membrane grafting is also performed if necessary. In 1953, Wullstein first used the term "tympanoplasty" and classified the surgery into type I to type V according to the status of the reconstructed hearing mechanism [1] (fig. 17). Type I restores the normal middle ear, maintaining the three ossicles and tympanic membrane in their original position. In type II, the ossicular chain is partially destroyed and the tympanic membrane is attached to the remaining ossicle(s). Type III tympanoplasty was originally a myringostapediopexy, in which the reconstructed tympanic membrane directly touches the stapes head. However, in cases in which there is a gap between the tympanic membrane and the stapes head, a small piece of bone, cartilage or artificial prosthesis called a "columella" is positioned to complete the sound conduction mechanism. (Details will be discussed in the following section.) Type IV tympanoplasty is the method used to protect the round window with a small tympanic cavity, leaving the mobile stapes footplate exposed. In type V, fenestration of the horizontal semicircular canal is made, protecting the round window in the same way as type IV. Nowadays, type I and III and their modified procedures are frequently performed, while type II, IV, and V are not commonly used. Thus, imaging after tympanoplasty is most important for type III, since the relationship between the newly formed tympanic membrane, the columella, and the stapes head or its footplate varies considerably from patient to patient.

Ossiculoplasty

For type I, the tympanic membrane and the ossicles are in their original locations and the imaging findings are almost the same as for those of normal ears. Therefore, type III tympanoplasty using a columella will be discussed in this section.

Type III tympanoplasty with a minor columella is performed when the superstructure of the stapes is present, while a major columella is required if the stapes superstructure is destroyed. The presence or absence of the malleus handle also affects the reconstruction procedure as well as its hearing results. The Austin's classification [2] of ossicular problems, which is based on the presence or absence of the malleus handle (M+, M−) and stapes superstructure (S+, S−) is therefore very useful. Ossicular defects are classified into four types: type A (M+, S+), type B (M+, S−), type C (M−, S+) and type D (M−, S−). Reconstruction procedures for each category of ossicular problems are illustrated in figure 18.

Good hearing results may depend on the materials used for the columella, columella placement for conducting adequate sound energy, and the airspace around the ossicular structure reconstructed [3]. From April 2004 to May 2011, 110 ears of 107 patients underwent type III tympanoplasty using columella in our department. All procedures were performed by the author (N.Y.). After excluding 9 patients with ossicular malformation, data from 101 ears of 99 patients (58 male and 41 female patients; age, 3–78 year old; mean age, 38 year old) were analyzed. All patients underwent type III tympanoplasty, with columella on stapes head performed on 74 ears and columella on stapes footplate performed on 27 ears. Fifty-one ears (50%) were pars flaccida type cholesteatoma, 25 ears (25%) were pars tensa type, combined, or secondary cholesteatoma, 13 ears (13%) were congenital cholesteatoma, and 13 ears (13%) were adhesive otitis media, tympanosclerosis, and others. Seventy-five ears (74%) underwent canal wall down mastoidectomy with soft wall reconstruction [4–6].

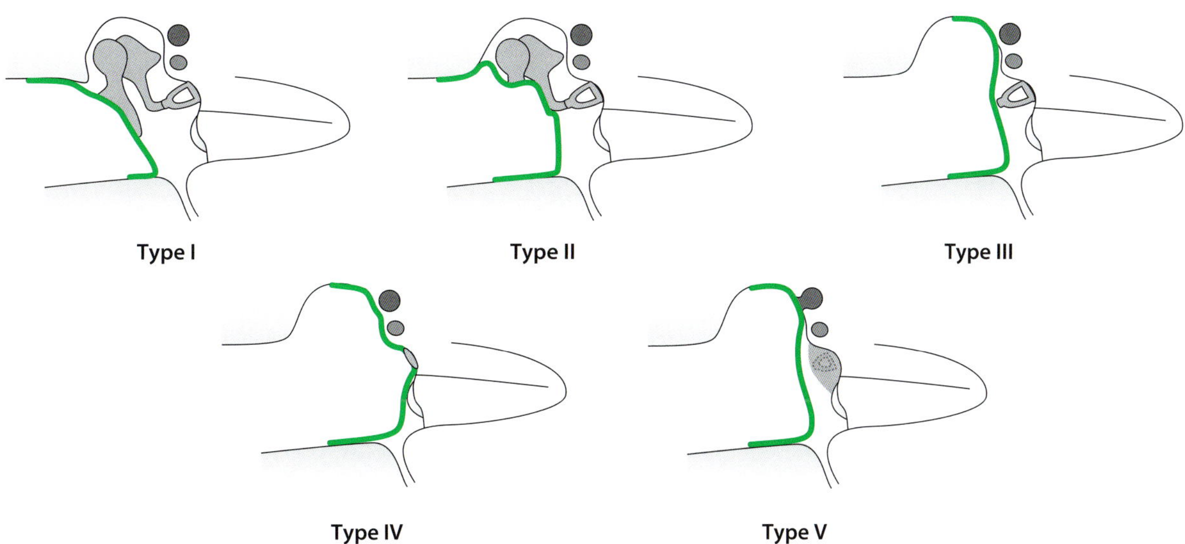

Fig. 17. Types of tympanoplasty introduced by Wullstein [1]

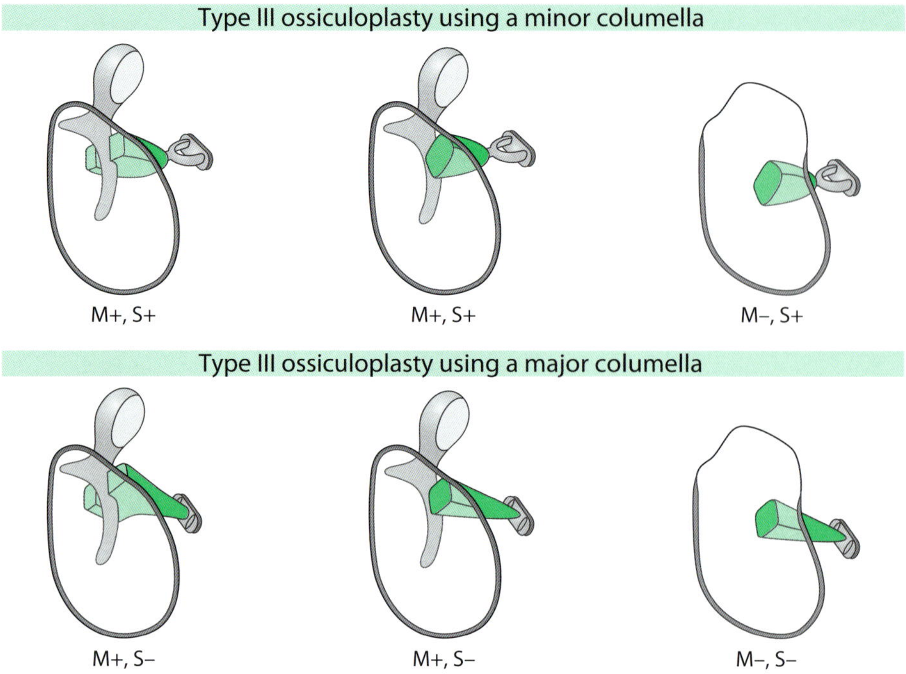

Type III ossiculoplasty using a minor columella

| M+, S+ | M+, S+ | M−, S+ |

Type III ossiculoplasty using a major columella

| M+, S− | M+, S− | M−, S− |

Fig. 18. Variations of type III ossiculoplasty according to ossicular defects. The Austin's classification of ossicular defects is used in this figure.

Evaluation of Postoperative Results

Hearing outcomes of ossiculoplasty are usually evaluated by postoperative pure-tone audiometric air-bone (A-B) gaps, and cases with A-B gap closure within 20 dB are generally regarded as a success. In our series of 101 ears that underwent type III ossiculoplasty, postoperative A-B gap within 20 dB was achieved in 81% for minor columella ossiculoplasty and 63% for major columella ossiculoplasty, which is in line with previous reports on ossiculoplasty results. The causes of failures (postoperative A-B gap wider than 20 dB) for tympanoplasties using a columella in our series are listed in table 1. Seventy-five percent of the failures were due to unfavorable conditions in the middle ear, while 25 % derived from problems of the columella itself.

Destruction of the stapes superstructure, which requires major columella ossiculoplasty, and persistent middle ear inflammation and Eustachian tube dysfunction may cause unfavorable postoperative hearing results. Cases with both successful and unsuccessful results will be shown in this chapter.

Table 1. Causes for failures in type III ossiculoplasty (*n=24*)

Causes for failures	n
Middle ear: *n=18 (75 %)*	
Eardrum retraction/adhesion Inflammation/fibrosis in the tympanic cavity	11
Tympanosclerosis, decreased stapes mobility	5
Eustachian tube dysfunction Sniffing habit, cleft palate	2
Columella: *n=6 (25%)*	
Displacement	2
Detachment from the eardrum/stapes head	2
Ankylosis	2

References

1 Wullstein H: Theory and practice of tympanoplasty. Laryngoscope 1956;66:1076-1093.
2 Austin DF: Ossicular reconstruction. Arch Otolaryngol 1971;94:525–535.
3 Merchant S, McKenna M, Mehta R et al: Middle ear mechanics of type III tympanoplasty (stapes columella): II. Clinical studies. Otol Neurotol 2003;24:186–194.
4 Hosoi H, Murata K: Tympanoplasty with reconstruction of soft posterior meatal wall in ears with cholesteatoma. Auris Nasus Larynx 1994;21:69–74.
5 Takahashi H, Hasebe S, Sudo M, et al: Soft-wall reconstruction for cholesteatoma surgery: reappraisal. Am J Otol 2000;21:28–31.
6 Haginomori S, Takamaki A, Nonaka R, et al: Postoperative aeration in the middle ear and hearing outcome after canal wall down tympanoplasty with soft-wall reconstruction for cholesteatoma. Otol Neurotol 2009;30:478–483.

Points

❶ Tympanoplasty is classified into type I to type V.

❷ In practice, type I and type III tympanoplasty are performed most often.

❸ The Austin's classification of ossicular problems, which is based on the presence or absence of the malleus handle and stapes superstructure, is practical and useful.

❹ Destruction of the stapes superstructure, persistent middle ear inflammation, and Eustachian tube dysfunction may cause unfavorable postoperative results.

Case 1 Cholesteatoma, 1: Good Aeration after Primary Operation

Subject: male, 16 years old

History and Clinical Findings

The subject had been aware for some time of slight hearing loss in the left ear, but had done nothing about it. When he visited a local otolaryngologist for mild tinnitus, the physician discovered a white mass in the pars flaccida of the left tympanic membrane and referred the patient to our department with suspected pars flaccida cholesteatoma. In our initial examination, pure tone audiometry was 8.3 dB right and 25.0 dB left, with a 13.7 dB air-bone gap in the left ear. In the temporal bone CT a pars flaccida cholesteatoma was confirmed in the epitympanum, but the cholesteatoma was limited to the epitympanum.

Primary Surgical Findings and Postoperative Course

For primary surgery on the left ear, a canal wall down tympanoplasty with soft wall reconstruction was performed. The posterior wall of the external auditory canal was excised and the incudostapedial joint confirmed and severed. Bone excision progressed into the epitympanum and the cholesteatoma was detached and extracted under clear view. The incus and head of the malleus were extracted. Silicon plates were placed in the tympanic cavity and the anterior and posterior tympanic isthmi, and surgery concluded with reconstruction of the pars flaccida using temporalis fascia.

Patient CT Findings

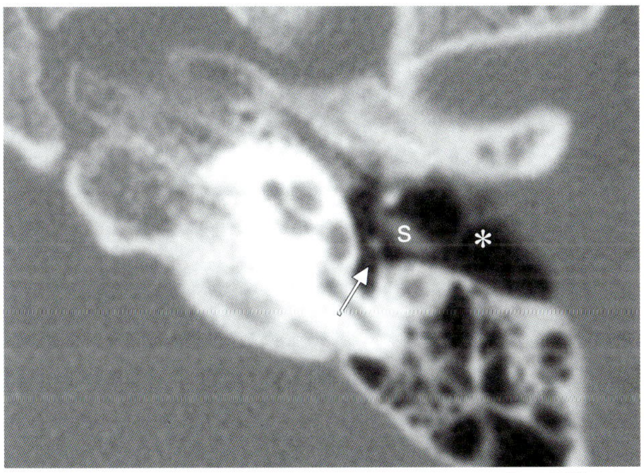

1. axial image

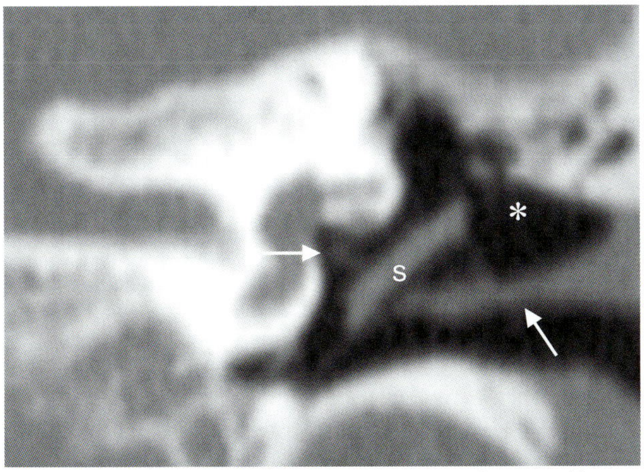

2. coronal image

Normal Control CT Findings

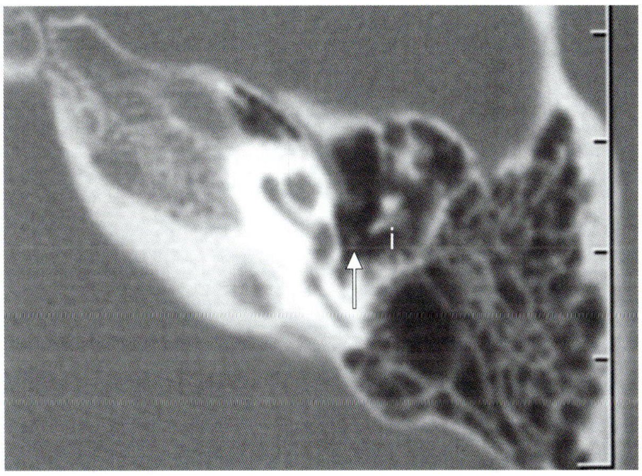

n1. axial image

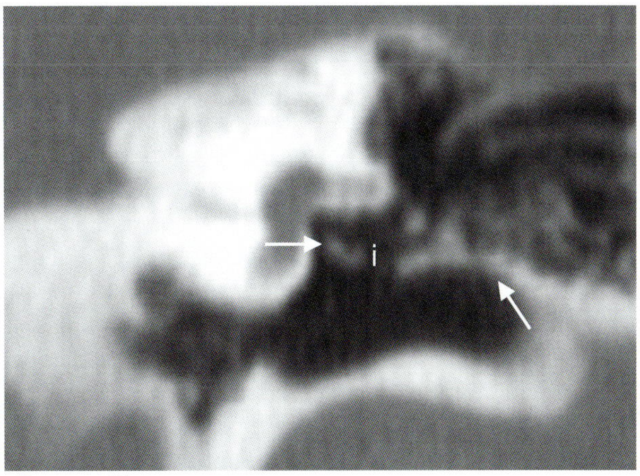

n2. coronal image

Fig. 19. (Case 1) Left ear CT: 8 months after primary operation

[Patient CT Findings]

These CT images are prior to second stage surgery, eight months after primary surgery. Mastoid air cell development and pneumatization are favorable (1, 2: ✻). The posterosuperior wall of the external auditory canal lateral to the epitympanum, which has been removed and reconstructed using the original EAC skin alone (2: ↖), displays a pneumatic cavity with no retraction (1, 2: ✻), forming a smooth external auditory canal. The head of the stapes can be confirmed (1, 2: ↗ ⇨), but the incus has been removed and the silicon plates left in the tympanic cavity and epitympanum are visible (1, 2: **s**). The normal control shows the bony wall of the EAC (n2: ↖) and the position of the head of the stapes (n1, n2: ⇧ ⇨) and the incus (n1, n2: **i**) for comparison.

■ Patient CT Findings Prior to Second Stage Surgery

These findings are prior to second stage surgery, eight months after primary surgery. Mastoid air cell development and pneumatization are favorable (fig. 19:1, 2). The posterosuperior wall of the external auditory canal lateral to the epitympanum, which has been removed and reconstructed using the original EAC skin alone (fig. 19:2), displays a pneumatic cavity with no retraction (fig. 19:1, 2), forming a smooth external auditory canal. The head of the stapes can be confirmed (fig. 19:1, 2), but the incus has been removed and the silicon plates left in the tympanic cavity and epitympanum are visible (fig. 19:1, 2). The position of the head of the stapes and the incus is shown in the normal control image (fig. 19:n1, n2) for comparison.

■ Second Stage Surgery and Postoperative Course

In second stage surgery to the left ear, first the silicon plates left in the primary surgery were removed and it was confirmed that no cholesteatoma persisted in the tympanic or mastoid cavities. Autologous cortical bone was formed into a columella in type III incus interposition ossiculoplasty. Mastoid cavity pneumatization was favorable, so the posterior wall of the external auditory canal was left as soft tissue, with no special reinforcement or obliteration. The postoperative pure tone audiometry for the left (affected) ear was as good as 12.5 dB.

■ Image Findings and Clinical Features

When performing staged surgery for middle ear cholesteatoma or adhesive otitis media, a temporal bone CT exam is also carried out before the second stage surgery. The purpose of this CT is to check for the residual cholesteatoma after primary surgery, pneumatization of the excised EAC posterosuperior wall, epitympanum, and mastoid, and the morphology of the external auditory canal and tympanic membrane. Residual cholesteatoma can be removed and essentially is not a major problem. Also, as in this case, so long as mastoid air cell development is reasonably favorable and there is no soft tissue density, progress after second stage surgery can be expected to be favorable. Problems arise when there is retraction of the tympanic membrane or expanded retraction in the external auditory canal, deficient pneumatization of the middle ear cavity, or fluid accumulation. Such cases require a variety of innovative techniques and countermeasures to prevent post second stage surgery cholesteatoma reformation in the long term. This is why I always conduct temporal bone CT exams, not just prior to the primary surgery, but prior to the second stage surgery as well.

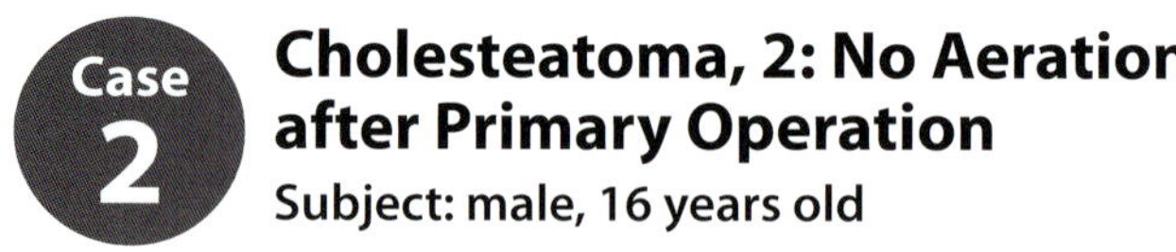

Case 2

Cholesteatoma, 2: No Aeration after Primary Operation

Subject: male, 16 years old

■ History and Clinical Findings

This case was covered in the previous section under "Cholesteatoma: pars flaccida cholesteatoma (2)" (p.137). In pre-primary surgical findings, the cholesteatoma was extensive and mastoid air cell development was poor, giving us concern that it would be a difficult case. A staged tympanoplasty (primary) was performed in the form of a canal wall down tympanoplasty with soft wall reconstruction, but half a year after primary surgery the epitympanum was broadly retracted.

■ Patient CT Findings

Figure 20 shows images prior to the primary operation (a), prior to the second stage operation (b), and normal control images (n). Comparing the images prior to the primary and second stage operations, first it is apparent that the lesion has been completely removed through surgery, and that there is no residual cholesteatoma. Examination of the axial image prior to the second stage operation (fig. 20:1b) reveals that the external auditory canal wall, which is formed only of skin, has become extremely thin and retracted (fig. 20:1b). However, there is some pneumatic cavity formation in the mastoid segment and no accumulation of effusion (fig. 20:1b). In the coronal section, compared to the superior wall of the external auditory canal in the normal control image (fig. 20:n2), the skin of the external auditory canal is considerably retracted and expands superiorly as far as the tegmen (fig. 20:2b). The plate-shaped soft tissue density present from the tympanic cavity to the epitympanum is the silicon plate.

■ Surgical Findings and Postoperative Course

In the second stage operation the three silicon plates were removed and absence of persistent cholesteatoma in the tympanic and mastoid cavities confirmed, then the preserved autologous incus bone was sculpted into a columella and type III incus interposition ossiculoplasty performed. The retracted skin area in the epitympanum was reinforced with auricular cartilage palisade. Postoperative pure tone audiometry in the left ear was 21.3 dB.

■ Image Findings and Clinical Features

This sort of case presents the most difficult challenge for those involved in ear surgery. First, in terms of imaging diagnosis, if the EAC wall is constructed with soft tissue alone during canal wall down tympanoplasty, the soft tissue is thick enough to be clearly depicted in CT imagery provided the external auditory canal does not expand postoperatively. However, observation via CT images becomes problematic if the skin becomes thinner and expands, as it did in this case, making it difficult to evaluate external auditory canal morphology.

In terms of controlling cholesteatoma, if the external auditory canal is removed, the epitympanum and posterosuperior wall may enlarge to form an excessive

Patient CT Findings

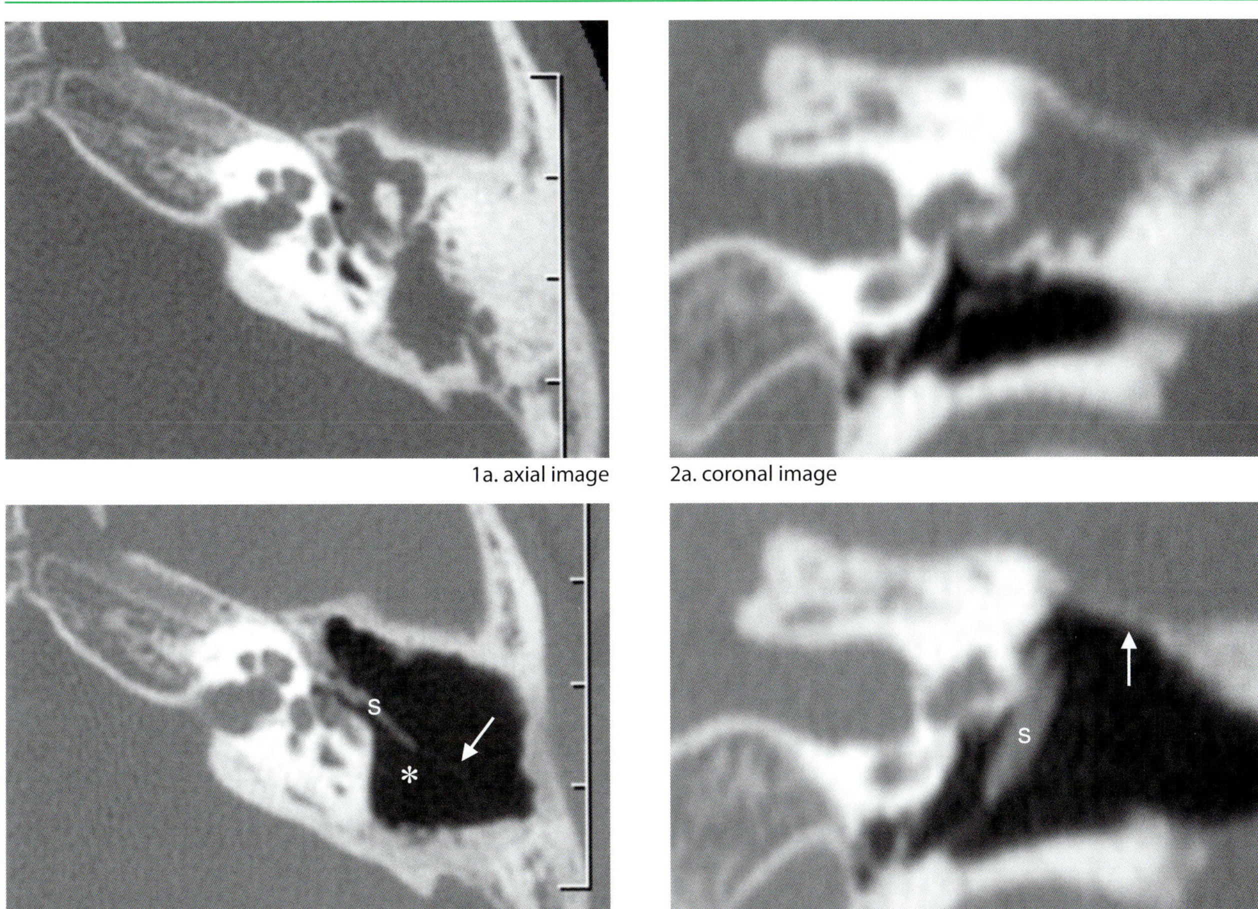

Normal Control CT Findings

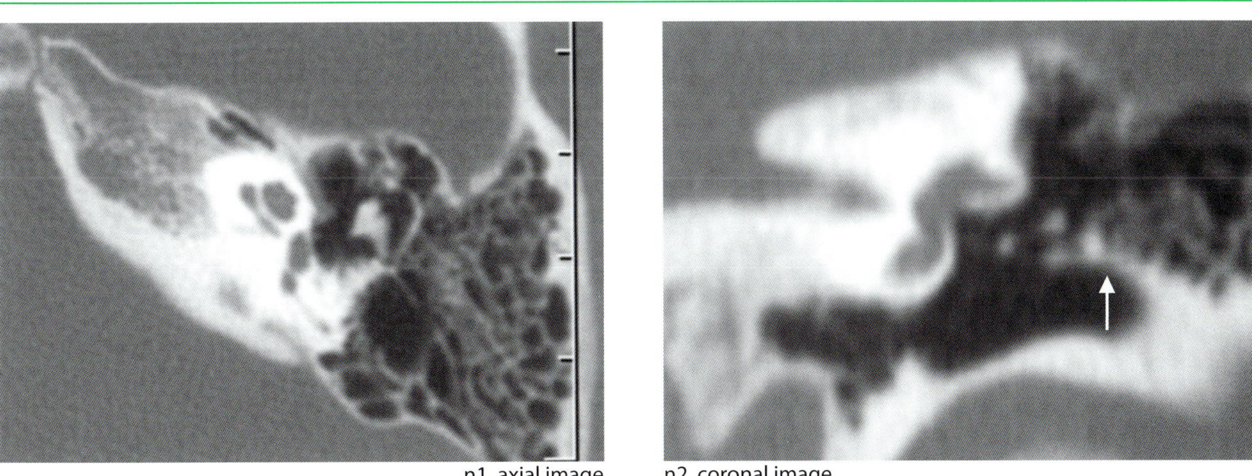

Fig. 20. (Case 2) Left ear CT: a=prior to primary operation; b=prior to second stage operation

[Patient CT Findings]

Images prior to the primary operation (a), prior to the second stage operation (b), and normal control images (n) are shown. Comparing the images prior to the primary and second stage operations, first it is apparent that the lesion has been completely removed through surgery, and that there is no residual cholesteatoma. Examination of the axial image prior to the second stage operation (1b) reveals that the external auditory canal wall, which is formed only of skin, has become retracted and extremely thin, making observation difficult (1b: ✐). However, there is some pneumatic cavity formation in the mastoid segment and no accumulation of effusion (1b: ❀). In the coronal section, compared to the superior wall of the external auditory canal in the normal control image (n2: ⇧), the skin of the external auditory canal is considerably retracted and expands superiorly as far as the tegmen (2b: ⇧). The plate-shaped soft tissue density present from the tympanic cavity to the epitympanum is the silicon plate (1b, 2b: **s**).

wound cavity, which creates the possibility of so-called cavity problem or re-formation of the cholesteatoma. This necessitates steps in the second stage operation such as reinforcement of the pars flaccida and posterior wall with cartilage, obliteration of the mastoid cavity with bone putty, and reinforcement of the posterior wall with a pedicle flap. On the other hand, in canal up surgery in which the EAC posterior wall is not removed, the physiological condition of the external auditory canal itself is preserved, but there is concern that in the long term the pars flaccida will become retracted again and the cholesteatoma re-form. Here also, a variety of countermeasures can be considered, including forming a tympanic membrane out of cartilage and obliterating the mastoid cavity. Yanagihara et al [1], based on long-term results from multiple cases of cholesteatoma surgeries, report favorable results combining a surgical microscope with an endoscope and performing canal up tympanoplasty, choosing to obliterate the mastoid cavity with either cartilage or bone putty as the case warrants. Either way, for the ear specialist, cholesteatoma surgery involving deficient eustachian tube function or mastoid air cell development is an area requiring the utmost effort, study, and perspicacity.

References

1 Yanagihara N, Komori M, Hinohira Y: Total mastoid obliteration in staged canal-up tympanoplasty for cholesteatoma facilitates tympanic aeration. Otol Neurotol 2009;30:760–770.

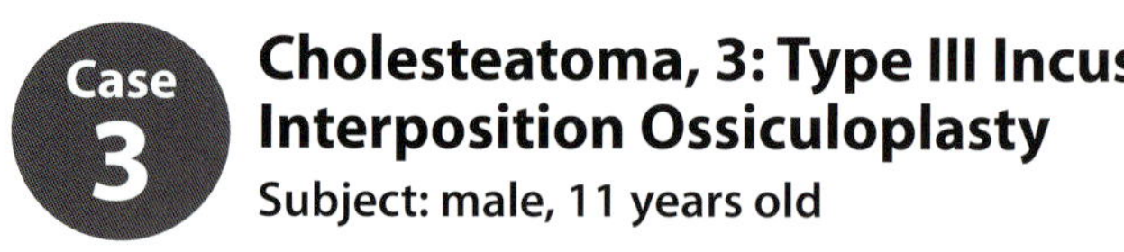

Case 3 — Cholesteatoma, 3: Type III Incus Interposition Ossiculoplasty

Subject: male, 11 years old

■ History and Clinical Findings

Right ear hearing loss was identified at a school health exam and the subject was referred to our department via a local physician. Right ear hearing at time of the initial exam was 46.7 dB (air-bone gap: 40.0 dB), with no stapedial reflex detected. In an exploratory tympanotomy of the right ear, an open congenital cholesteatoma was confirmed in the center of the posterosuperior tympanic cavity and the long process of the incus was deficient, but the lenticular process of the incus remained and no abnormalities were ascertained in the stapes. The incus and head of the malleus were extracted to secure a broad field of view and the cholesteatoma removed completely in a staged tympanoplasty (primary). The second stage operation was performed 13 months later. After confirming that there was no residual cholesteatoma, a type III incus interposition ossiculoplasty was performed using preserved autologous incus as a columella.

■ Patient CT Findings and Clinical Course

CT images taken prior to the primary surgery and after the second stage surgery are shown. Preoperatively, a cholesteatoma is present in the posterosuperior part of the tympanic cavity and the long process of the incus cannot be confirmed, but the incudostapedial joint is visible (fig. 21:1). Mastoid air cell development is moderate, with pneumatization, but there is soft tissue density on the margins of the air cells, suggesting the existence of inflammation and effusion.

Postoperatively, mastoid air cells lateral to the epitympanum have been excised and internal pneumatization is favorable, with no findings of residual cholesteatoma or effusion accumulation. The columella formed using autologous incus is positioned between the superstructure of the stapes and the handle of the malleus (fig. 21:2). Postoperatively, the external auditory canal and tympanic membrane developed favorably, with no retraction, and pure tone audiometry in the right (affected) ear was favorable at 13.8 dB.

■ Image Findings and Clinical Features

There are many methods for reconstruction of the ossicular chain during tympanoplasty. When the ossicular chain is reconstructed, rather than preserving their original form as in a type I ossiculoplasty, the most common approach is type III and its variations. If the stapes superstructure remains and the connection between the stapes or the malleus and the tympanic membrane is stable, hearing results are favorable on average. The surgeon wants to obtain stable vibration from the area on the tympanic membrane where vibration is greatest. I prefer to try for a type III incus interposition ossiculoplasty in which the head of the stapes is connected to the handle of the malleus using a columella as close to the tip as possible. In imaging diagnosis, it is important to focus on the interrelationship between the head of the stapes and the columella, the handle of the malleus, or the tympanic

Patient CT Findings

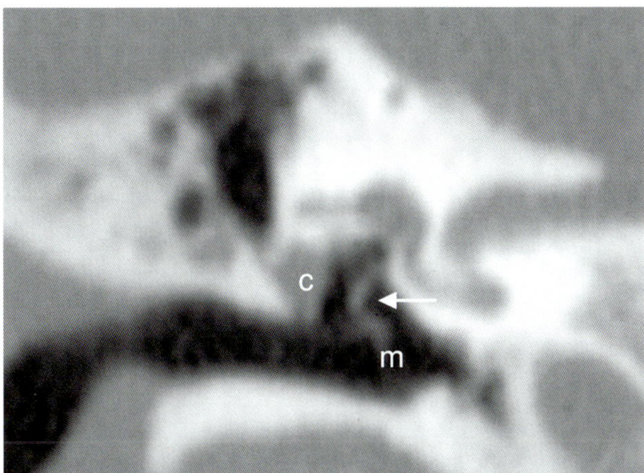

1. coronal image

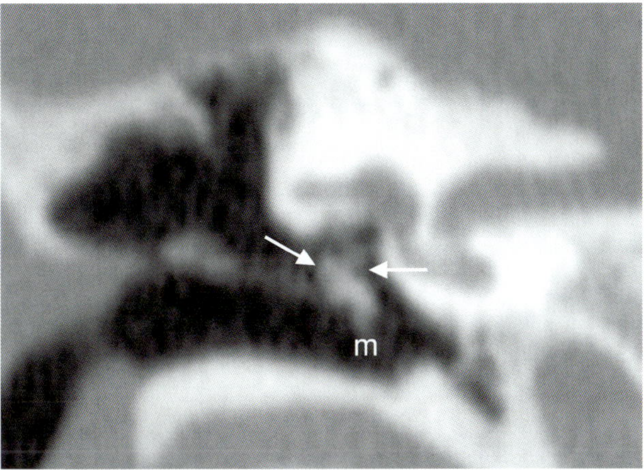

2. coronal image

Fig. 21. (Case 3) Right ear CT: 1=prior to primary operation; 2=post second stage operation

[Patient CT Findings]

CT images taken prior to the primary surgery (1) and after the second stage surgery (2) are shown. Preoperatively, a cholesteatoma is present in the posterosuperior part of the tympanic cavity (1: **c**) and the long process of the incus cannot be confirmed, but the incudostapedial joint is visible (1: ⇐). Mastoid air cell development is moderate, with pneumatization, but there is soft tissue density in the margins of the air cells, suggesting the existence of inflammation and effusion. The vicinity of the tip of the handle of the malleus is indicated with an " **m** ".

Postoperatively, mastoid air cells lateral to the epitympanum have been excised and internal pneumatization is favorable, with no findings of residual cholesteatoma or effusion accumulation. The columella formed using autologous incus (2: ↝) is positioned between the superstructure of the stapes (2: ⇐) and the handle of the malleus (2: **m**).

membrane itself. In the long term there is a chance that the columella will shift or drop out, so in the postoperative follow-up CT it is important to check the position of the columella in addition to checking for presence of cholesteatoma or inflammation.

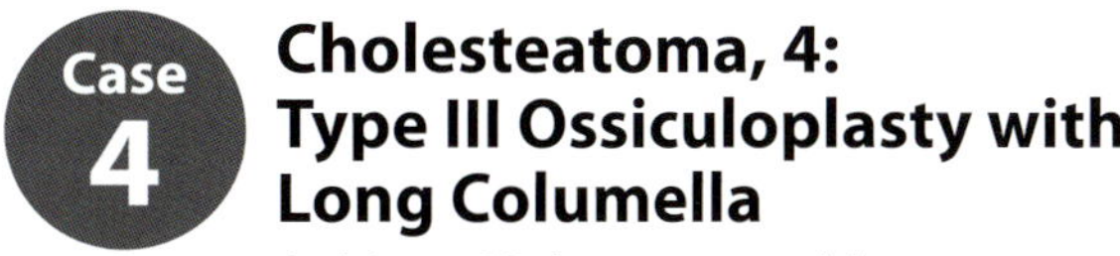

Cholesteatoma, 4: Type III Ossiculoplasty with Long Columella

Subject: Male, 9 years old

■ History and Clinical Findings

Left ear hearing loss was identified at a school health exam and the subject was referred to our department via a local physician. In our initial examination, pure tone audiometry was 7.5 dB right, 50.0 dB left (air-bone gap: 35.0 dB), and the stapedial reflex was absent in the left ear. An exploratory tympanotomy revealed an open type cholesteatoma in the posterosuperior part of the tympanic cavity and deficiency in the long process of the incus and superstructure of the stapes. A staged tympanoplasty (primary) was performed, extracting the incus and the head of the malleus and removing the cholesteatoma in its entirety. Nine months later in second stage surgery, after confirming that there was no residual cholesteatoma, a type III ossiculoplasty with long columella was performed using preserved autogenous incus as a columella. Because pneumatization of the mastoid cavity was favorable, no reinforcement of the posterior wall of the external auditory canal or obliteration of the mastoid cavity was carried out.

■ Patient CT Findings and Clinical Course after Second Stage Surgery

CT images taken after the second stage surgery are shown. Both mastoid air cell development and pneumatization are favorable and there is no soft tissue density. It is apparent that the medial tip of the columella formed from the incus bone is appropriately positioned near the center of the footplate of the stapes (fig. 22). Postoperative course was favorable, with no occurrence of otitis media or retraction of the tympanic membrane or external auditory canal, and pure tone audiometry in the left (affected) ear of 15.0 dB.

■ Image Findings and Clinical Features

Among the procedures for ossicular chain reconstruction employed during tympanoplasty, the success rate for type III ossiculoplasty with long columella is lower than for that with short columella, making it the most nerve-racking for the surgeon. If the medial tip of the columella is not correctly positioned in the central part of the footplate of the stapes, there is no hope of improvement to hearing. In long-term observation, hearing sometimes deteriorates due to gradual slipping of the columella or adhesion to the surrounding tissue. In such situations, it is important use CT imaging to accurately grasp the overall condition of the middle ear and the position of the columella. In cases in which there is a danger of re-retraction of the tympanic membrane, the epitympanum is often obliterated with bone putty, but caution is required when doing so as adhesion between the obliterating structure and the columella may cause deterioration of hearing.

Patient CT Findings

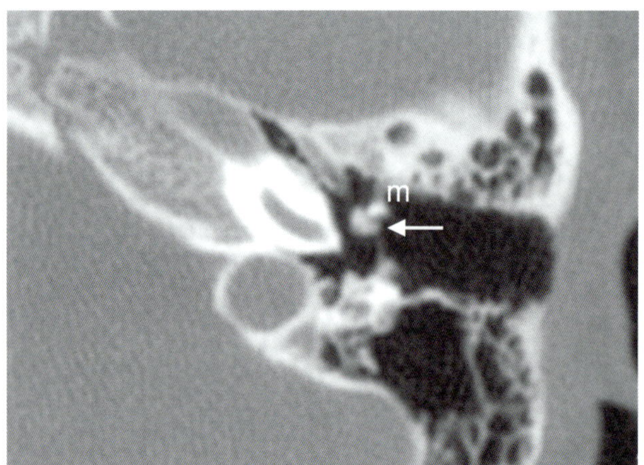

a1. axial image

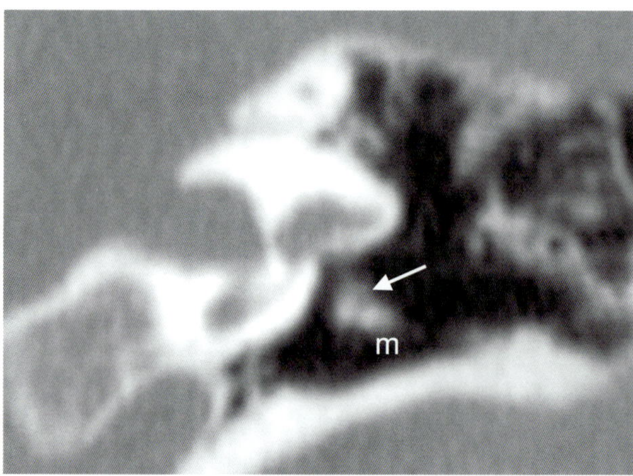

c1. coronal image

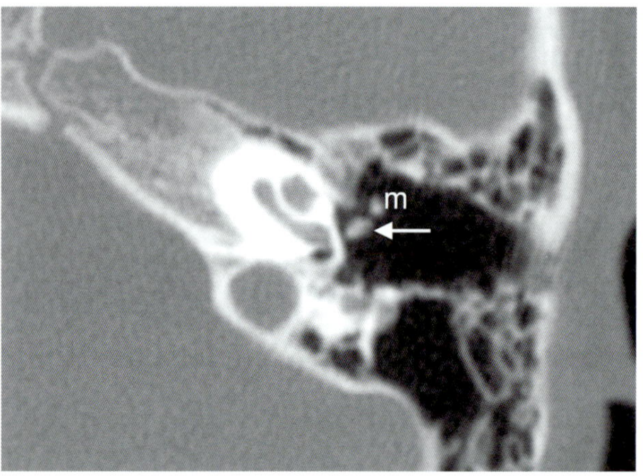

a2. axial image

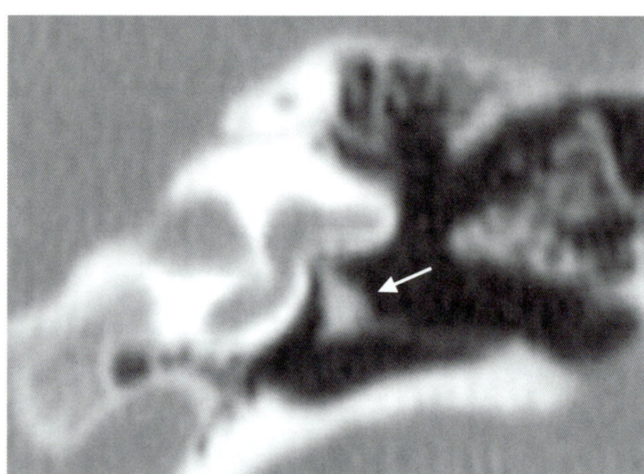

c2. coronal image

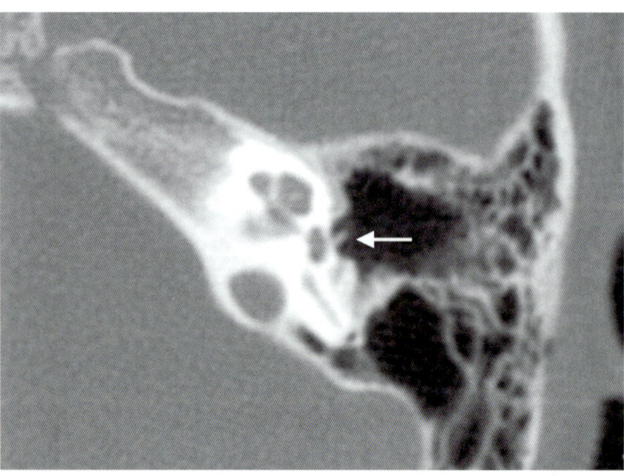

a3. axial image

Fig. 22. (Case 4) Left ear CT: after second stage operation

[Patient CT Findings]

CT images were taken after the second stage surgery. Both mastoid air cell development and pneumatization are favorable and there is no soft tissue density. It is apparent that the medial tip of the columella sculpted from the incus (a1–a3: ⟵ ; c1–c2: ⤶) is appropriately positioned near the center of the footplate of the stapes (a3, c2) and the lateral end is contacting the handle of the malleus (a1, c1: **m**).

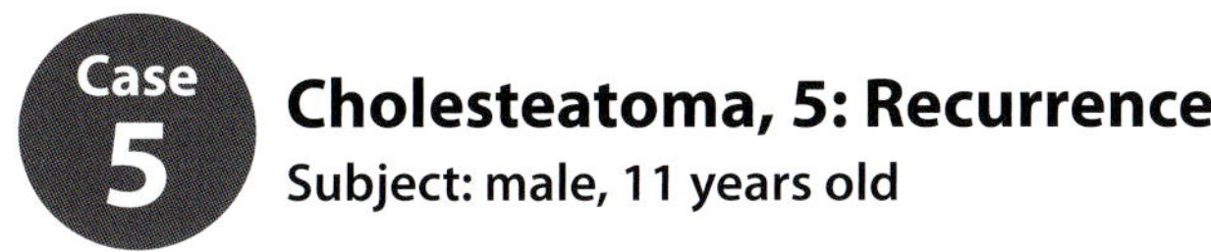

Cholesteatoma, 5: Recurrence
Subject: male, 11 years old

History and Clinical Findings

The subject had undergone canal wall down tympanoplasty with soft wall reconstruction (primary and secondary) for a right pars flaccida cholesteatoma. In the second stage surgery, a type III ossiculoplasty with long columella was performed and the posterior wall of the external auditory canal reconstructed with soft tissue only, with no particular reinforcement or obliteration of the mastoid. Starting around six months after surgery, the wound cavity gradually expanded and a difficult-to-clean buildup of cerumen appeared on the anterior part of the pars flaccida of the tympanic membrane, so reoperative surgery was performed four years after the second stage surgery for the previous operation. Pure tone audiometry prior to revision surgery was 48.8 dB right (air-bone gap: 28.8 dB) and 10.0 dB left.

Patient CT Findings

CT images for this case (fig. 23:1–3) and the normal control (fig. 23:n1–n3) are shown. Mastoid air cell development in this case is deficient, and even where air cells are barely discernible there is no pneumatization and the area is filled with soft tissue density. The axial section taken at the lateral semicircular canal level shows enlargement of the mastoid wound cavity from the external auditory canal, with the wound cavity reaching the anterior end of the epitympanum (fig. 23:1). Compared to the corresponding normal control image, it is apparent that this location was originally deep within the middle ear (fig. 23:n1). In the section superior to this, there is a mass of soft tissue density (fig. 23:2) in the area of retraction connected to the wound cavity, which is diagnosed as recurrence of the pars flaccida cholesteatoma. In the coronal section as well, one can observe that the retraction connected to the wound cavity progresses superiorly from the lateral semicircular canal level and has caused an accumulation of soft tissue (keratin debris) (fig. 23:3). Also, the columella (fig. 23:3) is contacting the facial canal. Originally, this area contained the tiny structures of the long and lenticular processes of the incus and superstructure of the stapes (fig. 23:n3), so it is understandable that positioning the columella so as to preserve the space between this and the surrounding area requires as delicate sculpting as possible.

Surgical Findings and Postoperative Course

Surgery was performed. After the postauricular incision, a connective tissue flap with a cephalad pedicle was formed from subcutaneous connective tissue. The skin that had retracted into the mastoid cavity was detached to reveal the interior of the tympanic cavity, where it was observed that the medial tip of the columella's pedicle was correctly positioned on the footplate of the stapes. However, the columella overall was angled cephalad and contacting the facial canal, so it was raised and attached to the medial surface of the tympanic membrane. The mastoid space was filled with bone putty and the aforementioned connective tissue flap. Postoperatively, there was no recurrence of retraction in the external auditory canal and pure tone audiometry in the right (affected) side improved to 28.8 dB.

■ Image Findings and Clinical Features

Postoperative relapse of middle ear cholesteatoma may be caused either by persistence, due to re-growth of the cholesteatoma from skin persisting after surgery, or by recurrence, due to formation of a new cholesteatoma that occurs when the formed tympanic membrane re-succumbs to retraction. A variety of surgical techniques have been tried to avoid both patterns of recurrence, but with current procedures a certain percentage of surgical cases will result in recurrence over the long term. Recurrence is thought to be brought on by multiple factors, but Moriyama [1] has shown that recurrence is more prone to occur when the cholesteatoma has progressed into the mastoid cavity. After surgery for middle ear cholesteatoma, progress should be observed over the long term and, if recurrence is suspected, it is necessary to observe the middle ear cavity using CT.

Echo-planar diffusion MRI can depict cholesteatoma as a high intensity mass, but its prominent artifact around the skull-base has been an obstacle for its routine use in cholesteatoma diagnosis. Non-echo-planar diffusion MRI, however, has significantly improved the image quality and spatial resolution, which might become a first choice modality for postoperative follow-up imaging of middle ear cholesteatoma [2].

References

1 Moriyama H: Chuji shinjushu no byotai to chiryo. Dai 105 kai Nihon jibiinkokagakkai sokai shukudai hokoku (Middle ear cholesteatoma; its pathology and treatment: Report on the issues raised at the 105th annual meeting of Oto-Rhino-Laryngological Society of Japan), 2004 (in Japanese.)
2 De Foer B, Vercruysse JP, Bernaerts A, et al: Middle ear cholesteatoma: non-echo-planar diffusion-weighted MR imaging versus delayed gadolinium-enhanced T1-weighted MR imaging—value in detection. Radiology 2010;255:866–872.

Points

❶ Recurrence refers to a cholesteatoma that forms after tympanoplasty when the tympanic membrane re-succumbs to retraction.

❷ Cases of recurrence arise with a background of deficient mastoid air cell development and deficient eustachian tube function.

❸ Cholesteatomas are formed from partial retraction of the external auditory canal, tympanic membrane, and wound cavity, along with debris accumulation.

❹ Procedures to prevent recurrence include reconstruction of the EAC wall or tympanic membrane using bone putty or auricular cartilage, obliterating and sealing the mastoid cavity, reinforcement of the EAC wall with a pedicle flap, and insertion of a tympanic membrane ventilation tube.

Patient CT Findings	**Normal Control CT Findings**

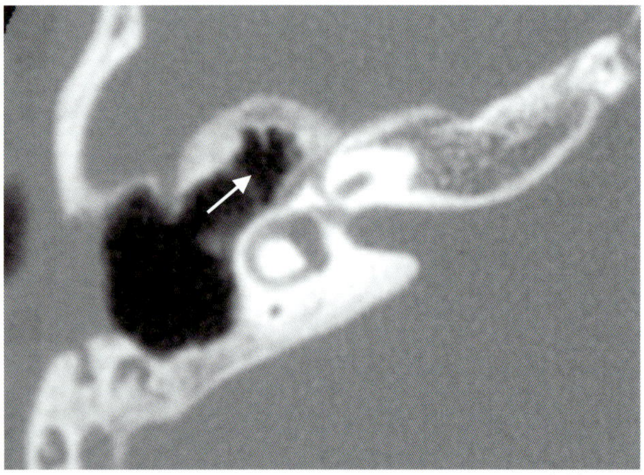

1. axial image 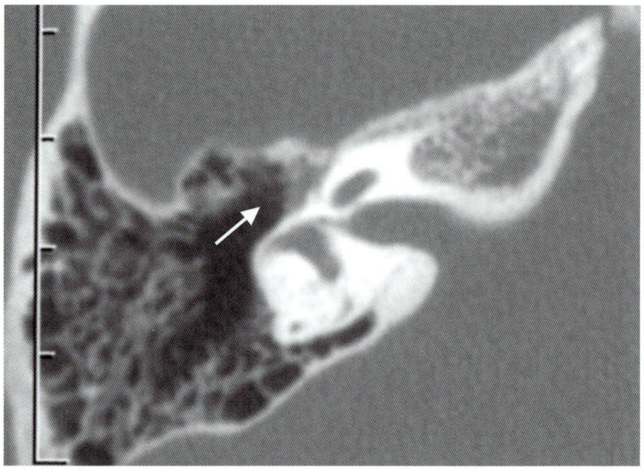   n1. axial image

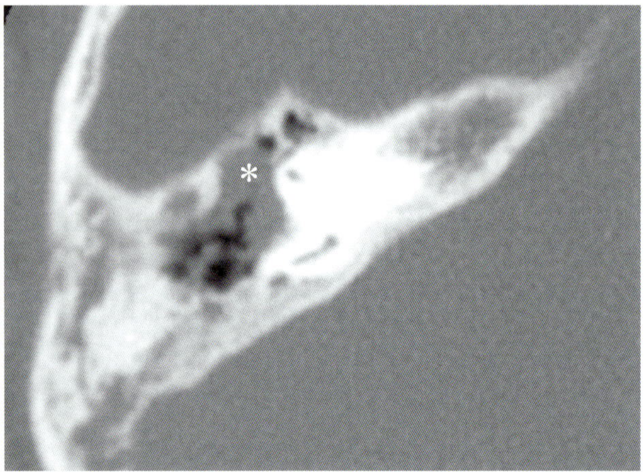

2. axial image 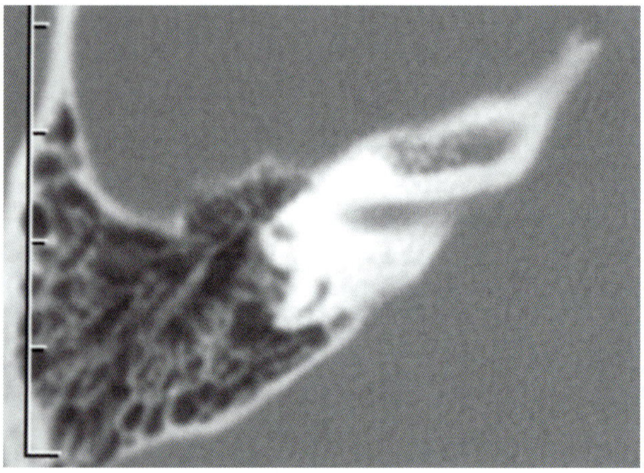   n2. axial image

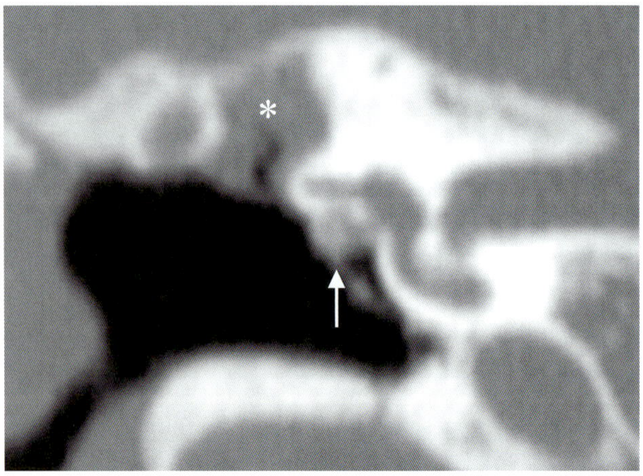

3. coronal image 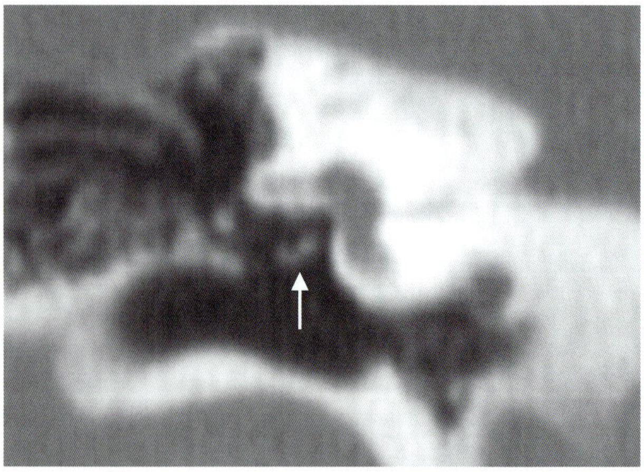   n3. coronal image

Fig. 23. (Case 5) Right ear CT: 4 years, 4 months after second stage surgery for previous operation

[Patient CT Findings]

CT images for this case (1–3) and the normal control (n1–n3) are shown. Mastoid air cell development in this case is deficient, and even where air cells are barely discernible there is no pneumatization and the area is filled with soft tissue density. The axial section taken at the lateral semicircular canal level shows enlargement of the mastoid wound cavity from the external auditory canal, with the wound cavity reaching the anterior end of the epitympanum (1: ↗). Compared to the normal control image, it is apparent that this location was originally deep within the middle ear (n1: ↗). In the section superior to this, there is a mass of soft tissue density (2: ✳) in the area of retraction connected to the wound cavity, which is diagnosed as recurrence of the pars flaccida cholesteatoma. In the coronal section as well, one can observe that the retraction connected to the wound cavity progresses superiorly from the lateral semicircular canal level and has caused an accumulation of soft tissue (keratin debris) (3: ✳). Also, the columella (3: ⇑) is contacting the facial canal. Originally, this area contained the tiny structures of the long and lenticular processes of the incus and superstructure of the stapes (n3: ⇑), so it is understandable that positioning the columella so as to preserve the space between this and the surrounding area requires as delicate sculpting as possible.

Pediatric Ear Diseases
Diagnostic Imaging Atlas and Case Reports

Other Ear Disorders

In this chapter, we will examine five cases that do not fall under the categories of either congenital anomaly or infectious disease, and cannot be grouped together as a single category. The first case is one of conductive hearing loss accompanied by low CT density in the vicinity of the cochlea, complicated by pervasive developmental disorder that made diagnosis of the pathology difficult. The relationship between image findings and hearing findings, including otosclerosis, is presented here. Cases 2 and 3 present traumatic injuries, one of typical middle ear trauma and the other a rarer case of trauma accompanied by cochlear implant trouble. The fourth case is one of severe hearing loss complicated by a difficult to treat middle ear cholesteatoma, requiring repeated operations ending in cochlear implant surgery. Case 5 presents an infant who suffered bilateral deafness brought on by bilateral labyrinthitis that occurred after a bout of meningitis.

In these cases, except for those of simple trauma, a response that takes both the primary disease and hearing into consideration is necessary; treatment of a single disease or condition in isolation will be unsuccessful in resolving the overall problem. It is my hope that these cases will provide a useful reference for those encountering similar diseases or pathologies.

Chapter 5

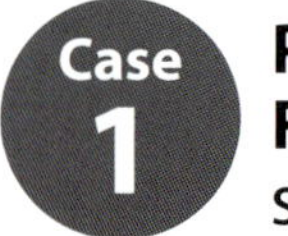

Case 1 · Pericochlear Hypoattenuating Foci and Stapes Fixation
Subject: male, 7 years, 3 months

■ History and Clinical Findings

The subject was under ongoing observation and guidance by a local physician due to pervasive developmental disorder, and his lack of language communication with those around him was thought to arise from his developmental disorder. However, the possibility of hearing loss was revealed at a school health exam and he was referred to our department. The subject was incompatible for pure tone audiometry due to his pervasive developmental disorder, but ASSR testing revealed findings of moderate hearing loss in both ears (fig. 1), while tympanogram results were type As for the right ear and type A for the left, with no stapedial reflex, leading us to suspect conductive hearing loss.

■ Patient CT Findings

CT temporal bone images for the right ear only are shown here (fig. 2, 3), as findings were roughly the same for both ears. Mastoid air cell development is favorable, with no abnormal soft tissue density, and no clear abnormal findings ascertained in the inner ear or internal auditory canal. However, decalcification can be ascertained in the vicinity of the cochlea and anterior portion of the oval window (fig. 2, 3). The head of the malleus and body of the incus show slight thickening with slight low-density

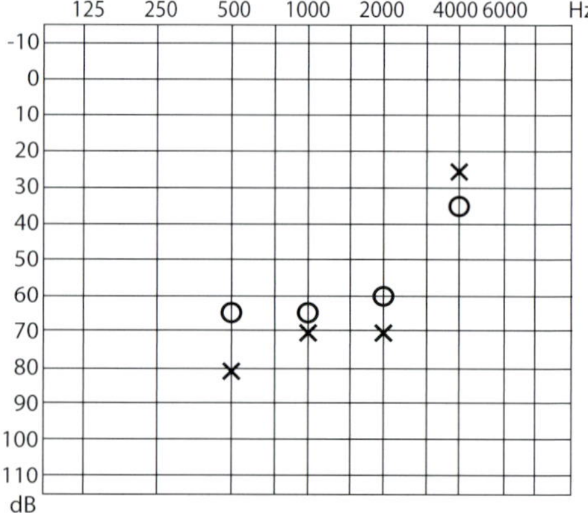

Fig. 1. (Case 1) ASSR testing

Patient CT Findings

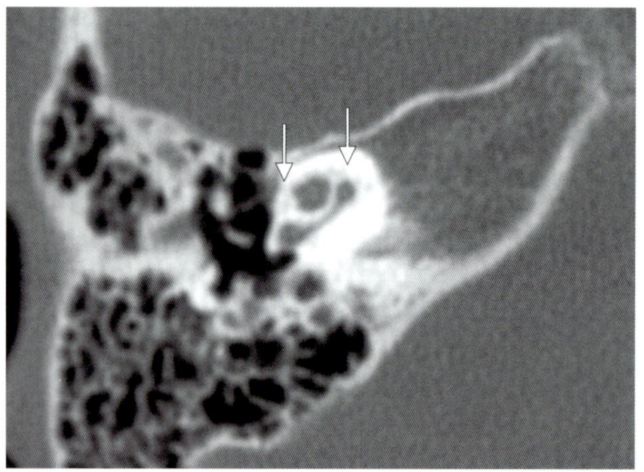

1. axial image

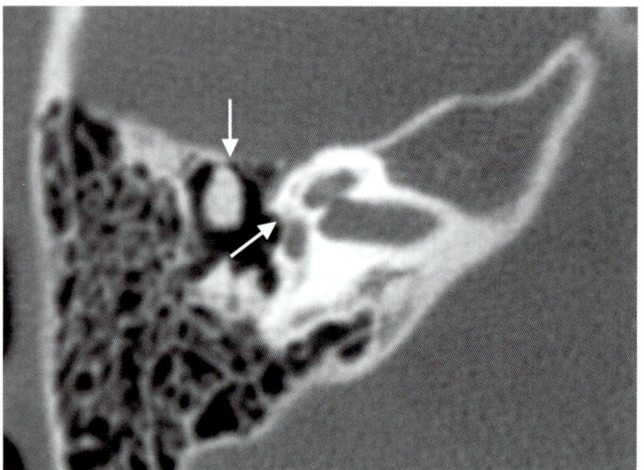

2. axial image

Fig. 2. (Case 1) Right ear CT

[Patient CT Findings]

Normal Control CT Findings

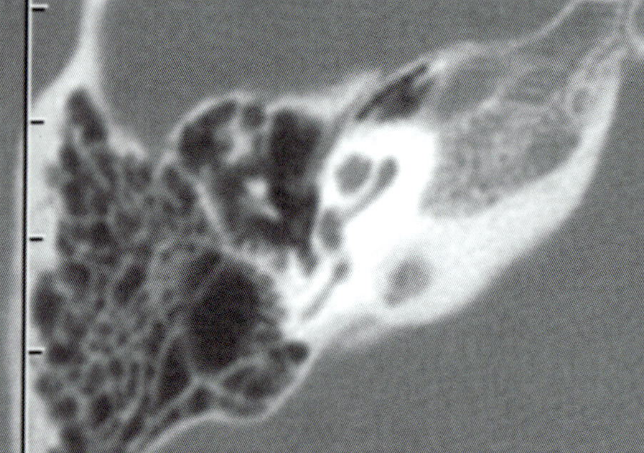

n1. axial image

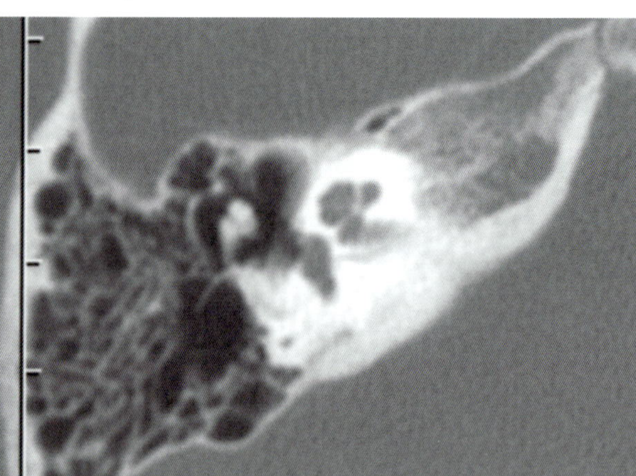

n2. axial image

Patient CT Findings

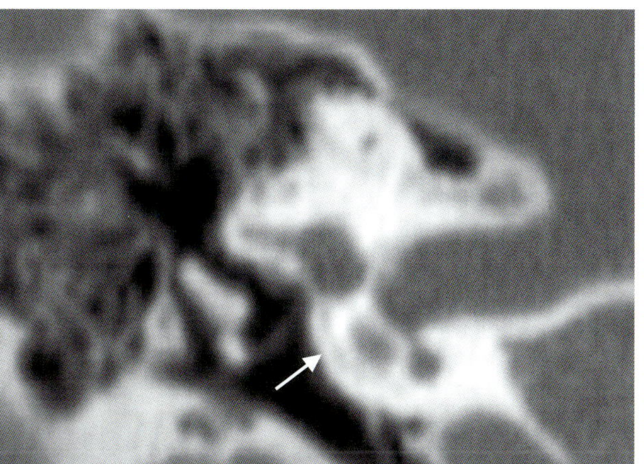

1. coronal image

2. coronal image

Normal Control CT Findings

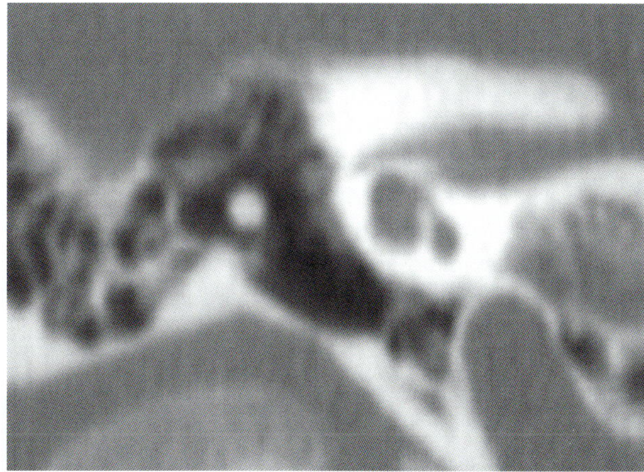

n1. coronal image

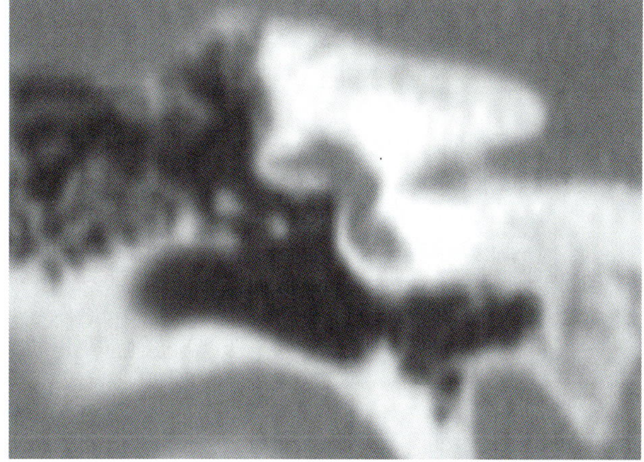

n2. coronal image

Fig. 3. (Case 1) Right ear CT

internally that suggests decalcification. Based on these findings, we considered the likely cause of hearing loss to be stapes fixation due to either otosclerosis or a similar pathology and decided to perform an exploratory tympanotomy, to be accompanied by stapes surgery if actual stapes fixation was confirmed.

■ Surgical Findings and Postoperative Course

Surgery was performed on the left ear first. Surgery was performed via postauricular rather than endaural incision, as we could not negate the possibility of abnormalities other than in the stapes. Observing the interior of the tympanic cavity, the long process of the incus showed slight thickening and the footplate of the stapes was completely fixed. Mobility of the malleus and incus was favorable. The superstructure of the stapes was removed, fenestration performed on the footplate of the stapes, and a Schuknecht teflon wire piston inserted and its wire fastened to the long process of the incus.

Postoperatively, response to environmental sound was favorable and activity during daily life improved. Pure tone audiometry became possible, with pure tone averages of 56.7 dB right and 21.7 dB left after left-ear surgery. When the same surgery was performed on the right ear eight months later, the same improvement to hearing was obtained as for the left ear. Figure 4 shows the results of pure tone audiometry conducted nine months after completion of surgery on both ears.

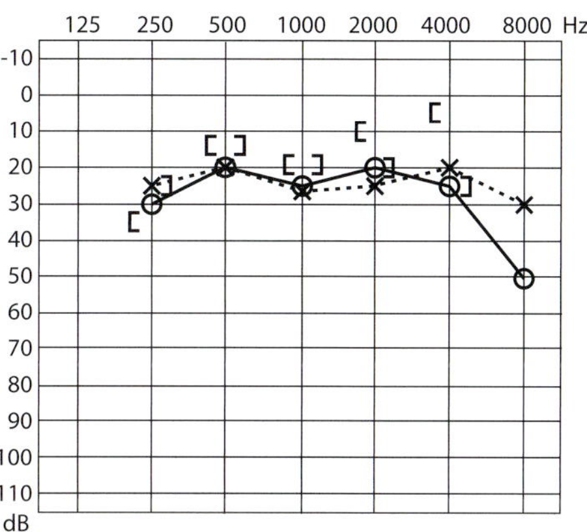

Fig. 4. (Case 1) Pure tone audiogram nine months after surgery

■ Image Findings and Clinical Features

The distinguishing feature in this case was the combined pervasive developmental disorder and hearing loss. It is common knowledge that pervasive developmental disorder is accompanied by impaired language development. Hearing loss is commonly suspected as a cause of delayed language development in children, but when there is a clear developmental disability that explains the delayed language development, confirmation of presence or absence of hearing loss may be delayed. During hearing evaluation for developmentally delayed children it is difficult to obtain the cooperation of the patient, making objective techniques such as ASSR, ABR, and stapedial reflex the main methods of evaluation. In cases of conductive hearing loss, such as this one, improvement through surgery is basically expected, so it is worth making the effort to conduct accurate hearing evaluations even in developmentally delayed children. Of course, improved hearing does nothing to treat the developmental delay itself, but in this case the subject obtained significant improvement in his ability to hear everyday sounds, facilitating easier communication with his family. The fact that he was able to respond to pure tone audiometry postoperatively, whereas before he could not, represented a significant step forward in hearing management.

Another major concern in this case is that the cause of the conductive hearing loss has still yet to be clearly determined. As is explained below, a linear low-density area is sometimes observed in the vicinity of the cochlea in small children and, while there is not yet a clear explanation for its presence, it is considered to be a physiological finding that depends on the degree of ossification of the cochlear bone capsule. On the other hand, cases have been reported in which this low-density area in the vicinity of the cochlea is accompanied by hearing loss. With the current subject, the linear low-density area in the vicinity of the cochlea extended to the anterior portion of the oval window, and stapes footplate fixation was actually confirmed. It would seem unreasonable to assert that these CT findings are unrelated to the stapes fixation. Also, the formation of the malleus and incus in this case was thicker than normal and there was a chance of slight ossicular malformation, but favorable mobility of the malleus and incus was confirmed during surgery, allowing us to discount any chance of fixation in the malleus or incus. Unfortunately, because no histological examination was performed on the stapes superstructure removed from this subject it is impossible to reach a definite conclusion, but the cause of disease in this case can be assumed to have been either a singular form of otosclerosis or some kind of congenital bone metabolism disorder that may include genetic abnormality.

■ Decalcification of the Cochlear Region in Children

A linear low-density area is sometimes observed in the vicinity of the cochlea in small children, which is considered to be a physiological finding that depends on the degree of ossification of the cochlear bone area [1]. On the other hand, cases have been reported in which this low-density area in the vicinity of the cochlea is accompanied by actual hearing loss [1]. In the case presented here, the appearance of the low-density area extending from the cochlear region to the anterior portion of the oval window, while differing somewhat from otosclerosis normally encountered, has a broader low-density area than physiological findings reported in the literature, and furthermore stapes fixation was actually confirmed. In cases where a low-density area is observed in the vicinity of the cochlea in temporal bone CT images, rather than simply concluding that it is a physiological finding seen in young children, one should consider the possibility of otosclerosis or some form of bone metabolism disorder.

Otosclerosis is a disease involving the decalcification and re-ossification of the cochlear bone capsule. Its cause is unknown, but possible causes that have been reported include genetic factors, viral infection, and metabolic disorders [2]. The lesion frequently involves decalcification and ossification around the anterior margin of the oval window, which leads to stapes fixation causing hearing loss. The hearing loss is essentially conductive, but frequently presents itself as mixed hearing loss due to the appearance of bone conduction deterioration. Otosclerosis mainly arises in adults, and occasionally in children, but with little opportunity for a definitive diagnosis it may remain classified as hearing loss of unknown origin for a long period of time.

Otosclerosis is more problematic in children than in adults. While rare, it does occur in children, who comprise around 5% of all patients, adults included [3]. Because severe hearing loss does not occur in the initial stages of otosclerosis, it is discovered later in children as symptoms are not readily apparent. In some cases, a definitive diagnosis is made only after a detailed examination occasioned by an infant or school entrance physical exam.

There is no treatment for otosclerosis itself, but hearing can be improved through stapes surgery. Previously with otosclerosis in infants, stapes surgery was usually not performed until the child became somewhat older, out of concern for maintaining inner ear function over the long term. However, reports have emerged indicating that pediatric cases present no specific safety concerns for stapes surgery when compared to adult cases [4], making surgery an option when one gives serious consideration to the circumstances of the child.

References

1 Pekkola J, Pitkaranta A, Jappel A, et al: Localized pericochlear hypoattenuating foci at temporal-bone thin-section CT in pediatric patients: nonpathologic differential diagnostic entity? Radiology 2004; 230:88–92.

2 Markou K, Goudakos J: An overview of the etiology of otosclerosis. Eur Arch Otorhinolaryngol 2009;266:25–35.

3 Lescanne E, Bakhos D, Metais JP, et al: Otosclerosis in children and adolescents: a clinical and CT-scan survey with review of the literature. Int J Pediatr Otorhinolaryngol 2008;72:147–152.

4 Vincent R, Sperling NM, Oates J, et al: Surgical findings and long-term hearing results in 3,050 stapedotomies for primary otosclerosis: a prospective study with the otology-neurotology database. Otol Neurotol 2006;27(8. Suppl 2):S25–S47.

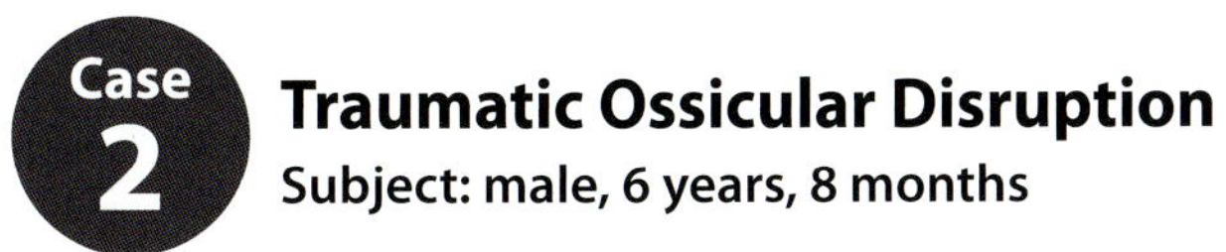

Traumatic Ossicular Disruption

Case 2

Subject: male, 6 years, 8 months

History and Clinical Findings

The subject suffered a blow to the left temporal region after falling from a 1.5 m high piece of playground equipment, which caused hemorrhaging of the left ear. No intracranial hemorrhaging was detected in a cranial CT taken by a neurosurgeon, but because there were symptoms of hearing loss and the ear continued to hemorrhage, the subject was examined by our department on the day following the injury.

Our initial examination indicated mixed hearing loss, with left-ear pure tone audiometry of 41.7 dB for air conduction and 16.7 dB for bone conduction. There were no abnormalities in the right ear. Pure tone audiometry two months post-trauma was 22.5 dB for air conduction and 6.7 dB for bone conduction, with the air-bone gap of 15.8 dB indicating residual conductive hearing loss. Tympanometry was type A for both ears.

Patient CT Findings

Figures 5 (1–3) and 6 (1–2) show left ear temporal bone CT images taken two months post-trauma. Both mastoid air cell development and pneumatization are favorable. In the axial section, fracturing of the bony segment of the external auditory canal can be ascertained (fig. 5:1). Observing the ossicular chain, the malleoincudal joint is disrupted and the body of the incus is displaced slightly laterally (fig. 5:3, fig. 6:1). The incudostapedial joint displays no clear abnormalities (fig. 5:2, fig. 6:2).

Surgical Findings and Postoperative Course

After a mastoidectomy, a posterior tympanotomy and epitympanotomy were performed to observe the interior of the tympanic cavity and the epitympanum (attic). The incus was displaced slightly posteriorly and laterally, and the malleoincudal joint was disrupted but held together with connective tissue. The head of the malleus was connected to the epitympanum with connective tissue. Also, the lenticular process of the incus was slightly flattened. There was no disruption of the incudostapedial joint and mobility of the footplate of the stapes was favorable. After severing the incudostapedial joint, we also severed the malleoincudal joint and temporarily extracted the incus. The connective tissue was thoroughly removed from the articular surfaces of both the malleus and the stapes and the incus returned to its original position and fixed in place with fibrin glue. Three months postoperatively, average air conduction hearing was 7.5 dB.

Postoperative CT Findings

CT images taken five months postoperatively are shown in figure 5, post-1–3 and figure 6, post-1 and post-2. The space can be confirmed via mastoidectomy and posterior tympanotomy (fig. 5: post-1, post-2). The incus is repositioned in its proper place and the malleoincudal joint is no longer detached (fig. 5: post-3; fig. 6: post-1).

Image Findings and Clinical Features

This case is a typical example of temporal bone fracture and ossicular chain disruption due to cranial contusion. So long as it is not a major injury involving extensive skull base fracture, the temporal bone fracture itself essentially does not involve significant bone displacement even with a fracture line present, and requires only prevention of infection and ongoing observation for recovery. Treatment is required if the fracture extends to the inner ear and causes leakage of perilymph or cerebrospinal fluid, but for non life-threatening injuries such as ossicular chain disruption the first priority is treatment of serious injury, as the problem can easily be dealt with after the patient's overall physical condition has stabilized. In this case, connective tissue builds up on the original articular surfaces with passage of time after the injury, and unless this connective tissue is thoroughly removed and cleaned, proper repositioning will be impossible. Also, in the case presented here there was no displacement of the malleus, allowing the ossicular chain to be completely repositioned by returning the incus to its original place, but if the external force is sufficient, the malleus may also be displaced. If the position or direction of the malleus is affected, it will be difficult to properly connect the incudostapedial joint if the incus is closely aligned with the malleoincudal joint. In this case, rather than performing a type I reconstruction, better results can be obtained by sculpting the incus into a columella and performing a type III incus interposition ossiculoplasty.

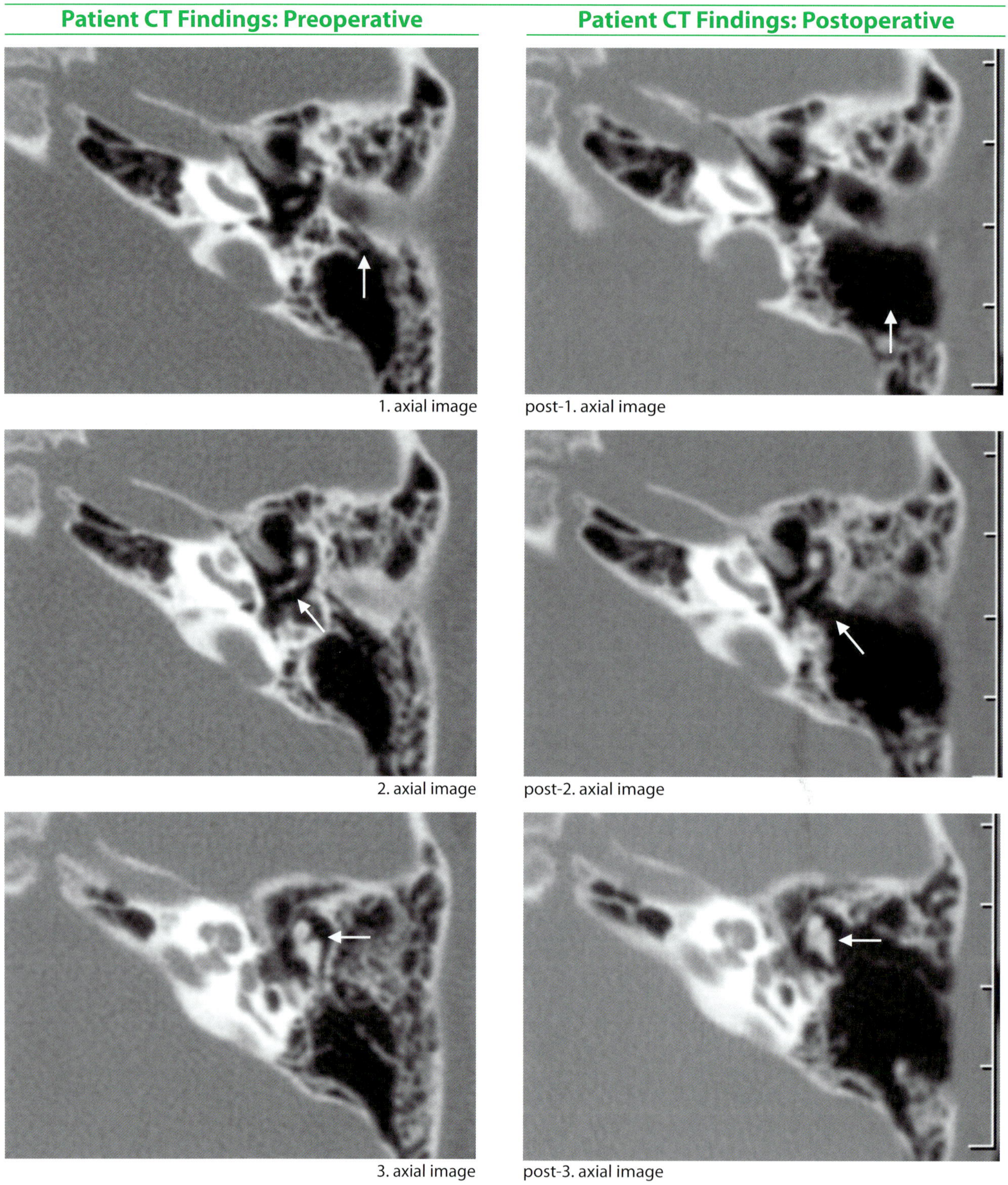

Patient CT Findings: Preoperative

Patient CT Findings: Postoperative

1. axial image   post-1. axial image

2. axial image   post-2. axial image

3. axial image   post-3. axial image

Fig. 5. (Case 2) Left ear CT: 1–3 = two months post-trauma; post-1–3 = postoperative

〖Patient CT Findings〗

Axial section temporal bone CT images show the ossicles before and after repositioning. Both mastoid air cell development and pneumatization are favorable. In the preoperative images shown on the left (taken two months post-trauma), fracturing of the bony part of the external auditory canal can be ascertained (1: ⇑), the malleoincudal joint is disrupted and the body of the incus is displaced slightly laterally (3: ⇐). The incudostapedial joint displays no clear abnormalities (2: ↖).

The postoperative images on the right show the condition after the mastoidectomy (post-1: ⇑) and posterior tympanotomy (post-2: ↖). The incus is repositioned in its proper place and the malleoincudal joint is no longer detached (post-3: ⇐).

Patient CT Findings: Preoperative

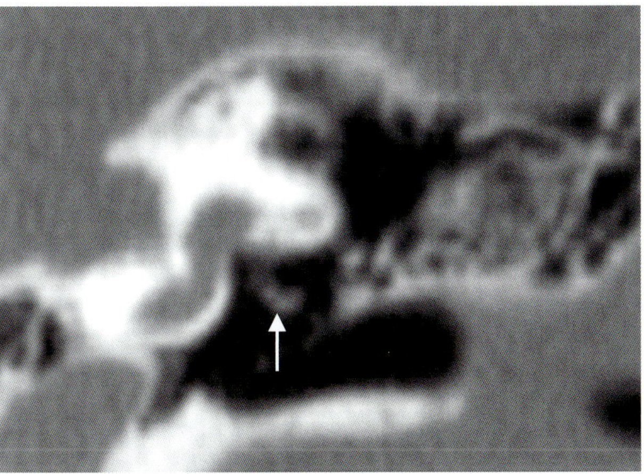

1. coronal image

2. coronal image

Patient CT Findings: Postoperative

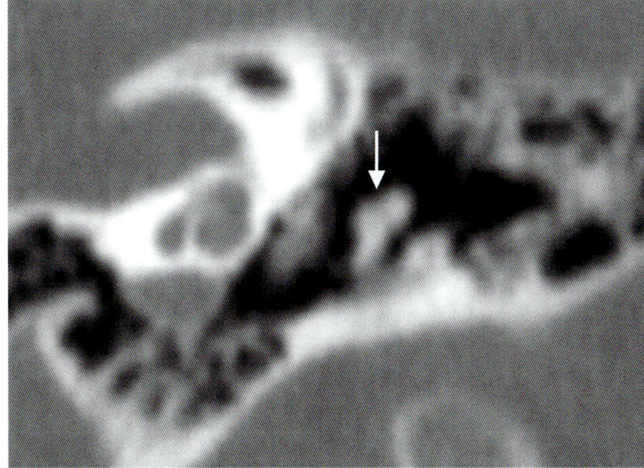

post-1. coronal image

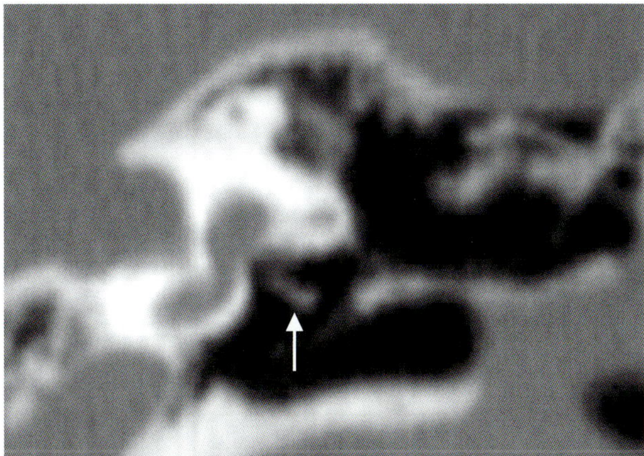

post-2. coronal image

Fig. 6. (Case2) Left ear CT: 1, 2 = two months post-trauma; post-1, 2 = postoperative

[Patient CT Findings]

Coronal section temporal bone CT images for this case are shown here. In the preoperative CT images shown on the left, the malleoincudal joint is disrupted and the body of the incus is displaced slightly laterally (1: ⇓), but the incudostapedial joint displays no clear abnormalities (2: ⇑).

The postoperative images on the right show that repositioning of the incus has caused the gap between the head of the malleus and the body of the incus to disappear (post-1: ⇓). During surgery the incus was temporarily extracted then returned to its original position, but the incudostapedial joint has properly reconnected (post-2: ⇑).

Points

❶ In head injuries, priority is on critical care; treatment of ossicular chain disruption and so on can wait until after the more serious injuries have been treated.

❷ A temporal bone CT is used for detailed inspection of the ossicular chain and the overall condition of the temporal bone. Functional testing is used to assess auditory function.

❸ In blows to the temporal region, longitudinal fractures are frequent and injuries occur mainly to the ossicular chain and the facial nerve, whereas in frontal or occipital blows, transverse fractures often result in severe inner ear damage, which frequently occurs bilaterally.

❹ The incus has less peripheral support than the malleus or stapes and is relatively heavier (25 mg), and therefore is most easily displaced by trauma.

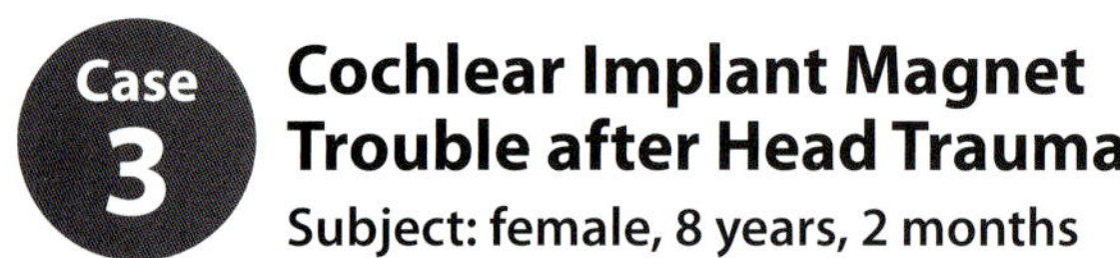

Case 3

Cochlear Implant Magnet Trouble after Head Trauma

Subject: female, 8 years, 2 months

■ History and Clinical Findings

The subject had suffered from progressive hearing loss due to incomplete partition type II inner ear malformation with enlarged vestibular aqueduct, for which cochlear implantation surgery had been performed four years ago with favorable results. However, since hitting her head on a metal towel rack three days previously, changes had occurred in cochlear implant function, including intermittent sound interruption and rapid battery depletion. At time of re-examination by our department there was only mild swelling at the site of the contusion, but because redness and swelling worsened over the area corresponding to the implant site of the cochlear implant magnet in the temporal region (fig. 7), we decided to investigate further using temporal bone CT imaging.

■ Patient CT Findings

Three-dimensional reconstructed images of the temporal bone CT are shown (fig. 8). It is apparent that the button magnet, which should be located in the center of the receiver/stimulator unit coil (the cochlear implant's implanted component), has become dislodged and displaced into an anteroinferior (fig. 8:a) and shallow (fig. 8:b) position.

■ Surgical Findings and Postoperative Course

With the subject under general anesthesia, an incision was made in the skin behind the receiver/stimulator unit for subcutaneous observation. The magnet had become dislodged from the silicon pocket at the center of coil of the cochlear implant's implanted component and displaced anteriorly, so it was extracted and a new magnet

inserted into the pocket. The postoperative course was favorable and hearing restored to its former level.

■ Image Findings and Clinical Features

There are many different types of cochlear implant, but there have been several reports of magnet dislodging due to trauma in types with replaceable internal magnets that have an external transmitter coil stabilized in optimum position relative to the internal receiver coil [1, 2]. In cases such as this, it is possible to surmise through palpation alone that the magnet may be dislodged from the center of the receiver coil, but as was shown in this case, a 3-dimensional reconstructed image makes it readily apparent and is useful when considering surgical procedures.

References

1 Wilkinson EP, Dogru S, Meyer TA, Gantz BJ: Case Report: Cochlear implant magnet migration. Laryngoscope 2004;114:2009–2011.
2 Posner D, Scott A, Polite C, et al: External Magnet Displacement in Cochlear Implants: Causes and Management. Otol Neurotol 2010; 31:88–93.

Patient 3-Dimensional Reconstructed CT Findings

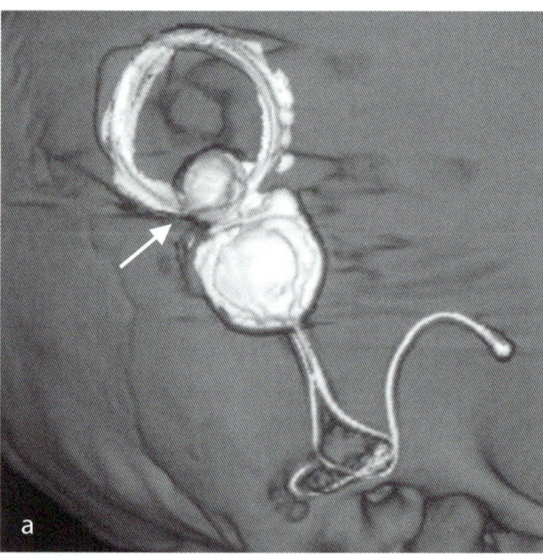

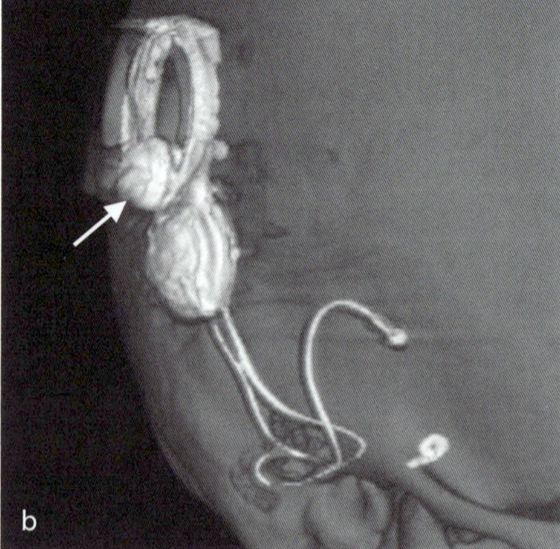

Fig. 8. (Case 3) 3-dimensional reconstructed images of the temporal bone CT

[Patient 3-Dimensional Reconstructed CT Findings]

Three-dimensional reconstructed images of the temporal bone CT are shown. It is apparent that the button magnet, which should be located in the center of the receiver/stimulator unit coil (the cochlear implant's implanted component), has become dislodged and displaced into an anteroinferior (a: ↗) and shallow (b: ↗) position.

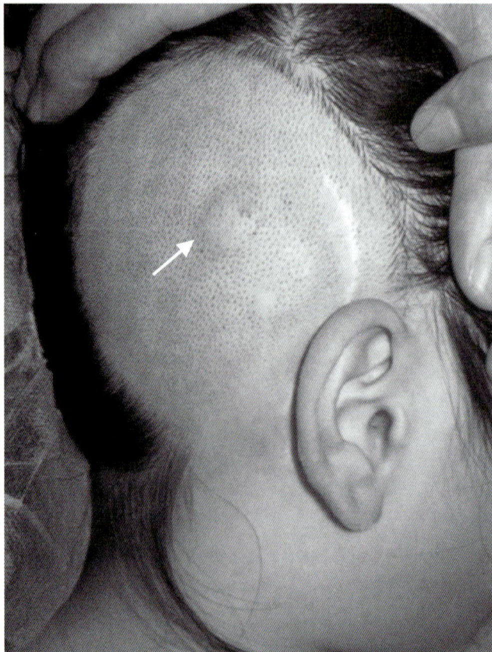

Fig. 7. (Case 3) The displaced button magnet can be palpated under the skin of the swollen area on the temporal region (↗).

Case 4
Cochlear Implantation in an Ear with Extensive Cholesteatoma
Subject: male, 10 years, 1 month

History and Clinical Findings

The subject had bilateral severe congenital hearing loss and had been wearing a hearing aid in the right ear since one year old. In the left ear, he had suffered from recurrent infections of acute otitis media, also since around one year old, and later formed middle ear cholesteatoma. The cholesteatoma was intractable and had not been completely cured even after two tympanoplasties by the previous physician, whereupon it had been decided to observe its progress as further treatment would be difficult. The subject's parents consulted our department hoping for a cure for the left cholesteatoma and an opinion on indication for cochlear implant surgery. At time of our initial examination, pure tone thresholds were 91.7 dB right and 113.3 dB left (fig. 9), with a maximum speech perception score of 35% right (100 dB) and 0% left. The left ear was filled with cholesteatoma debris to the external auditory canal, accompanied by infection and pus discharge. *Pseudomonas aeruginosa* was detected in bacterial testing of the otorrhea discharge. No abnormalities were ascertained in the right tympanic membrane. Since cochlear implant surgery could not be performed while the cholesteatoma otitis media remained, it was decided to first perform radical surgical therapy on the cholesteatoma.

Preoperative CT Findings

Observing the left temporal bone CT taken at time of initial examination (fig. 10), there is no mastoid air cell development whatsoever, with the area between the tympanic cavity and the mastoid filled with a large, continuous area of soft tissue density (fig. 10:a1, a2, c1, c2). There is destruction of the superior wall of the external auditory canal (fig. 10:c1), and a portion of the posterior wall is destroyed and retracted (fig. 10:a1).

Surgical Findings and Postoperative Course

A left radical mastoidectomy was performed with the objective of curing the cholesteatoma. The mastoid wound cavity was entered via postauricular incision and the debris that filled the cavity removed, then the epithelium of the cholesteatoma detached and extracted. The posterior wall of the external auditory canal was also removed. Since there was no bone conduction hearing in the left ear, ossicular chain reconstruction was not performed. To prevent reoccurrence, and also in preparation for future cochlear implant surgery, the tympanic membrane was formed in a much more shallow position than usual.

There were no problems for some time after surgery, but later the subject once again contracted otitis media and otorrhea was observed. Six months after the initial surgery by our department, upon performance of a second left radical mastoidectomy it was discovered that epithelial tissue had once again invaded the wound cavity through a perforation in the tympanic membrane and had formed a cholesteatoma, which was cleaned and removed along with granulation tissue. This time, the external auditory canal was sutured shut at the cartilaginous part immediately medial to the external acoustic aperture. Nine months later a third surgery was performed, at which time there was no infection in the wound cavity, which formed a broad, clean pneumatic cavity. However, there was a large, persistent recurrent cholesteatoma, so this was removed and another staged surgery performed to be absolutely certain. This is because it would be extremely difficult to treat a cholesteatoma should it reoccur after cochlear implantation.

Post Cholesteatoma Recovery: CT Images before and after Cochlear Implant Surgery

In the temporal bone CT taken immediately prior to cochlear implant surgery six months after the third surgery performed by our department, a broad, single mastoid cavity can be observed (fig. 11: pre-1–3), with no soft tissue density due to residual cholesteatoma. The external auditory canal, which underwent blind-sac closure, is thickly ossified (fig. 11: pre-3).

Left cochlear implant surgery was performed. When observed at time of surgery, the mastoid cavity was broadly pneumatized, with no sign of infection or residual cholesteatoma, so the basal turn of the cochlea was fenestrated in the wound cavity and the cochlear implant electrode inserted. Insertion of the electrode itself was unproblematic, and the surplus conducting wire was looped and stored in the mastoid cavity.

One year and two months after the cochlear implant surgery, postoperative course was favorable, but because the external auditory canal was closed and the condition of the middle ear could not be evaluated via the tympanic membrane, follow-up CT examination was performed. The wound cavity was broadly pneumatized and there were no findings of inflammation or cholesteatoma recurrence. There were no problems with the electrode in the cochlea (fig. 11: post-1, post-3), and the conducting wire at the base of the cochlear implant was looped inside the wound space with no observable tendency to become displaced laterally.

Postoperative Course Following Cochlear Implant Surgery

Following cochlear implant surgery, the left ear implant was used together with a hearing aid in the right ear. Whereas vowel discrimination using the right ear hearing aid alone was 90% and consonant discrimination 29%, they were 100% and 53%, respectively, when using the left ear cochlear implant alone. Furthermore, when using

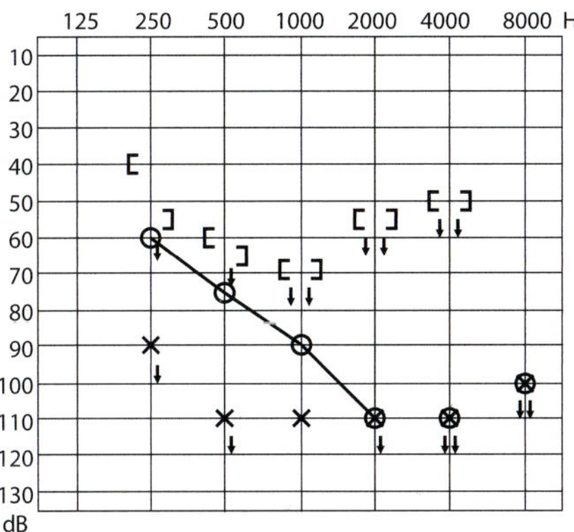

Fig. 9. (Case 4) Pure tone audiogram at time of initial examination

Patient CT Findings

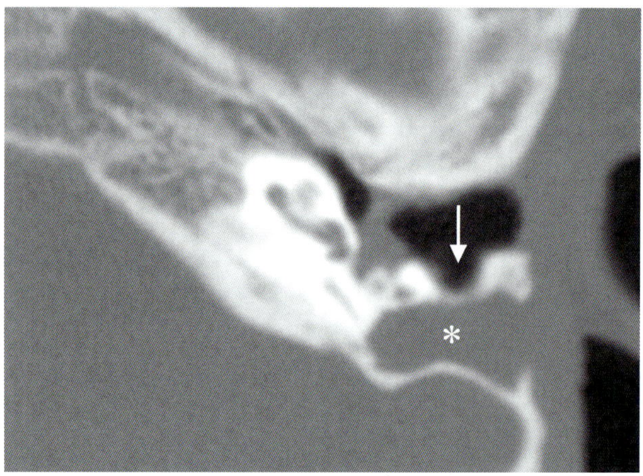

a1. axial image

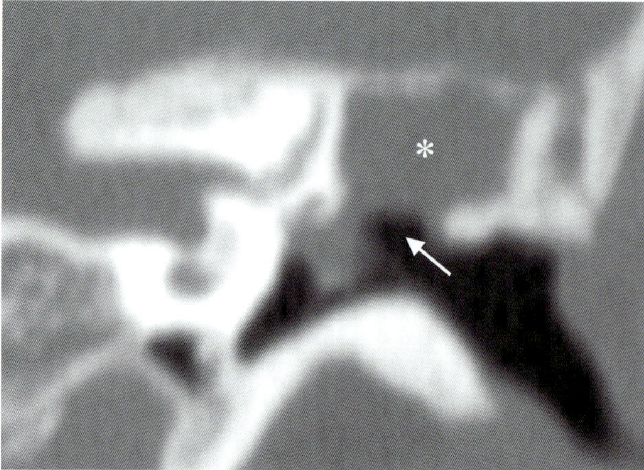

c1. coronal image

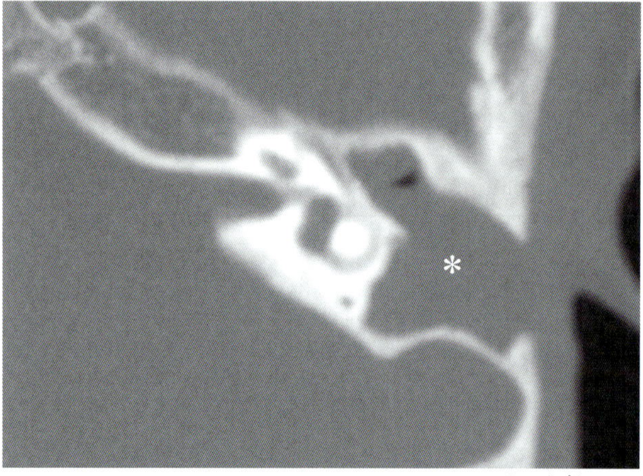

a2. axial image

c2. coronal image

Fig. 10. (Case 4) Left ear CT: initial examination

[Patient CT Findings]

Left temporal bone CT axial sections (a1, a2) and coronal sections (c1, c2) taken at time of initial examination are shown. There is no mastoid air cell development whatsoever, with the area between the tympanic cavity and the mastoid filled with a large, continuous area of soft tissue density (a1, a2, c1, c2: ✳). There is destruction of the superior wall of the external auditory canal (c1: ↖), and a portion of the posterior wall is destroyed and retracted (a1: ⇓).

both the right ear hearing aid and the left ear cochlear implant together, vowel discrimination improved to 100% and consonant discrimination to 64%. The subject in this case was twelve years, five months old when he underwent cochlear implant surgery, which is fairly old, but it may be that he was able to attain better language hearing capability with the cochlear implant than with the hearing aid alone because he initially had hearing in his left ear, and also maintained a steady level of spoken language acquisition using the hearing aid in the opposite ear.

■ Image Findings and Clinical Features

Cholesteatomas reoccur more easily in children than in adults and, as in this case, sometimes take as many as several surgeries to cure. In addition, in this case the subject suffered from bilateral severe to profound hearing loss and, through use of a hearing aid in the right ear, had barely acquired the language skills to communicate with those around him. In such a situation, there is a problem as to which to pursue first, treatment of the cholesteatoma or cochlear implant surgery. In this case, though, the cholesteatoma was in an advanced stage of development and we felt there was a risk of intracranial complications arising if we left it too long, and so proceeded with the cholesteatoma surgery first. Three surgeries were required at this hospital alone, but fortunately the cholesteatoma was cured completely. There were two reasons the external auditory canal was closed during cholesteatoma surgery: to prevent re-formation of the cholesteatoma due to re-retraction of the tympanic membrane; and to ensure that, when cochlear implant surgery was performed, the conducting wire would not become exposed to the external auditory canal. The cochlear implant is an artificial device, and frequently requires extraction and re-implantation when infection occurs around it. Also, if the electrode is exposed to the external auditory canal, this provides a pathway for infection and invasion of the epidermis into the middle ear. I personally have experienced difficult cases involving infection and cholesteatoma formation relating to cochlear implants, and in the long term the safest method is to use staged surgery to completely cure the cholesteatoma, then prevent any chance of electrode exposure by thoroughly closing the external auditory canal.

From his earliest awareness until our surgical treatment was complete, the child in question had never experienced a day without otorrhea in his left ear, and the

Patient CT Findings: Preoperative	**Patient CT Findings: Postoperative**

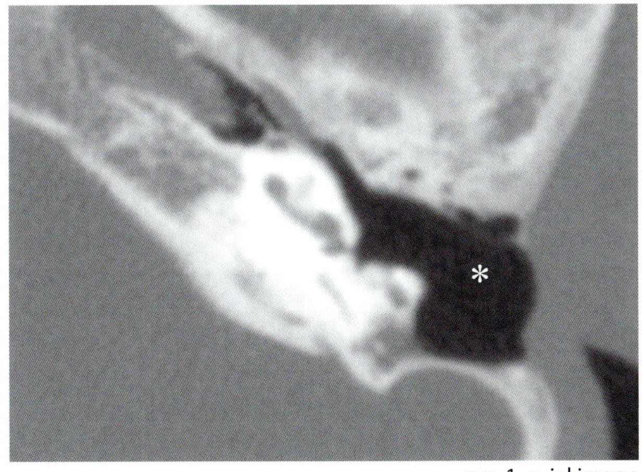

pre-1. axial image

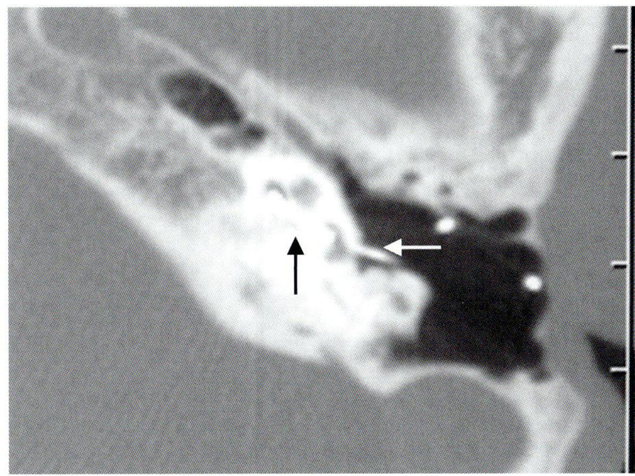

post-1. axial image

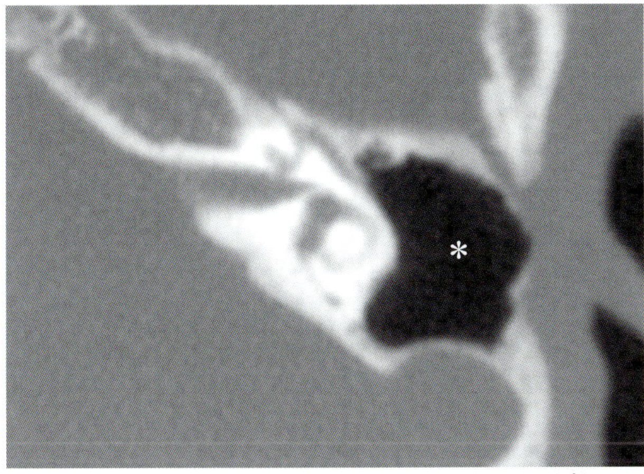

pre-2. axial image

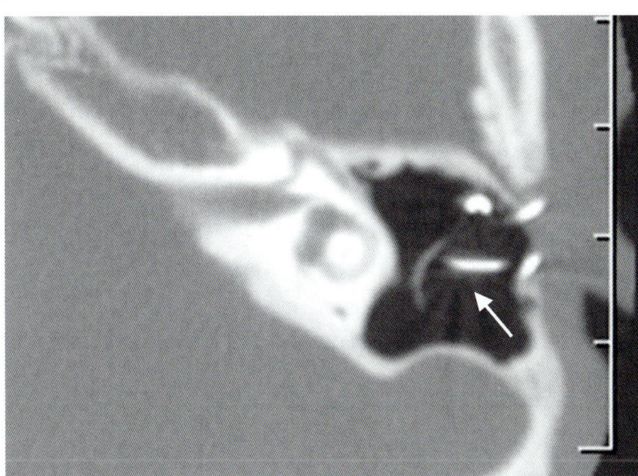

post-2. axial image

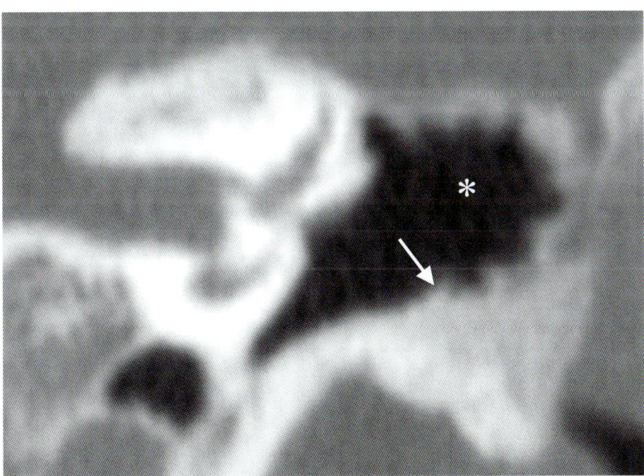

pre-3. coronal image

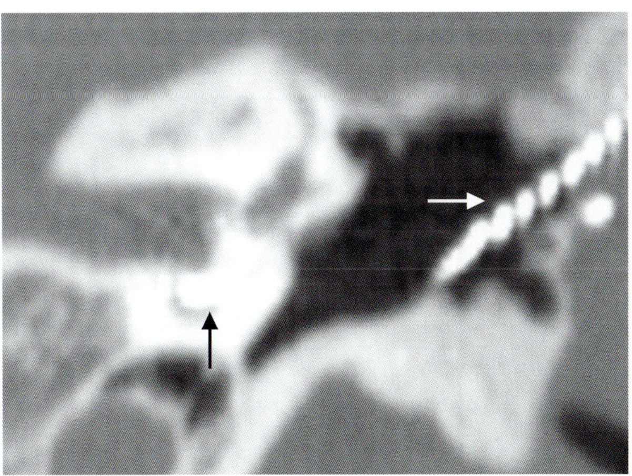

post-3. coronal image

Fig. 11. (Case 4) left ear CT: pre-1–3 = preoperative; post-1–3 = 1 year, 2 months after cochlear implant surgery

〖Patient CT Findings〗

In the CT image taken immediately prior to cochlear implant surgery after the cholesteatoma was cured (pre-1–3:1 and 2 are axial sections; 3 is a coronal section), a broad, single mastoid cavity can be observed (pre-1–3: ✿), with no soft tissue density due to residual cholesteatoma. The external auditory canal, which had been closed, is thickly ossified (pre-3: ✎).

One year, two months after the cochlear implant surgery, follow up CT testing was performed (post 1 3:1 and 2 are axial sections; 3 is a coronal section). The wound cavity is broadly pneumatized and there are no findings of inflammation or residual cholesteatoma. There are no problems with the electrode in the cochlea (post-1, post-3:↑), and the conducting wire at the base of the cochlear implant is looped inside the wound space (post-2: ✎) with no observable tendency to become displaced laterally. The entranceways of both the electrode into the cochlea (post-1: ⬅) and the base conducting wire into the mastoid cavity (post-3: ⤳) can be clearly observed.

longstanding symptoms of the otitis media that had been caused by the cholesteatoma had had a significant impact on his daily life. While it goes without saying that he benefited from improved speech perception with the cochlear implant, most impressive was the great relief both the boy and his family experienced at regaining a basically healthy ear as a result of eliminating the cholesteatoma.

Case 5

Meningitic Labyrinthitis
Subject: male, 8 months old

■ History and Clinical Findings

Eight months after birth, the subject presented light nasal discharge and a cough, then two weeks later suddenly developed a fever of 39 °C. The following morning, he was limp and vomiting, and was admitted to our hospital on the same day after being examined by the pediatric department. Test results were as follows. Blood test: white blood cell count: 5,400/µl; CRP: 26.1 mg/dl. Spinal fluid test: cell count: 30,976/3 mm³; glucose: 46 mg/dl; protein: 160 mg/dl. Culture test: positive for *Streptococcus pneumoniae*. Based on these findings, the subject was diagnosed with meningitis due to *Streptococcus pneumoniae*. Also, when examined by an otolaryngologist during hospital admission, findings of left acute otitis media were observed. The subject received antimicrobials and steroid treatment and showed gradual improvement in his overall physical condition, but in ABR testing conducted both at five days and at 14 days after onset of symptoms there was a complete lack of response on both sides, and he was referred to our department for consultation. At our initial examination we observed mild reddening of the left tympanic membrane and fluid retention in the tympanic cavity, but no abnormalities in the right ear. We decided to conduct temporal bone CT and MRI examination.

■ Patient CT Findings

Because the patient is only eight months old mastoid air cell development is understandably limited, but on comparison of the two sides, air cell development on the left is slightly deficient and the left middle ear cavity is filled with soft tissue density (fig. 12). The right side contains no clear abnormalities. There are no abnormalities in the soft tissue density inside the cochlea, and no ossification can be confirmed on the images. Enlargement of the hiatus for the greater petrosal nerve is also visible.

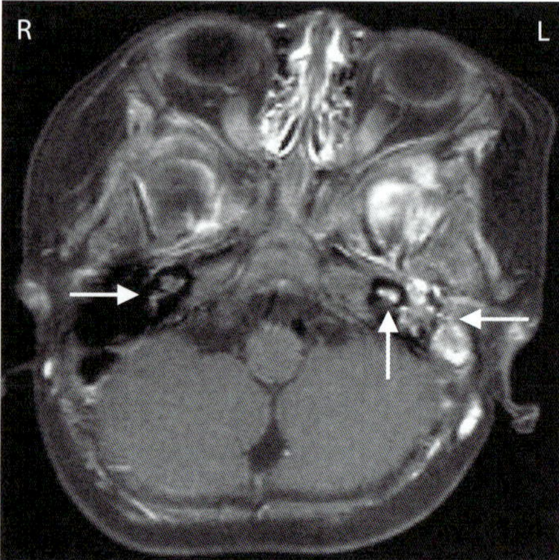

Fig. 13. (Case 5)   Contrast-enhanced MRI

[Patient MRI Findings]

The left mastoid segment is filled with soft tissue, with a particularly strong contrast enhancement on the margin of the mastoid air cells (⇐). The left cochlea exhibits strong contrast enhancement (⇑), but on close observation the right cochlea's signal is also slightly elevated and is clearly higher than the signal intensity for cerebrospinal fluid (⇢).

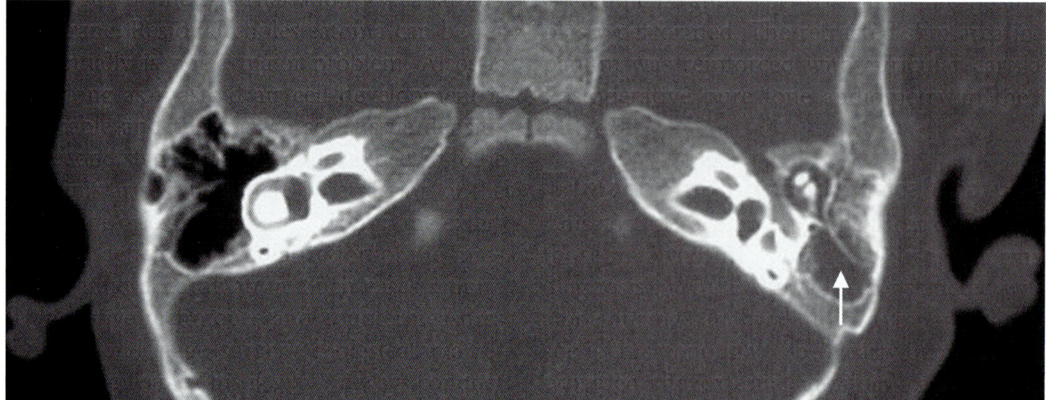

Fig. 12. (Case 5) Non-contrast CT axial section of cranium, including temporal bone

[Patient CT Findings]

Comparing the two sides, air cell development on the left is slightly deficient and the left middle ear cavity is filled with soft tissue density (⇑). The right side contains no clear abnormalities. There are no abnormalities in the soft tissue density inside the cochlea, and no ossification can be confirmed on the images. Enlargement of the hiatus for the greater petrosal nerve is also visible.

Patient MRI Findings

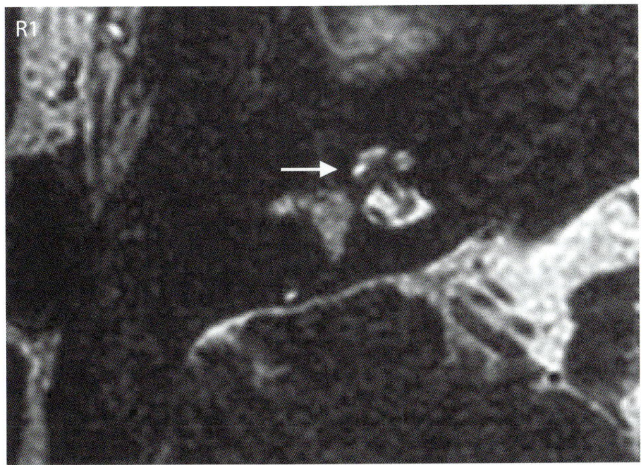

R1. coronal image

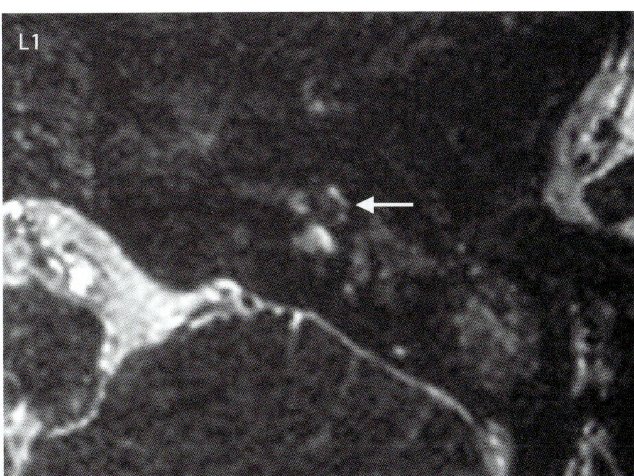

L1. coronal image

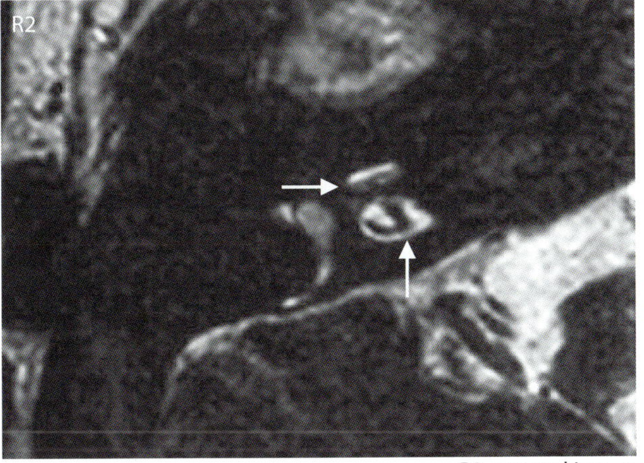

R2. coronal image

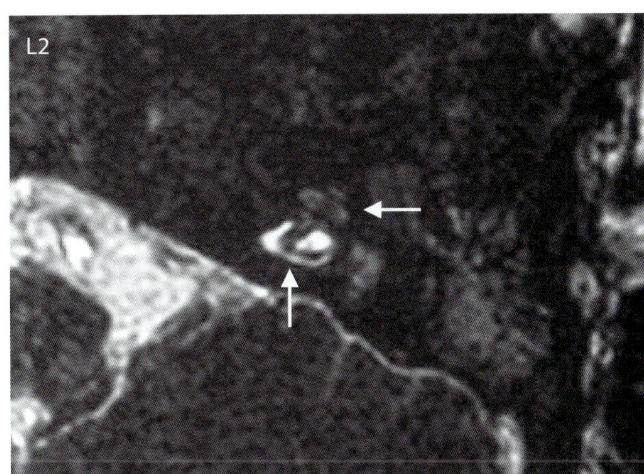

L2. coronal image

Fig. 14. (Case 5) High-resolution heavy T2 weighted MRI

Patient MRI Findings

Observing the contrast-enhanced MRI, the left mastoid segment is filled with soft tissue, with a particularly strong contrast enhancement on the margin of the mastoid air cells (fig. 13). The left cochlea exhibits strong contrast enhancement (fig. 13), but on close observation the right cochlea's signal intensity is also slightly elevated and is clearly higher than the signal intensity for cerebrospinal fluid.

Observing the high-resolution heavy T2 weighted MRI, signal intensity for the left cochlea is reduced (fig. 14:L1, L2), but the cochlear nerve within the internal auditory canal is clearly depicted and there are no abnormalities to its thickness (fig. 14:L2). On the other hand, observing the right cochlea, while not to the same extent as the left, signal intensity is lower and, on closer inspection, within the cochlea the scala media and scala vestibuli have higher signal intensity than the scala tympani (fig. 14: R1, R2). The cochlear nerve within the internal auditory canal is clearly seen, as on the left side, and displays no abnormalities (fig. 14: R2).

From the above findings, it was probable that the subject had bilateral labyrinthitis, resulting in inner ear fibrosis that was more pronounced in the left ear.

Further Developments

The subject experienced bilateral profound hearing loss due to bilateral labyrinthitis accompanying meningitis, and in this case the probability of recovery of hearing is virtually none. We thought that cochlear implant surgery ought to be considered before inner ear fibrosis and ossification progress and explained this to the parents, but they wanted to hear other opinions and treatment options and were referred to another hospital.

Image Findings and Clinical Features

Hearing loss in this case occurred bilaterally, not just in the left ear with otitis media, so there is a high probability that it was due to labyrinthitis accompanying meningitis. As described above, post-meningitic labyrinthitis frequently leads to fibrosis and even ossification, making accurate evaluation of inner ear using CT and MRI examination important. Once inner ear fibrosis and ossification has occurred, even if cochlear implant surgery is later performed it is more problematic and, if the number of electrodes that can be inserted is limited due to ossification, hearing results are unfavorable [1]. Also, it is already commonly accepted that better results can be obtained using bilateral cochlear implants, and if cochlear ossification occurs in even one side while keeping the patient under observation this reduces the possibility of being able to use bilateral cochlear implants. Thus, in cases of post-meningitic hearing loss, a decision that takes the patient's future into account must be made in a limited time, and is fraught with difficulties.

References

1 Philippon D, Bergeron F, Ferron P, et al: Cochlear implantation in postmeningitic deafness. Otol Neurotol 2010;31:83–87.

Index

Note: Colored page numbers indicate figures

Author

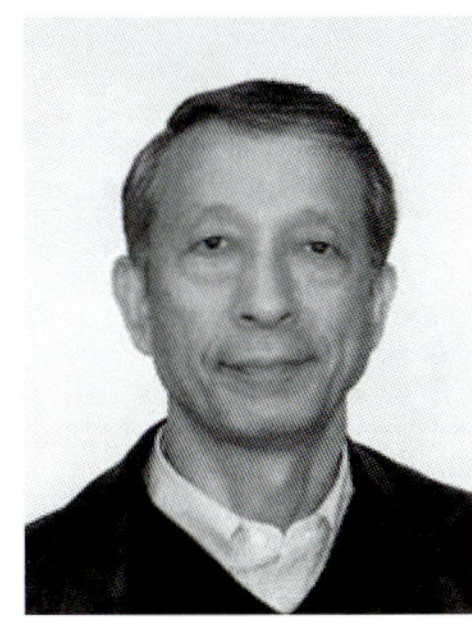

Yasushi Naito, M.D.

1980 Resident, Dept. of Otolaryngology, Kyoto University Hospital
1981 Staff, Dept. of Otolaryngology, Kyoto National Hospital
1990 Visiting Scholar, UCLA School of Medicine, Prof. Vicente Honrubia
1992 Lecturer, Dept. of Otolaryngology, Kyoto University School of Medicine
2004 Director of Otolaryngology, Kobe City Medical Center General Hospital
       Clinical Professor of Otolaryngology-Head and Neck Surgery, Kyoto University
2009 Vice President for Research and Education,
       Kobe City Medical Center General Hospital

Memberships:
Oto-Rhino-Laryngological Society of Japan (Councilor)
Japan Otological Society (Councilor)
Japan Audiological Society (Board Member)
Japan Society for Equilibrium Research (Board Member)
Association for Research in Otolaryngology (USA)
Collegium Oto-Rhino-Laryngologicum Amicitiae Sacrum (CORLAS)
Barany Society

Acknowledgments

The Japanese edition of this book was published in April 2011. A section on incomplete partition type III anomaly of the inner ear was added for the current English edition. Some clinical studies in this book were supported by Grants-in-Aid for Scientific Research (C) 22591894 from the Japan Ministry of Education, Science and Culture.

I acknowledge with gratitude the contribution of Dr. Levent Sennaroglu, Professor of Otolaryngology, Hacettepe University, Turkey, not only for writing a special article on IP-III for this book, but also for his epoch-making scientific achievement in the classification of inner ear anomalies, which greatly helped in making the description of inner ear anomalies in this book more lucid and systematic.

I am indebted to Dr. Iwao Honjo, Professor Emeritus of Kyoto University, for supervising the first edition of the Japanese version of this book, and Dr. Kimitaka Kaga, Professor Emeritus of Tokyo University, for his warm support concerning the publication of this book. I offer my sincere gratitude to Mr. Atsushi Moriyama, of International Medical Publishers Ltd., who realized the publication of both the Japanese and English editions of this book, and Mr. Peter Roth, of Karger Medical and Scientific Publishers, for helping us to create the English edition. I thank Drs. Kyo Ito and Sho Koyasu, Department of Radiology, Kobe City Medical Center General Hospital, for their great help in clinical imaging, the members of Hyogo Otolaryngologist Society for introducing important patients who appear in this book, and the editorial staff of International Medical Publishers Ltd., for their professionalism in editing this book. I am grateful to Dr. Toru Kita, President of Kobe City Medical Center General Hospital, Dr. Haruhiko Kikuchi, Board Chairman of Kobe City Hospital Organization, and Dr. Juichi Ito, Professor of Otolaryngology-Head and Neck Surgery, Kyoto University, for their continuous support and supervision on clinical works and research in the hospital.

Finally, I want to thank my colleagues in our department: Drs. Shogo Shinohara, Yosaku Shiomi, Keizo Fujiwara, Masahiro Kikuchi, Hiroshi Yamazaki, Yuji Kanazawa, Risa Kurihara, Ippei Kishimoto, Hiroyuki Harada, Satoshi Kakutani, Tsunemichi Adachi, Shin-ya Hori, Yosuke Tona; speech therapists Saburo Moroto, Tomoko Yamazaki, and Rinko Yamamoto; and department secretary Noriyo Sakamoto.